Fifth Edition — Illustrated

Dental Anatomy, Physiology and Occlusion

RUSSELL C. WHEELER, D.D.S., F.A.C.D.

Washington University School of Dentistry
Instructor, Crown and Bridge Prosthesis, 1924 - 1927
Instructor, Dental Anatomy and Prosthetic Art, 1927 - 1935
Assistant Professor, Oral Anatomy, 1936
St. Louis University School of Dentistry
Associate Professor of Dental Anatomy, Human and Comparative,
Chairman of Department, 1937 - 1944
Washington University School of Dentistry
Associate Professor of Anatomy, 1945 - 1951
Research Professor, Dental Anatomy and Physiology, 1971—

W. B. SAUNDERS COMPANY · Philadelphia · London · Toronto

W. B. Saunders Company: West Washington Square
Philadelphia, PA 19105

1 St. Anne's Road
Eastbourne, East Sussex BN21 3UN, England

1 Goldthorne Avenue
Toronto, Ontario M8Z 5T9, Canada

Listed here is the latest translated edition of this book together

with the language of the translation and the publisher.

Italian (*5th Edition*) — Edizioni Ermes, Milan, Italy

Spanish (*5th Edition*) — Nueva Editorial Interamericana S.A. de C.V.
Mexico City, Mexico

Dental Anatomy, Physiology and Occlusion   ISBN 0-7216-9262-1

Last digit is the print number: 18   17   16   15   14   13   12   11   10

DEDICATED TO
Those interested in Dental Practice
and Associated Research,
which necessarily involves a scientific approach
toward the subject of Dental Maintenance.

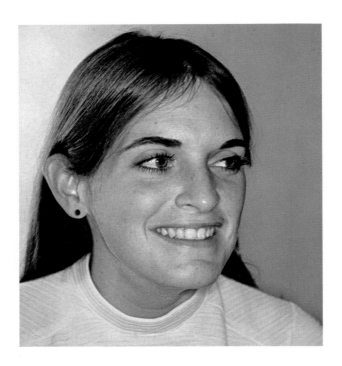

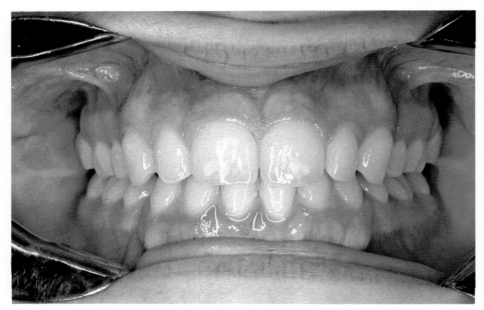

"The face is man's most individual characteristic. The jaws and teeth comprise two-thirds of its structure."

"Normal occlusion of the teeth and jaws is essential to a pleasing appearance of the entire face and to efficiency in mastication."*

*(From Massler and Schour, "Atlas of the Mouth." American Dental Association)

Foreword

The Arrangement of the Teeth and Occlusion

The teeth of man perform *two* major functions in life:

1. The teeth incise and reduce food material during the masticatory process, an activity which sustains the life of the host, but the teeth themselves would be short-lived without a second characteristic which they possess that is functional and most important.

2. The teeth help sustain themselves in the dental arches by assisting in the development and the protection of the tissues that support them. The static form of the individual tooth contributes to the protection of the investing tissues and to the stabilization of dental arch alignment; to its alignment with neighbors in the same jaw; and to the normal development of the jaws. Finally, dental maintenance is assisted by normal alignment and occlusion of the teeth in the two dental arches. Good occlusion stabilizes jaw relations during functional movements.

Preface
to the Fifth Edition

Thirty-four years after *A Textbook of Dental Anatomy and Physiology* was published in the year 1940, the title of the book has been changed. Although none of the fundamental subject matter in the initial chapters has been eliminated, the work is no longer called a textbook, because it has advanced beyond the category of undergraduate training. Since there has been a continuous demand by practitioners and teachers for more information on the science of dental occlusion, the words "A Textbook of" have been eliminated; the word "Occlusion" has been added. The title of the fifth revision is now *Dental Anatomy, Physiology and Occlusion*.

The old term, "dental anatomy," used to describe a course of study in the dental curriculum, is passé. Formerly the complete discipline was a technical study of art forms in the laboratory and of surveys made in dental dissection studies. The laboratory discipline, although still important, is now but a part of the science discipline of Dental Anatomy, Physiology and Occlusion.

If the scope of the subject could be described in one sentence it might be described thus: *functional dental units are formed into two dental arches, which in turn become combination units working together to create a required functional activity called occlusion.* The development of the temporomandibular joints, the musculature and the ligamentous attachments of the jaws are affected accordingly. The details of design involved in the plan of occlusion are to be found in the teeth themselves; the plan of occlusion is there, and not in the movable parts of jaw articulation. The maturation of tooth parts antedates the maturation of associated parts.

The study of dental physiology and dental maintenance is very elaborate and has become recognized as such over the last 30 years; every group in dentistry must be made aware of this fact. Tooth form and function should be thoroughly understood by every operator from dental hygienist to oral surgeon; from periodontist to the designer of fixed appliances, to name a few. No one associated with dental practice may be released from the obligation.

The fifth edition has been revised more extensively than has any former revision. This was possible because the author was able to devote full time to research and revision for two years prior to publication. Observations made during that time have convinced the author that what he had thought all along was pertinent: research in his subject has been neglected, possibly in part because research in other fields has been made more attractive.

Research is needed in macroscopic dental anatomy associated with research in jaw development. In the future the study should receive more emphasis so that young people in dentistry will become involved in it. In recent years, experience has proved that people possessing high potential in their abilities are apt to favor certain areas in dentistry of special interest to them. Many, while still in school, are attracted to phases of practice with popular appeal, especially those leading to the practice of specialties. Occasionally these students err by associating the manual arts and manual dexterity with manual labor, feeling somehow that such aptitudes are below the intellectual level usually attributed to the professional person. Thinking in this manner, they opt to by-pass the "manual art" pursuits in the dental curriculum whenever it seems convenient. Unfortunately, many instructors share the same point of view because their preceptors, in turn, did not hold the dental laboratory courses in high regard. This attitude is supported by the tendency of many dental schools to neglect the technical laboratories by not insisting on their maintenance being equal to that of other science laboratories. Neither faculty nor students will respect any department that is unattractive, especially if lack of cleanliness is a factor.

The subject of dental anatomy and physiology and occlusion needs to be considered in depth in any subject that involves the oral cavity and the head and neck.

In recent years in dental education there has been a singular lack of attention given to technical reviews of tooth form in most schools. This occurs in spite of the general acceptance of high-speed instruments which can be destructive in the hands of poorly trained persons. The added interest also in the problems of occlusion should have been accompanied by an added interest in the basic science of dental anatomy and physiology, which emphasizes the fundamental principles of form. Training in the subject must include laboratory and classroom work in tooth form drawing and carving. There is no other way for an individual to accumulate the information necessary for diagnostic skill, or for a scientific clinical approach to treatment.

Throughout human history, understanding or conscious insight in scientific studies has been gained in part through two-dimensional (drawing) and three-dimensional records (forming or carving). Among other beneficial aspects, the activity stimulates one to observe details, and this in turn stimulates the mind, making it conscious of its ability to create. To look upon this learning process as being below the intellectual level of a learned profession is unintelligent.

An artist uses his many skills to achieve effect. The achievement at the same time of functional accuracy is ordinarily of little interest to him. (However, the ancient Greek sculptors were very conscientious and learned in their accurate portrayals of functional anatomy!) In dentistry our approach to this matter must be the scientific one and should not foster mere figments of the imagination. Functional form should be the final goal of our efforts, while at the same time we make use of "art" training. The requirements for competence in the work are exacting, and even the most talented cannot expect to succeed without effort.

In the preface to the fifth edition, repetition is avoided by keeping the preface to the fourth edition intact. It explains the book's original plan and also some major changes in makeup that seemed desirable for publication in 1965.

Major and minor changes and improvements will be noted throughout the 16 chapters of the book. One improvement common to all: Figures and legends will be numbered by chapters. As an example, Figure 6–15 will refer to Chapter 6, Figure 15, and so forth. This arrangement obviates the search for an illustration which does not indicate the chapter number at the same time.

Whenever illustrations could be made more graphic, this was done. Innumerable enlargements were made where it seemed advisable, many originals were replaced and new figures were added. The six chapters on permanent teeth have new layouts; all of the illustrations were improved. It is doubtful whether these illustrations of prime tooth collections can be matched anywhere else in dental literature.

From the beginning it was the aim of this book to assist those in dentistry who accepted the responsibility for dental maintenance. With that thought in mind, Chapter 13, "The Pulp Cavities of the Permanent Teeth," was completely revised. Although the chapter was always *avant-garde* in its liberal display of natural tooth sections, there was no attempt to coordinate the photographic records with an approach to endodontic treatment. The spread of interest in endodontics has developed in a spectacular fashion in recent years, so in the chapter some suggestions are made regarding anatomical considerations in the manipulation and in the approach to pulp cavities. Some fundamentals only are discussed, because a separate book, not just a chapter in one, would be required to cover the subject completely. Nevertheless, anyone interested in endodontics should find Chapter 13 helpful.

In Chapter 14, "Dento-osseous Structures," an addition to the publication was made that should please those interested in treatment or in clinical instruction. Under the heading "Landmarks and Bony Processes of Both Jaws," some graphic illustrations borrowed from "X-rays in Dentistry," published by the Eastman Kodak Company in 1972, point out areas and landmarks of clinical interest. The illustrations are remarkable in this and as numbered will aid in making referrals to more detailed anatomy of the specific areas.

Chapter 16, the concluding chapter, is actually a summarization of all the material in preceding chapters. Because of the chapter's significance, "The Arrangement of the Teeth and Occlusion" was revised extensively and enlarged considerably. Because it was decided to feature the word occlusion in the book's new title, every effort was made to have the chapter qualify as outstanding in its approach to the subject. So many changes were made in composition and illustration that listing them here is out of the question.

One observation may be in order: in Chapter 16, when the fundamentals of occlusal contacts are to be discussed and illustrated, the traditional approach to the subject is discarded; traditional, that is, in most dental literature where treatment is discussed and promulgated. In composing the chapter, all thoughts of inclined planes or of fixed occlusal surfaces sliding up and down over each other during occlusal movements were rejected. The principles of occlusion that are featured are those described by paleontologists in their writings, which refer to comparative studies of dental structures and dental anatomy *i.e.*, (Gregory and Hellman). Paleontologists were active many years ago in research intended to explain dental development in man and lower animals. In tracing the processes of evolution, principles of occlusion dependent on that development were presented. It was realized that there were different types of occlusion. The types varied with tooth development. Joint and jaw development followed, conforming to the dental plan.

Concluding the preface, the author extends special words of appreciation to Mr. Spencer T. Olin of St. Louis, whose sponsorship has made possible two years of work on this fifth edition. All others who assisted in the production of this edition are to be given proper credit in illustration or text. Their kind cooperation is appreciated. Washington University in St. Louis, and the publishers, W. B. Saunders Company, must be included in the group.

RUSSELL C. WHEELER

Preface
to the Fourth Edition

TWENTY-FIVE years have elapsed since this book went to press for the first time. Increased public interest in dentistry has stimulated new developments in dental education since then. Dentistry is recognized as a major division of the complete health service, and dental schools and complete dental clinics are being included as functioning departments of medical centers.

It is the author's opinion, however, that although this situation is satisfying, there is some danger that students of dentistry may forget their primary duties and the way in which they will become most valuable to the public in their future life in dentistry. With the present emphasis on research in teaching, students tend to pursue attractive "mirages" of subjects usually associated with the practice of various fields of medicine.

Actually, in recent years the dental profession has come to realize that no other group enjoys a more advantageous position in scientific pursuit, now or in the future. Graduate students and undergraduate students should accept this truth also: there is no other profession capable of assuming the duties involved in the diagnosis and treatment of dental problems. Basically, these duties involve care during development as well as the maintenance of the normal function of the teeth and jaws after maturity. The teeth and jaws are the foundation tissues of the oral cavity.

It is now common knowledge that the health and welfare of the human being must wait upon the health and welfare of the "portal" of his body, his mouth. This fact promotes emphasis on the most important single subject in the dental curriculum: Dental Anatomy and Physiology.

Teeth are unique in that their static outside form is functional. They are incapable of readaptation in case of wear or accident; neither are they capable of recovery when they are partially destroyed by disease. Any dental treatment, general or specialized, requires an intimate and detailed knowledge of dental anatomy and physiology. Only dentists, among those in the health sciences, have the knowledge or the skills needed to care for the mouth; they must therefore apply themselves dutifully to this basic need.

Each new edition of this book was revised to keep up with the times and to cooperate with those who were interested enough to contribute constructive criticism. In this fourth edition, more changes in text and illustration have been made than in any previous revision.

The overall teaching plan has not been changed except to include the chapter on deciduous teeth within the first three chapters; these chapters are considered elementary instruction. It was thought that instruction in development, calcification and eruption should be closely followed by information concerning the deciduous dentition; that all of this information was really one phase of instruction.

The first twelve chapters are intended for first year work in dental school, with portions of Chapter XVI (the last chapter) on occlusion to be assigned at the instructor's discretion. The major portion of the material in the last four chapters, XIII to XVI, is intended for more advanced students and for postgraduate instruction.

If separate instruction in drawing and carving of teeth is required for laboratory reference, it is recommended that the student obtain "An Atlas of Tooth Form" (W. B. Saunders Co.), a book designed for that purpose. It is a useful companion to this text.

The new frontispiece of the textbook illustrates graphically the principles followed in making new half page figures for chapters VI through XII. These figures are enlargements of photographs of specimens of the permanent dentition, illustrating true anatomy from five aspects, obviating misrepresentation or errors in observation which might be registered in artist's drawings. Most of the illustrations in the seven chapters are new reproductions from new prints and photographs. An additional feature is the inclusion of full page figures of graph drawings facing full page figures of shaded drawings with three dimensional quality. These illustrations represent the eight typical tooth forms.

There has been some criticism from instructors that there was too much descriptive detail in the text. The author understands such criticism, but insists that there will always be a need for reference works in dental anatomy and physiology. Elaborate detail is necessary in a subject of this sort; this is true of most scientific disciplines! Let the student absorb as much as he can, for what he does retain may be the foundation for his success in practice.

Chapter XIII on pulp cavities in permanent teeth is probably more complete in anatomical description and illustration than material found in any other textbook at present writing. All illustrations are actual photographs of sectioned teeth or illustrations copied from photographs. Illustrations of cross sections which portray angles which cannot be obtained in radiographic examination are so labeled. This chapter should be of interest to endodontists in practice as well as upper classmen in dental school.

Particular attention should be paid to Chapter XIV on dento-osseous structures. Description of the maxilla and mandible must include the normally developed framework encompassing the teeth in complete dental arches. *This establishes the teeth as foundation tissues to be included with the bones for proper jaw relations and as integral parts of the important framework which supports the mobile portion of the face.* The size and angulation of the root forms of the teeth will govern the shape of the alveoli in the jaws, and this, in turn, shapes the contour of the dento-osseous portions facially.

The realization of these facts should have considerable influence in the diagnosis and prognosis of cases in Orthodontics. For instance, the premolars are succedaneous to the deciduous molars in identical sections of the maxillae and mandible. These sections are valuable combinations during development and after maturity. See "Dental Arch Formation," Chapter XVI. No other tooth combinations can serve as a substitute for the combined form of the premolars or the form of their osseous sections as completed around them. These beautiful and important teeth should not be sacrificed unless the patient's welfare demands it without question. The loss of any of the teeth brings about an atrophic reduction of valuable portions of the maxilla and mandible, a fact which adds disfigurement and psychological injury to the more obvious one of masticatory malfunction.

Chapter XV now includes new illustrations of the muscles of mastication, with illustrations of the muscles of facial expression.

The final chapter, Chapter XVI, on "Arrangement of the Teeth and Occlusion," has been carefully re-edited with figures placed in a manner which improves clarity and readability. Exercises have been suggested in chart tracing to be associated with simultaneous observation of three dimensional models or skulls.

The printed text on occlusion of the teeth is detailed. There is no "short cut" to the description of normal occlusal contacts during the various jaw movements. The student in dentistry must realize that normal occlusion of the teeth in his patients is the ultimate goal of the dental practitioner. All of his treatment plans, in dental development, in dental maintenance and in dental restoration, are to be devoted to that end.

The study of dental anatomy and physiology furnishes the *key* to that end; without it, there can be no real understanding of occlusion.

RUSSELL C. WHEELER

Contents

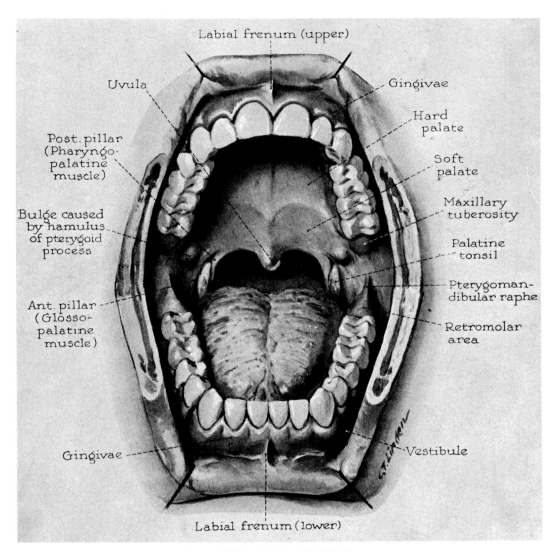

Labial frenum (upper)

Uvula

Post. pillar
(Pharyngo-
palatine
muscle)

Bulge caused
by hamulus
of pterygoid
process

Ant. pillar
(Glosso-
palatine
muscle)

Gingivae

Gingivae

Hard
palate

Soft
palate

Maxillary
tuberosity

Palatine
tonsil

Pterygoman-
dibular raphe

Retromolar
area

Vestibule

Labial frenum (lower)

THE ORAL CAVITY

(TAKEN FROM "ATLAS OF THE MOUTH," BY MASSLER AND SCHOUR.
AMERICAN DENTAL ASSOCIATION BUREAU OF PUBLIC RELATIONS.)

Nomenclature and
General Considerations

In order to obtain a comprehensive view of any subject, one must learn the nomenclature and a general outline of what the subject includes. This can be done by reading an abstract or outline of the material that names and illustrates the terms. Chapters 1, 2, 3, 4 and 5 will cover such an outline. When a term is used for the first time it is emphasized in italics. If the definition is not clear at the time it is read in the text, further description may be found in proximate illustrations or elsewhere in the book. (Consult the index.)

NOMENCLATURE

THE DECIDUOUS TEETH

At birth, the individual has no functioning teeth in the mouth. Radiograms of the infant's jaws, however, show many teeth in various stages of the process of formation. The diet in early infancy is fluid or semifluid; therefore teeth are unnecessary until the reduction of solid food is required. Usually, at the age of two years or thereabout the *deciduous dentition* is complete.

The denomination and number of teeth for all Mammalia are expressed by formulae. The denomination of each tooth is represented by its initial letter, I for *incisor*, C for *canine*, P for *premolar*, M for *molar;* each letter is followed by a horizontal line, and the number of each type of tooth is placed above the line for the *maxilla* (upper jaw) and below the line for the *mandible* (lower jaw). The formula includes one side only.

The deciduous dental formula of man is:

$$I \frac{2}{2} C \frac{1}{1} M \frac{2}{2} = 10$$

This formula should be read thus: Incisors, two maxillary and two mandibular; canines, one maxillary and one mandibular; molars, two maxillary and two mandibular—or ten altogether on one side, right or left (Fig. 1–1, A).

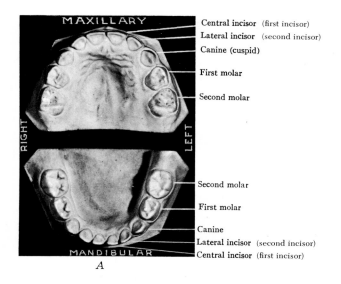

MAXILLARY

Central incisor (first incisor)
Lateral incisor (second incisor)
Canine (cuspid)

First molar

Second molar

RIGHT

LEFT

Second molar

First molar

Canine
Lateral incisor (second incisor)
Central incisor (first incisor)

MANDIBULAR

A

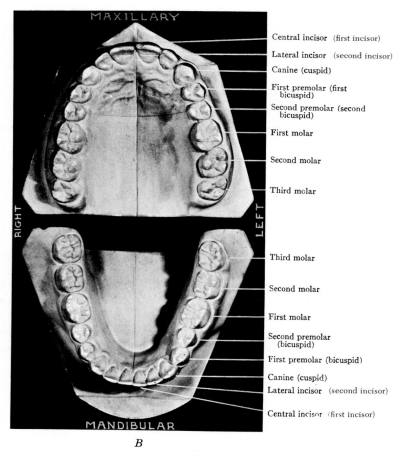

MAXILLARY

Central incisor (first incisor)
Lateral incisor (second incisor)
Canine (cuspid)
First premolar (first bicuspid)
Second premolar (second bicuspid)
First molar

Second molar

Third molar

RIGHT

LEFT

Third molar

Second molar

First molar

Second premolar (bicuspid)

First premolar (bicuspid)
Canine (cuspid)
Lateral incisor (second incisor)

Central incisor (first incisor)

MANDIBULAR

B

Figure 1–1. *A,* Casts of deciduous or primary dentition. *B,* Casts of permanent dentition.

The incisors are cutting teeth, the canines have a pointed cusp for tearing and incision, whereas the molars have broad occlusal surfaces with multiple cusps which break up food material as an aid in the digestive process.

THE PERMANENT TEETH

By the time the child is about six years of age, the first permanent teeth (the first molars) appear in the maxilla and mandible, which have now become large enough to accommodate them. These teeth take their position *posterior* to the deciduous teeth. One by one the deciduous teeth are exfoliated, from the seventh year on, by a natural process brought about by *resorption* of their roots. *Succedaneous* permanent teeth take their places at the proper time. When the jaws have grown sufficiently, two additional molars are added posteriorly to the first molars.

The *permanent dental formula* of man is:

$$I \frac{2}{2} \, C \frac{1}{1} \, P \frac{2}{2} \, M \frac{3}{3} = 16$$

Premolars have now been added to the formula, two maxillary and two mandibular, and a third molar has been added, one maxillary and one mandibular (Fig. 1–1, *B*).

From the above we make the observation that the child has twenty deciduous teeth, and the adult thirty-two permanent teeth.

THE CROWN AND ROOT

Each tooth has a *crown and root* portion. The crown is covered with *enamel,* and the root portion is covered with *cementum.* The crown and root join at the *cementoenamel* junction. This junction, also called the *cervical line* (Fig. 1–2), is plainly visible on a specimen tooth. The main bulk of the tooth is composed of *dentin,* which is clear in a cross section of the tooth. This cross section displays a *pulp chamber* and a

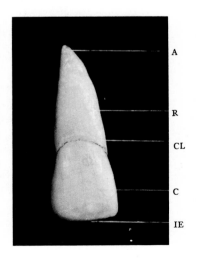

Figure 1–2. Maxillary central incisor (labial aspect). *A,* apex of root; *R,* root; *CL,* cervical line; *C,* crown; *IE,* incisal edge.

A

R

CL

C

IE

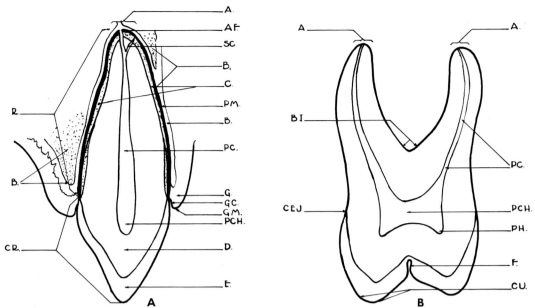

Figure 1–3.   Schematic drawings of cross sections of an anterior and a posterior tooth. *A,* Anterior tooth. *A,* apex; *AF,* apical foramen; *SC,* supplementary canal; *C,* cementum; *PM,* periodontal membrane; *B,* bone; *PC,* pulp canal; *G,* gingiva; *GC,* gingival crevice; *GM,* gingival margin; *PCH,* pulp chamber; *D,* dentin; *E,* enamel; *CR,* crown; *R,* root. *B,* Posterior tooth. *A,* apices; *PC,* pulp canal; *PCH,* pulp chamber; *PH,* pulp horn; *F,* fissure; *CU,* cusp; *CEJ,* cementoenamel junction; *BI,* bifurcation of roots.

pulp canal which normally contain the *pulp tissue.* The pulp chamber is in the crown portion mainly, and the pulp canal is in the root (Fig. 1–3). The spaces are continuous with each other and are spoken of collectively as the *pulp cavity.*

The four tooth tissues are *enamel, cementum, dentin* and *pulp.* The first three are known as *hard tissues,* the last as *soft tissue.* The pulp tissue furnishes the blood and nerve supply to the tooth.

The *crown* of an incisor tooth may have an incisal *ridge* or edge, as in the *central* and *lateral incisors;* a single *cusp,* as in the canines; or two or more cusps, as on premolars and molars. Incisal ridges and cusps form the cutting surfaces on tooth crowns.

The *root* portion of the tooth may be *single,* with one *apex* or terminal end, as usually found in *anterior* teeth and some of the premolars; or *multiple,* with a *bifurcation* or *trifurcation* dividing the root portion into two or more extensions or roots with their *apices* or terminal ends, as found on all molars and in some premolars.

The *root* portion of the tooth is firmly fixed in the bony process of the jaw, so that each tooth is held in its position relative to the others in the *dental arch.* That portion of the jaw which serves as a support for the tooth is called the *alveolar process.* The bone of the tooth socket is called the *alveolus* (plural, *alveoli)* (Fig. 1–6).

The crown portion is never covered by bone tissue after it is fully erupted, but it is partly covered at the *cervical third* in young adults by soft tissue of the mouth known as the *gingiva* or *gingival tissue,* or *gum tissue.* In older persons all of the enamel may be exposed in the oral cavity, and frequently some cervical cementum.

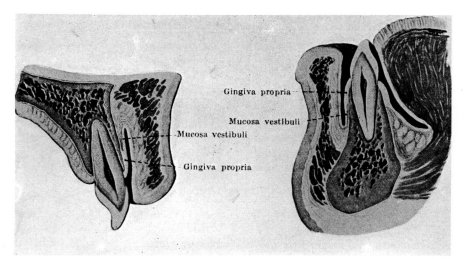

Figure 1–4. Sagittal sections through the central incisors and adjacent tissues (maxillary and mandibular). (Sicher, *Oral Anatomy,* The C. V. Mosby Company.)

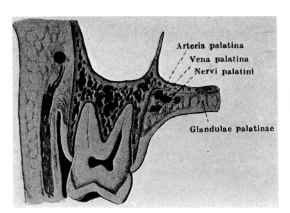

Figure 1–5. Vertical section through the second maxillary molar and adjacent tissues. (Sicher, *Oral Anatomy,* The C. V. Mosby Company.)

Figure 1–6. Left maxillary bone showing the alveolar process with three molars in place, and the alveoli of the central incisor, lateral incisor, canine, first and second premolars. Note the opening at the bottom of the canine alveolus, an opening which accommodates the nutrient blood and nerve supply to the tooth in life. Although they do not show in the photograph, the other alveoli present the same arrangement.

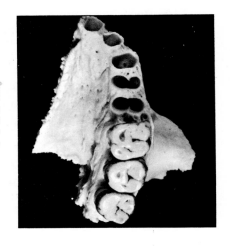

SURFACES AND RIDGES

The crowns of the incisors and canines have four surfaces and a ridge, and the crowns of the premolars and molars have five surfaces. The surfaces are named according to their positions and uses (Fig. 1–7). In the incisors and canines the surfaces toward the lips are called *labial surfaces*, and in the premolars and molars those facing the cheek are the *buccal surfaces*. When labial and buccal surfaces are spoken of collectively they are called *facial surfaces*. All surfaces facing toward the tongue are called *lingual surfaces*. The surfaces of the premolars and molars which come in contact with those in the opposite jaw during the act of closure (called *occlusion*) are called *occlusal surfaces*. In incisors and canines, those surfaces are called *incisal surfaces*.

The surfaces of the teeth facing toward adjoining teeth in the same dental arch are called *proximal* or *proximate surfaces*. The proximal surfaces may be called either *mesial* or *distal*. These terms have special reference to the position of the surface relative to the *median line* of the face. This line is drawn vertically through the center of the face, passing between the central incisors at their point of contact with each other

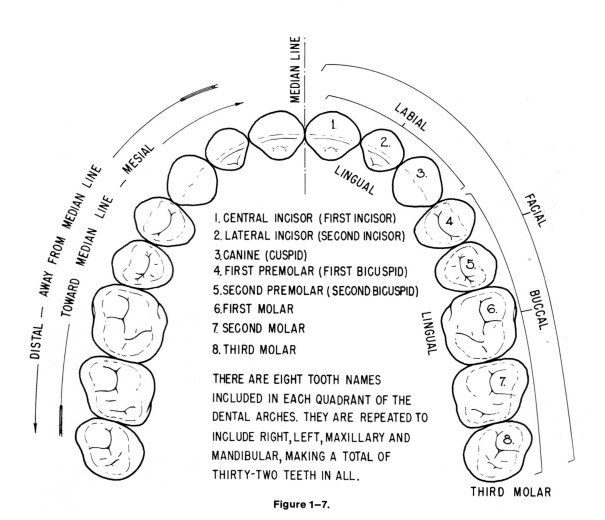

1. CENTRAL INCISOR (FIRST INCISOR)
2. LATERAL INCISOR (SECOND INCISOR)
3. CANINE (CUSPID)
4. FIRST PREMOLAR (FIRST BICUSPID)
5. SECOND PREMOLAR (SECOND BICUSPID)
6. FIRST MOLAR
7. SECOND MOLAR
8. THIRD MOLAR

THERE ARE EIGHT TOOTH NAMES INCLUDED IN EACH QUADRANT OF THE DENTAL ARCHES. THEY ARE REPEATED TO INCLUDE RIGHT, LEFT, MAXILLARY AND MANDIBULAR, MAKING A TOTAL OF THIRTY-TWO TEETH IN ALL.

Figure 1–7.

in both the maxilla and the mandible. Those proximal surfaces which, following the curve of the arch, are faced toward the median line, are called *mesial surfaces,* and those most distant from the median line are called *distal surfaces.*

Four teeth have mesial surfaces which contact each other: the maxillary and mandibular central incisors. In all other instances the mesial surface of one tooth contacts the distal surface of its neighbor, except for the distal surfaces of third molars of permanent teeth and distal surfaces of second molars in deciduous teeth, which have no teeth distal to them. The area of the mesial or distal surface of a tooth which touches its neighbor in the arch is called the *contact area.*

Central and lateral incisors and canines as a group are called *anterior teeth;* premolars and molars as a group, *posterior teeth.*

OTHER LANDMARKS

In order to study an individual tooth intelligently one must be able to recognize all landmarks of importance by name. Therefore at this point it will be necessary to become familiar with additional terms such as:

cusp	triangular ridge	developmental groove
tubercle	transverse ridge	supplemental groove
cingulum	oblique ridge	pit
ridge	fossa	lobe
marginal ridge	sulcus	

A *cusp* is an elevation or mound on the crown portion of a tooth making up a divisional part of the occlusal surface (Figs. 1–3 and 1–8).

A *tubercle* is a smaller elevation on some portion of the crown produced by an extra formation of enamel (Fig. 4–25, A, Chapter 4). These are deviations from the typical form.

A *cingulum* is the lingual lobe of an anterior tooth. It makes up the bulk of the cervical third of the lingual surface. Its convexity mesiodistally resembles a girdle (cingulum is the Latin for girdle) encircling the lingual surface at the cervical third (Fig. 1–10 and Fig. 4–23, A, Chapter 4).

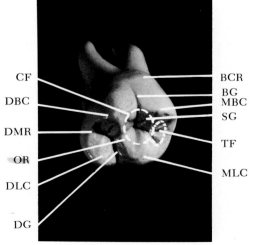

Figure 1–8. Some landmarks on the maxillary first molar. *BG*, buccal groove; *MBC*, mesiobuccal cusp; *SG*, supplemental groove; *TF*, triangular fossa; *MLC*, mesiolingual cusp; *DG*, developmental groove; *DLC*, distolingual cusp; *OR*, oblique ridge; *DMR*, distal marginal ridge; *DBC*, distobuccal cusp; *CF*, central fossa; *BCR*, buccocervical ridge.

CF
DBC
DMR
OR
DLC
DG

BCR
BG
MBC
SG
TF
MLC

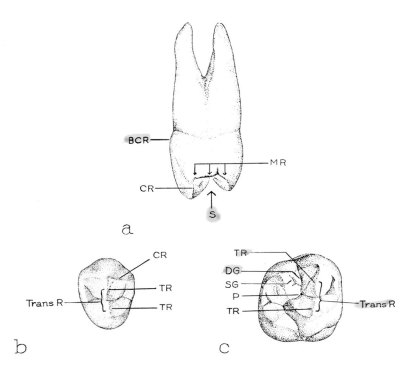

Figure 1-9. *a,* Mesial view of a maxillary right first premolar. *S,* sulcus traversing occlusal surface; *MT,* marginal ridge; *CR,* cusp ridge; *BCR,* buccocervical ridge. *b,* Occlusal view of maxillary right first premolar, *CR,* cusp ridge; *TR,* triangular ridges; *Trans R,* transverse ridge, formed by two triangular ridges crossing the tooth transversely. *c,* Occlusal view of a maxillary right first molar. *TR,* triangular ridge; *DG,* developmental groove; *SG,* supplemental groove; *P,* pit formed by junction of developmental grooves; *TR,* triangular ridge; *Trans R,* transverse ridge.

A *ridge* is any linear elevation on the surface of a tooth and is named according to its location: *buccal* ridge, *incisal* ridge, *marginal* ridge, etc.

Marginal ridges are those rounded borders of the enamel which form the mesial and distal margins of the occlusal surfaces of premolars and molars and the mesial and distal margins of the lingual surfaces of the incisors and canines (Fig. 1-9, *A* and Fig. 1-10).

Triangular ridges are those ridges which descend from the tips of the cusps of molars and premolars toward the central part of the occlusal surfaces. They are so named because the slopes of each side of the ridge are inclined to resemble two sides of a triangle (Fig. 1-9, *B* and *C*, and Fig. 1-11). They are named after the cusps to

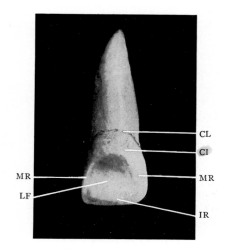

Figure 1-10. Maxillary right central incisor (lingual aspect).*
CL, cervical line; *CI,* cingulum, also called linguocervical ridge; *MR,* marginal ridge; *IR,* incisal ridge; *LF,* lingual fossa.

*For further graphic imformation on landmarks see Figs. 3-27, 6-1, 7-1, 8-1, 8-3, 9-1, 9-15, 10-1, 11-1 to 11-7 and 12-1 to 12-6.

Figure 1–11. Mandibular right first molar. *MLC*, mesio-lingual cusp; *MMR*, mesial marginal ridge; *MBC*, mesiobuccal cusp; *MBG*, mesiobuccal groove; *CF*, central fossa; *DBG*, disto-buccal groove; *DBC*, distobuccal cusp; *DC*, distal cusp; *TR*, triangular ridge; *DLC*, distolingual cusp; *TRR*, transverse ridge; *BCR*, buccocervical ridge.

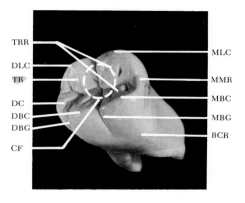

which they belong—e.g., triangular ridge of the buccal cusp of the maxillary first premolar.

When a buccal and a lingual triangular ridge join, they form a *transverse ridge*. A transverse ridge is the union of two triangular ridges crossing transversely the surface of a posterior tooth (Fig. 1–9, *B* and *C*).

The *oblique ridge* is a variable ridge crossing obliquely the occlusal surfaces of maxillary molars. It, too, is formed by the union of two triangular ridges (Fig. 1–8).

A *fossa* is an irregular depression or concavity. *Lingual* fossae are on the lingual surface of incisors. *Central* fossae are on the occlusal surface of molars. They are formed by the converging of ridges terminating at a central point in the bottom of the depression, where there is a junction of grooves. *Triangular* fossae are found on molars and premolars on the occlusal surfaces mesial or distal to marginal ridges. They are sometimes found on the lingual surfaces of maxillary incisors at the edge of the lingual fossae where the marginal ridges and the cingulum meet (Fig. 4–24, *A*, p. 94).

A *sulcus* is a long depression or valley in the surface of a tooth between ridges and cusps, the inclines of which meet at an angle. A sulcus has a developmental groove at the junction of its inclines. (The term "sulcus" must not be confused with the term *groove*.)

A *developmental groove* is a shallow groove or line between the primary parts of the crown or root. A *supplemental groove*, less distinct, is also a shallow linear depression on the surface of a tooth, but it is supplemental to a developmental groove and does not mark the junction of primary parts. *Buccal* and *lingual grooves* are developmental grooves found on the buccal and lingual surfaces of posterior teeth (Figs. 1–8 and 1–11).

Pits are small pinpoint depressions located at the junction of developmental grooves or at terminals of those grooves. For instance, *central pit* is a term used to describe a landmark in the central fossa of molars where developmental grooves join (Fig. 1–9, *C*).

A *lobe* is one of the primary sections of formation in the development of the crown. Cusps and mamelons are representative of lobes. A *mamelon* is any one of the three rounded protuberances found on the incisal ridges of newly erupted incisor teeth (Fig. 4–5, Chapter 4). (For further description of lobes see Figs. 4–23, 4–24 and 4–25, Chapter 4.)

The *roots* of the teeth may be single or multiple. Both maxillary and mandibular anterior teeth have only one root each. Mandibular first and second premolars and the maxillary second premolar are single-rooted, but the maxillary first premolar has two roots in most cases, one buccal and one lingual. Maxillary molars have three roots, one mesiobuccal, one distobuccal and one lingual. Mandibular molars have two roots, one mesial and one distal. It must be understood that description in anatomy can never follow a hard and fast rule. Variations frequently occur. This is especially true regarding tooth roots.

DIVISION INTO THIRDS, LINE ANGLES AND POINT ANGLES

For purposes of description the crowns and roots of teeth have been divided into thirds, and junctions of the crown surfaces are described as *line angles* and *point angles*. Actually, there are no angles or points or plane surfaces on the teeth anywhere except those which appear from wear, or *abrasion*, or from accidental fracture. The terms "line angle" and "point angle" are used only as descriptive terms to indicate a location.

When the surfaces of the crown and root portions are divided into *thirds*, these thirds are named according to their location. Looking at the tooth from the *labial* or *buccal* aspect, one sees that the crown and root may be divided into thirds from the incisal or occlusal surface of the crown to the apex of the root (Fig. 1–12). The *crown* is divided into an incisal or occlusal third, a middle third and a cervical third. The *root* is divided into a cervical third, middle third and apical third.

The crown may be divided into thirds in three directions: inciso- or occlusocervically, mesiodistally, or labio- or buccolingually. Mesiodistally it is divided into the mesial, middle and distal thirds. Labio- or buccolingually it is divided into labial or buccal, middle and lingual thirds. Each of the five surfaces of a crown may be so divided. There will be one middle third and two other thirds, which are named according to their location as cervical, occlusal, mesial, lingual, etc.

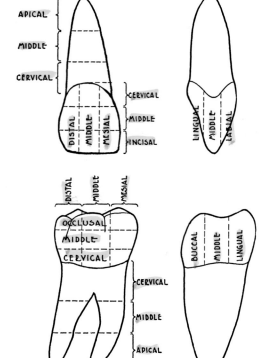

Figure 1–12.   Division into thirds.

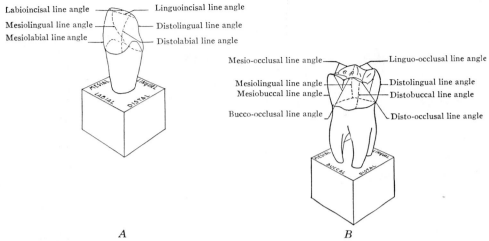

Figure 1–13.   Line angles.

A *line angle* is formed by the junction of two surfaces and derives its name from the combination of the two surfaces that join. For instance, on an anterior tooth, the junction of the mesial and labial surfaces is called the "mesiolabial line angle" (Fig. 1–13, *A*).

The *line angles* of the *anterior teeth* are:

mesiolabial   distolingual
distolabial   labioincisal
mesiolingual   linguoincisal

Because the mesial and distal incisal angles of anterior teeth are rounded, *mesioincisal line angles* and *distoincisal line angles* are usually considered nonexistent. They are spoken of as *mesial* and *distal incisal* angles only.

The *line angles* of the *posterior teeth* are:

mesiobuccal   distolingual   bucco-occlusal
distobuccal   mesio-occlusal   linguo-occlusal
mesiolingual   disto-occlusal

A *point angle* is formed by the junction of three surfaces. The point angle also derives its name from the combination of the names of the surfaces forming it. For example, the junction of the mesial, buccal and occlusal surfaces of a molar is called the "mesiobucco-occlusal point angle" (Fig. 1–14, *B*).

The *point angles* of the *anterior teeth* are:

mesiolabioincisal   mesiolinguoincisal
distolabioincisal   distolinguoincisal

The *point angles* of the *posterior teeth* are:

mesiobucco-occlusal   mesiolinguo-occlusal
distobucco-occlusal   distolinguo-occlusal

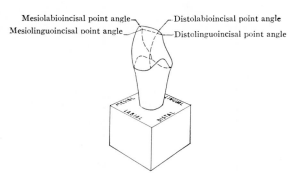

Mesiolabioincisal point angle — Distolabioincisal point angle
Mesiolinguoincisal point angle — Distolinguoincisal point angle

A. Anterior tooth.

Figure 1–14. Point angles.

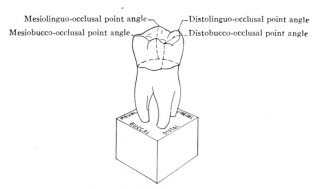

Mesiolinguo-occlusal point angle — Distolinguo-occlusal point angle
Mesiobucco-occlusal point angle — Distobucco-occlusal point angle

B. Posterior tooth.

TOOTH FORM DRAWING AND CARVING

The subject of tooth drawing and carving is being introduced at this point because it has been found through experience that a laboratory course in tooth morphology (dissection, drawing and carving) should be carried on simultaneously with lectures and reference work on the subject of dental anatomy. Illustrations and instruction in tooth form drawing and carving will not, however, be included in this volume. A manual covering the subject is published in a separate binding (*An Atlas of Tooth Form,* W. B. Saunders Company).

Since form and function are allied so closely, the smallest details in dental anatomy are important. If restoration in operative dentistry is to be done scientifically, conscientious study through continuous close observation is necessary.

In an effort to establish more accuracy in restoration, an attempt was started some years ago to improve the teaching of tooth form by means of drawing to scale and carving to scale.

The author's plans and specifications for drawings and carvings of a complete model of dental arches began with the use of Dr. Greene Vardiman Black's table of average measurements for permanent teeth as a basis. It was found, however, that teeth drawn or carved to those dimensions would not give what was wanted. Adjoining teeth in either of the dental arches were not always in good proportion, and opposing teeth in the opposite arch would not occlude properly when carvings were set up and occluded. Also, carving teeth natural size calibrated to tenths of a millimeter was found impracticable. Dr. Black's table being used as a starting point, therefore, deviation was made only when it seemed necessary to create the approach to the idealized norm. The only fractions listed in the model table are five-tenths of a millimeter and three-tenths of a millimeter, the latter in a few instances only. Fractions were avoided wherever possible in order to facilitate familiarity with the table and to avoid confusion.

Carvings were completed that corresponded to the adjusted measurements; they were set up and occluded on an articulator in "balanced" occlusion. The carvings placed in "ideal" alignment proved the advisability of the tooth form in the carvings and the efficacy of the suggested table of measurements. (Figs. 1–17, 1–18, and 1–19).

A table of measurements must be arbitrarily agreed upon, so that a reasonable comparison can be made when appraising the dimensions of any one aspect of one tooth in the mouth with that of another. It has been found that the projected table functions well in that way. For instance, if the mesiodistal measurement of the maxillary central incisor is 8.5 millimeters, the canine will be approximately one millimeter narrower in that measurement; if by chance the central incisor is wider or narrower than 8.5 millimeters, the canine measurement will correspond proportionately.

Photographs of the five aspects of each tooth (mesial, distal, labial or buccal, lingual and incisal or occlusal) were taken with a lens capable of two diameter registrations. In short, the photographs show each tooth with its dimensions squared. These photographs were superimposed on squared millimeter cross section paper, obtainable from engineers' supply firms, which was a practical help in standardizing the relative positions of the tooth outlines on a given background. This procedure reduced the tooth outlines of each aspect to an accurate graph, so that it was possible to compare and record the contours (Figs. 1–15 and 1–16).

Close observation of the outlines of the squared backgrounds shows the relationship of crown to root, extent of curvatures at various points, inclination of roots, relative widths of occlusal surfaces, height of marginal ridges, contact areas, and so on. The *Atlas*, illustrating the methods of drawing and carving teeth, makes use of the scientific information discovered through these investigations.

Although there is no such thing as an established invariable norm in nature, in the study of anatomy it is necessary that there be a starting point; therefore we must begin with an *arbitrary criterion*, accepted after experimentation and due consideration. Since restorative work in dentistry is a manual art which must approach the scientific as closely as manual dexterity will allow, models, plans, photographs and natural specimens should be given preference over the written text in this subject.

Every curve and segment of a normal tooth has some functional basis, and it is important to reproduce them. *It is to be hoped that dental restoration will continue to develop as a science to restore function and not as a manual art to provide mere substitutes for lost tissue.*

"Art and Science have their meeting point in method." With that thought in mind, these plans with a finished model are presented. The successful operator in dentistry or, for that matter, any designer of dental restorations should be able to create pictures in his mind of the teeth from any aspect. Complete pictures can be formed only when one is familiar with all details in tooth form.

One should find it possible to draw reasonably well an outline of any aspect of any tooth in the mouth. It should be in good proportion without reference to another drawing or three-dimensional model. If drawings are mastered, tooth carving in three dimensions will follow successfully without incident. The fact is, if drawing in two dimensions is found to be difficult, carving the same subject in three dimensions will prove to be much more so.

Dental restoration must be approached from the engineer's viewpoint. Therefore the study of tooth reproduction must have a plan, and details of reconstruction should

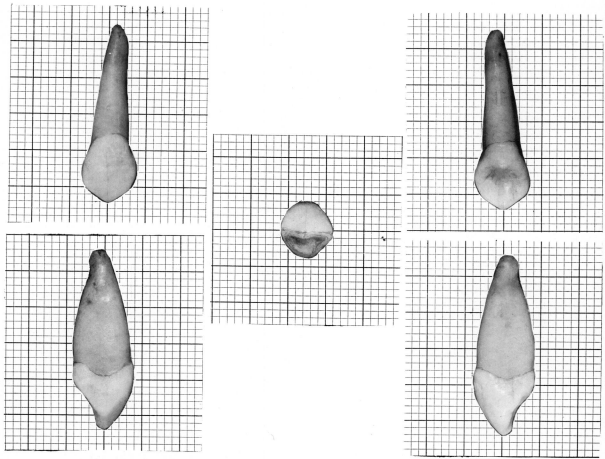

Figure 1–15. Maxillary left canine. When viewing the mesial and distal aspects, note the curvature or bulge on the crown at the cervical third below the cementoenamel junction. This is called the *cervical ridge,* or the *cervicoenamel ridge.*

comply with the plan at all times. While it is impossible for the dentist to work with the precision of a mechanic operating a machine, and since the dentist's work must finally be the result of the coordination of hand and eye only, nevertheless, the engineer's viewpoint will give the operator an attitude of approach which will make him dissatisfied with anything less than logical sequence and good finish in technique.

Acute observation comes only after habitual study of detail. With the necessary application and interest, any dental operator can train himself to be an authority on the anatomy of the teeth—and that is the first step in becoming a master operator. To be a finished operator on human teeth, the observer must absorb every detail of dental anatomy.

For excellence, an observer must:

1. *Become so familiar with the table of measurements that it is possible to make instant comparisons mentally of the proportion of one tooth to another from any aspect.*
2. *Learn to draw accurate outlines of any aspect of any tooth.*

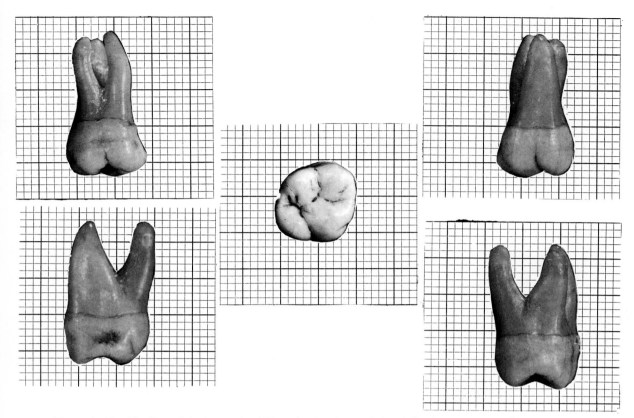

Figure 1–16. Maxillary right first molar. When viewing the mesial and distal aspects, note the curvature or bulge on the crown at the cervical third below the cementoenamel junction. This is called the *cervical ridge,* or the *cervicoenamel ridge.*

3. *Learn to carve with precision any design one can illustrate with line drawings.*

Although many individuals find the drawing and carving of teeth relatively easy, it is extremely difficult for others. It must also be remembered that a carving showing considerable skill and a beautiful finish often will fail to pass a rigid inspection with the caliper. Since this is a *scientific* course as well as an *art* course, *accuracy of outline* is paramount. Remember, *tooth contours affect function.*

When one is studying the *form* of anything, work will be facilitated by having a standard for comparative purposes. Since skulls and extracted teeth show so many variations and anomalies, an arbitrary norm for individual teeth had to be established for comparative study. Hence the thirty-two teeth were carved, natural size, in normal alignment and occlusion, and from the model a table of measurements was drafted. (Figs. 1–17, 1–18, 1–19.)

Although no claim is made that the table of measurements established by the carvings proves an average norm for tooth measurements which must be recognized as such, carvings and drawings made according to the measurements will illustrate teeth which will be accepted generally as close to the average in dimensions; close enough to prove observations on proportion in the study of form.

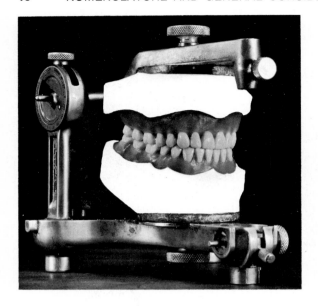

Figure 1–17. Carvings in Ivorine of individual teeth made according to the table of measurements on page 20. These models of teeth are set up into complete dental arches on an anatomic articulator. They have "balance" in lateral and protrusive movements, as well as good centric relation.

If the reader is not familiar with the *Boley gauge,* he should study its use before reading the following instructions on the use of the table of measurements.

In order to understand the table, let us demonstrate the calibrations as recorded and the landmarks they encompass. There are *eight calibrations* of each tooth to be remembered. These measurements are shown in the accompanying example for the maxillary central incisor.

The method of measuring an *anterior* tooth will be shown first, then a posterior one will be used for illustration.

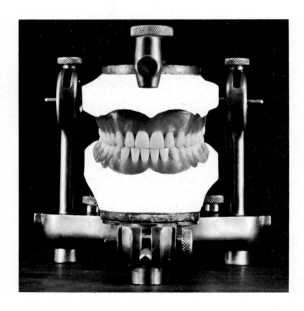

Figure 1–18. Another view of the models shown in Figure 1–17.

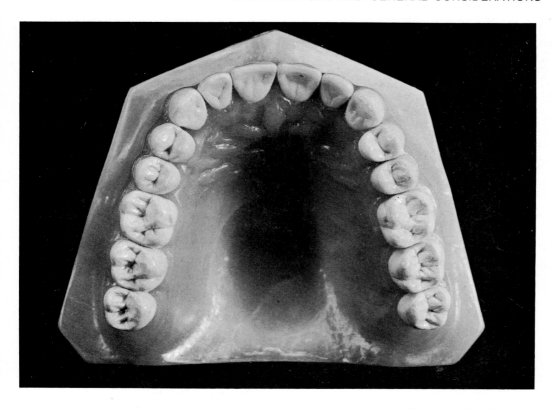

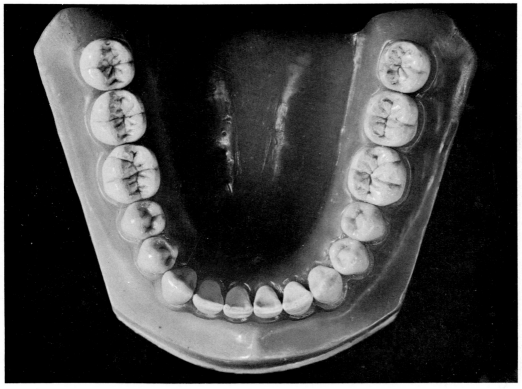

Figure 1–19.   Occlusal view of the models shown in Figures 1–17 and 1–18.

Measurements of the Teeth—Millimeters: Specifications for Drawing and Carving Teeth of Average Size (This table was "proved" by carvings shown in Figures 1–17 and 1–18 and elsewhere in this book.)

Maxillary Teeth	Length of Crown	Length of Root	Mesio-distal Diameter of Crown°	Mesio-Distal Diameter at Cervix	Labio- or Bucco-lingual Diameter	Labio- or Bucco-lingual Diameter at Cervix	Curvature of Cervical Line—Mesial	Curvature of Cervical Line—Distal
Central Incisor	10.5	13.0	8.5	7.0	7.0	6.0	3.5	2.5
Lateral Incisor	9.0	13.0	6.5	5.0	6.0	5.0	3.0	2.0
Canine	10.0	17.0	7.5	5.5	8.0	7.0	2.5	1.5
1st Premolar	8.5	14.0	7.0	5.0	9.0	8.0	1.0	0.0
2d Premolar	8.5	14.0	7.0	5.0	9.0	8.0	1.0	0.0
First Molar	7.5	b 12 l 13	10.0	8.0	11.0	10.0	1.0	0.0
Second Molar	7.0	b 11 l 12	9.0	7.0	11.0	10.0	1.0	0.0
Third Molar	6.5	11.0	8.5	6.5	10.0	9.5	1.0	0.0
Mandibular Teeth								
Central Incisor	9.0†	12.5	5.0	3.5	6.0	5.3	3.0	2.0
Lateral Incisor	9.5†	14.0	5.5	4.0	6.5	5.8	3.0	2.0
Canine	11.0	16.0	7.0	5.5	7.5	7.0	2.5	1.0
1st Premolar	8.5	14.0	7.0	5.0	7.5	6.5	1.0	0.0
2d Premolar	8.0	14.5	7.0	5.0	8.0	7.0	1.0	0.0
First Molar	7.5	14.0	11.0	9.0	10.5	9.0	1.0	0.0
Second Molar	7.0	13.0	10.5	8.0	10.0	9.0	1.0	0.0
Third Molar	7.0	11.0	10.0	7.5	9.5	9.0	1.0	0.0

°The sum of the mesiodistal diameters, both right and left, which gives the arch length, is: maxillary 128 mm., mandibular 126 mm.

†Lingual measurement approximately 0.5 mm. longer.

Measurements of the Teeth—Millimeters: Example

Maxillary Teeth	Length of Crown	Length of Root	Mesio-distal Diameter of Crown	Mesio-distal Diameter of Crown at Cervix	Labio- or Bucco-lingual Diameter of Crown	Labio- or Bucco-lingual Diameter at Cervix	Curvature of Cervical Line—Mesial	Curvature of Cervical Line—Distal
Central Incisor	10.5	13.0	8.5	7.0	7.0	6.0	3.5	2.5

Method of Measuring an Anterior Tooth

(Keep the long axis of the tooth vertical.)

1. Length of Crown (Labial)*

Measurement
{
Crest of curvature at cemento-enamel junction

Incisal edge
}

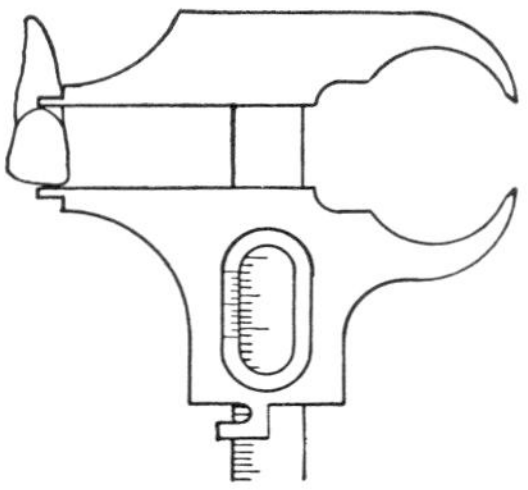

Figure 1–20. Length of crown.

2. Length of Root

Measurement
{
Apex

Crest of curvature at crown cervix
}

Figure 1–21. Length of root.

3. Mesiodistal Diameter of Crown

Measurement
{
Crest of curvature on the mesial surface (mesial contact area)

Crest of curvature on the distal surface (distal contact area)
}

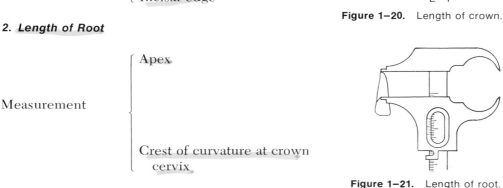

4. Mesiodistal Diameter of Crown at the Cervix

Figure 1–22. Mesiodistal diameter of crown.

Measurement
{
Junction of crown and root on mesial surface

Junction of crown and root on distal surface (use caliper jaws of Boley gauge in this instance instead of parallel beaks)
}

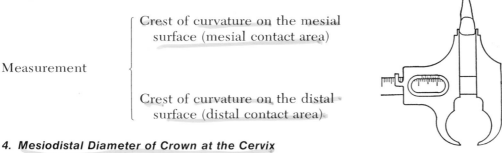

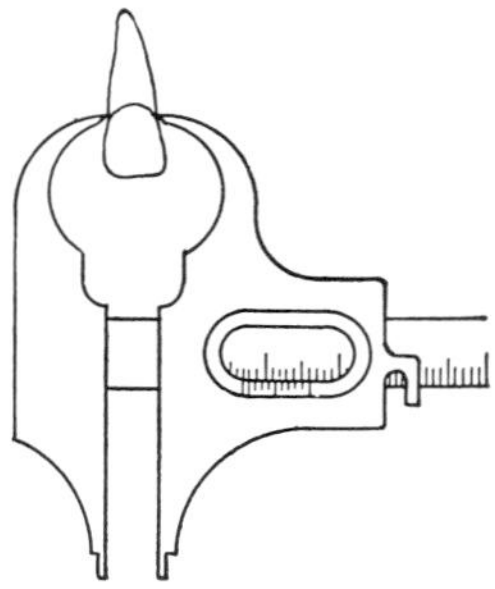

Figure 1–23. Mesiodistal diameter of crown at cervix.

---

*Use the parallel beaks of the Boley gauge for measurements whenever feasible. The contrast of the various curvatures with the straight edges will help to make the close observer more familiar with tooth outlines.

5. *Labiolingual Diameter of Crown*

Measurement
{
Crest of curvature on the labial surface

Crest of curvature on the lingual surface
}

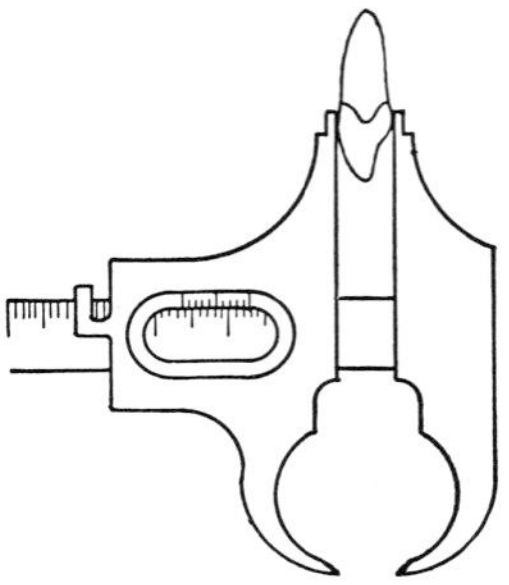

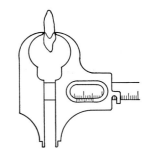

Figure 1–24. Labiolingual diameter of crown.

6. *Labiolingual Diameter of Crown at the Cervix*

Measurement
{
Junction of crown and root on labial surface

Junction of crown and root on lingual surface (use caliper jaws in this instance also)
}

Figure 1–25. Labiolingual diameter of cervix.

7. *Curvature of Cementoenamel Junction on Mesial**

Measurement
{
Crest of curvature of cemento-enamel junction, labial and lingual surface

Crest of curvature of cemento-enamel junction on the mesial surface
}

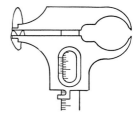

Figure 1–26. Curvature of cementoenamel junction on mesial.

8. *Curvature of Cementoenamel Junction on the Distal*

(Turn the tooth around and calibrate as in Fig. 1–26.)

Measurement
{
Crest of curvature of cemento-enamel junction on the labial and lingual surfaces

Crest of curvature of cemento-enamel junction on the distal surface
}

---

*This measurement is most important because, normally, it represents the extent of curvature approximately of the periodontal attachment when the tooth is in situ.

Method of Measuring a Posterior Tooth

(Keep the long axis of the tooth vertical.)

1. Length of Crown (Buccal)

Measurement
{
Crest of buccal cusp or cusps

Crest of curvature at cemento-
    enamel junction
}

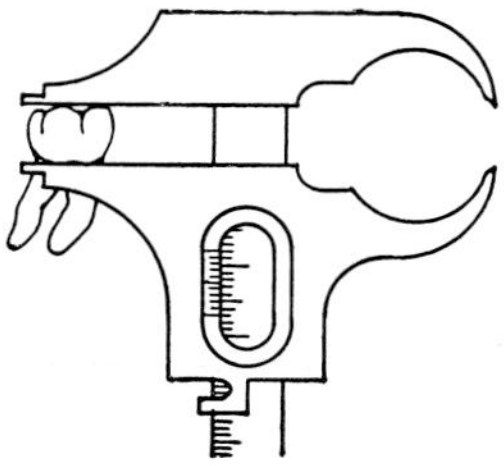

Figure 1–27. Length of crown.

2. Length of Root

Measurement
{
Crest of curvature at crown
    cervix

Apex of root
}

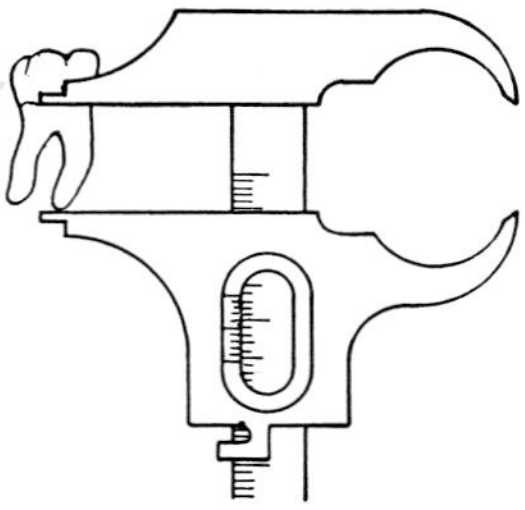

Figure 1–28. Length of root.

3. Mesiodistal Diameter of Crown

Measurement
{
Crest of curvature on mesial
    surface (mesial contact area)

Crest of curvature on distal sur-
    face (distal contact area)
}

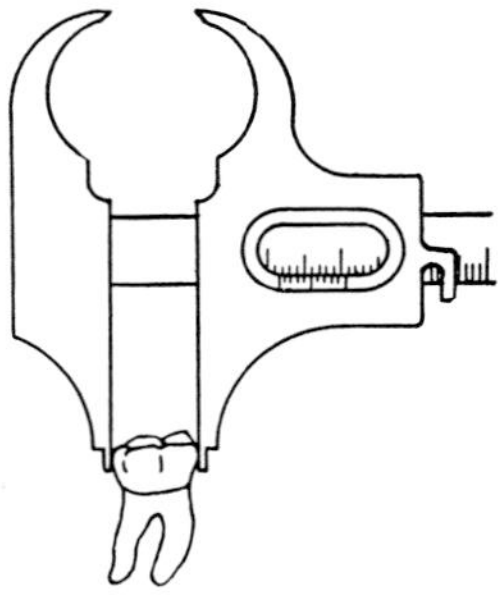

Figure 1–29. Mesiodistal diameter of crown.

4. Mesiodistal Diameter of Crown at the Cervix

Measurement
{
Junction of crown and root on
    mesial surface

Junction of crown and root on
    distal surface (use caliper jaws
    of Boley gauge instead of
    parallel beaks)
}

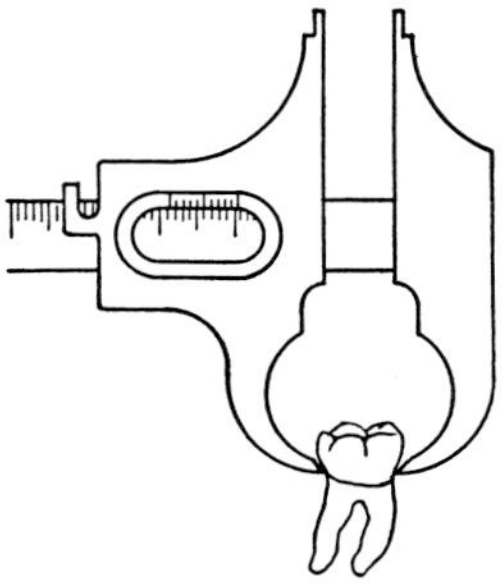

Figure 1–30. Mesiodistal diameter of crown at cervix.

5. *Buccolingual Diameter of Crown*

Measurement
{
Crest of curvature on the buccal surface

Crest of curvature on the lingual surface
}

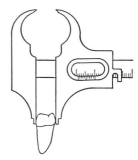

Figure 1–31. Buccolingual diameter of crown.

6. *Buccolingual Diameter of Crown at the Cervix*

Measurement
{
Junction of crown and root on buccal surface

Junction of crown and root on lingual surface. (use caliper jaws)
}

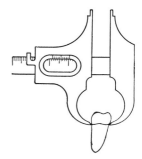

Figure 1–32. Buccolingual diameter of crown at cervix.

7. *Curvature of Cementoenamel Junction on Mesial*

Measurement
{
Crest of curvature of cemento-enamel junction on the mesial surface

Crest of curvature of cemento-enamel junction, buccal and lingual surfaces
}

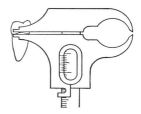

Figure 1–33. Curvature of cementoenamel junction on mesial.

8. *Curvature of Cementoenamel Junction on the Distal*

(Turn tooth around and measure as in Fig. 1–33.)

Measurement
{
Crest of curvature of cemento-enamel junction on the distal surface

Crest of curvature of cemento-enamel junction on the buccal and lingual surfaces
}

2

Development of the Teeth, Calcification and Eruption

The crown and part of the root of a tooth are formed before emergence into the mouth. The crown is formed first; the root follows.

THE DECIDUOUS DENTITION

Calcification of the deciduous teeth begins about the fourth month of fetal life; near the end of the sixth month all of the deciduous teeth have begun to develop. Normally, at birth no teeth are visible in the mouth; occasionally, however, infants are born with erupted mandibular incisors. Such prematurely erupted teeth are usually lost soon after birth because of the incomplete development of the root attachment.

It must be emphasized at this point that all eruption schedules (and this includes calcification) must of necessity be approximate, because no two individuals are exactly alike in their development. Nevertheless, an approximation of averages in an eruption schedule can be a very valuable asset in diagnosis during the developmental years.

According to Schour, "It must be pointed out that the tooth is more than an organ of mastication. During the development of its enamel and dentin the tooth is also a biologic recorder of health and disease, especially of alterations in mineral metabolism. The incremental layer of enamel and dentin reflect metabolic fluctuations just as the growth rings of a tree reflect its life history (weather, nutrition, etc.)."

The deciduous *mandibular central incisors* appear in the mouth at the age of approximately six months. They are followed a month or so later by the *maxillary central incisors*. About two months elapse before the *maxillary lateral incisors* appear. The *mandibular lateral incisors* usually emerge a little earlier than maxillary laterals; in fact, to illustrate the variance in sequence in individuals, babies are often seen displaying four mandibular incisors and no maxillary teeth at all. However, the general rule to be kept in mind is that individual mandibular teeth usually precede the maxillary teeth in the process of eruption, and the teeth in both jaws erupt in *pairs*, one right and one left.

At the age of one year or a little later, the first deciduous molars erupt. The

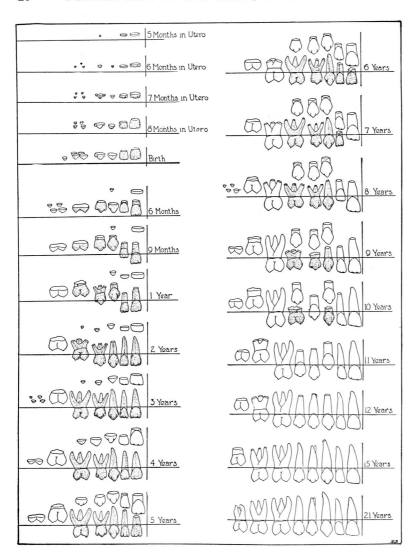

Figure 2–1. The chronology of the upper dentition. (Deciduous teeth stippled.) (From Noyes, Schour and Noyes, *Dental Histology and Embryology,* Lea & Febiger.) Refer also to Figures 2–2 and 2–3.

deciduous canines appear at about sixteen months. When the child is two or two and a half years of age, all of the deciduous teeth are expected to be in use. (Figs. 3–34 and 3–35, Chapter 3.)

To repeat the usual order of appearance of the deciduous teeth in the mouth:

1. Central incisors
2. Lateral incisors
3. First molars
4. Canines
5. Second molars

Mandibular teeth usually precede the maxillary teeth in the order of appearance.

By the time the child is five years old or before, the jaw growth is made manifest by some separation of the deciduous teeth (Fig. 3–2, Chapter 3).

A common impression, which is still widespread, is that the deciduous teeth are not to be taken seriously, since they will be lost at an early age in the process of making way for the permanent teeth. Many therefore think that since these deciduous teeth are to be replaced, any damage done them, or their premature loss, is not important. This is an erroneous view and one that has dire possibilities in the dental development of children. Possibly because they have been called "baby teeth" or "milk teeth," the laity at times regard the deciduous teeth as being temporary. That is not the case. All of the deciduous teeth are in use from the age of two until the age of seven years, or five years in all. Some of the deciduous teeth are in use from six months until twelve years of age, or eleven and a half years in all. The actual situation is, then, that these teeth are in use, contributing to the health and well-being of the individual, during his first years of greatest development, physically and mentally. With premature loss of deciduous teeth, normal jaw development may not take place. Unless the deciduous dental arches remain intact, therefore, the first permanent molars may not be guided into their normal position to act as "cornerstones" for the permanent dentition.

What is just as important to assure sufficient development for maturity, is normal function on both sides of the dental arches. Normal growth and development cannot take place without daily exercise and the use of both jaws. Without the comfortable activity of either side, one side will be favored to the detriment of normal formation.

PERMANENT DENTITION

The first teeth of the permanent dentition to emerge into the oral cavity are the *first molars*. They make their appearance immediately distal to the deciduous second molars at the age of approximately six years (Fig. 3–3, page 45). As a consequence, these teeth are often called the "six-year molars." They begin to calcify during the first month of life. They are much larger than any of the deciduous teeth and cannot make their entry until the jaw growth has progressed sufficiently to allow the space.

The second permanent tooth to take its place in the arch is the central incisor, which appears when the child is between six and seven years of age. As in the deciduous dentition, the mandibular permanent teeth tend to precede the maxillary teeth in the process of eruption. The mandibular central incisors usually show themselves some months previous to the maxillary central incisors. Often they erupt simultaneously with, or even previous to, the mandibular first molars and are often accompanied by the mandibular lateral incisors.

Before the permanent central incisor can come into position, the deciduous central incisor must be exfoliated. This is brought about by the phenomenon called *resorption* of the deciduous roots. The permanent tooth in its follicle attempts to force its way into the position held by its predecessor. The pressure brought to bear against the deciduous root evidently causes resorption of the root which continues until the deciduous crown has lost its anchorage, becomes loose and is finally exfoliated (Fig. 2–14). In the meantime, the permanent tooth has moved occlusally, so that when the deciduous tooth is lost, the permanent one is at the point of eruption and in proper position to succeed its predecessor.

The *follicles* of the developing *incisors* and *canines* are in a position lingual to the deciduous roots (Fig. 3–4). The developing *premolars* which are to take the place of deciduous molars are within the bifurcation of deciduous molar roots (Figs. 2–11 and 2–12). The permanent incisors, canines and premolars are called *succedaneous teeth*, since they take the place of their deciduous predecessors.

Root resorption sometimes does not follow the routine procedure, with the result that the permanent tooth cannot emerge or else is kept out of its normal place. The

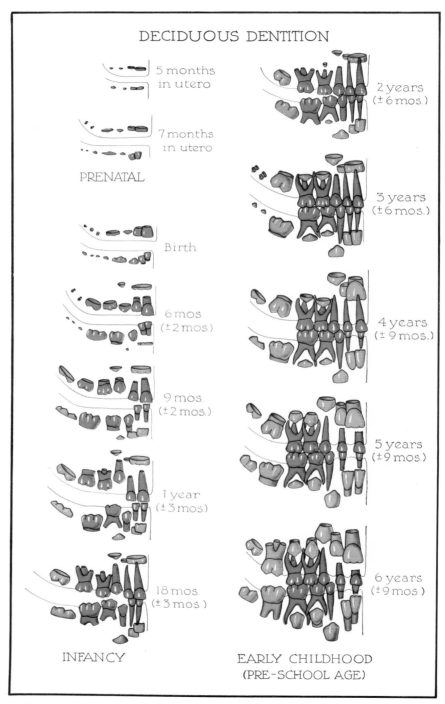

Figure 2–2. Development of the human dentition to the sixth year. The deciduous or primary teeth are the darker ones in the illustration. (I. Schour and M. Massler, University of Illinois College of Dentistry.)

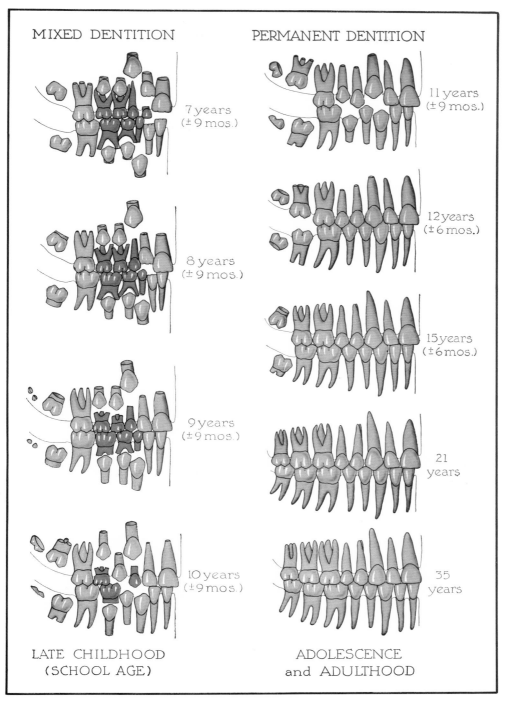

MIXED DENTITION   PERMANENT DENTITION

7 years (±9 mos.)

8 years (±9 mos.)

9 years (±9 mos.)

10 years (±9 mos.)

11 years (±9 mos.)

12 years (±6 mos.)

15 years (±6 mos.)

21 years

35 years

LATE CHILDHOOD (SCHOOL AGE)   ADOLESCENCE and ADULTHOOD

Figure 2–3. Development of the human dentition from the seventh year to maturity. Note the displacement of deciduous teeth by succedaneous permanent teeth. (I. Schour and M. Massler, University of Illinois College of Dentistry.)

Chronology of the Human Dentition (Logan and Kronfeld, slightly modified by Schour)

		Tooth	First Evidence of Calcification	Crown Completed	Eruption	Root Completed
Deciduous dentition	Upper jaw	Central incisor	3–4 mos. *in utero*	4 mos.	7½ mos.	1½–2 yrs.
		Lateral incisor	4½ mos. *in utero*	5 mos.	8 mos.	1½–2 yrs.
		Canine	5¼ mos. *in utero*	9 mos.	16–20 mos.	2½–3 yrs.
		First molar	5 mos. *in utero*	6 mos.	12–16 mos.	2–2½ yrs.
		Second molar	6 mos. *in utero*	10–12 mos.	20–30 mos.	3 yrs.
	Lower jaw	Central incisor	4½ mos. *in utero*	4 mos.	6½ mos.	1½–2 yrs.
		Lateral incisor	4½ mos. *in utero*	4¼ mos.	7 mos.	1½–2 yrs.
		Canine	5 mos. *in utero*	9 mos.	16–20 mos.	2½–3 yrs.
		First molar	5 mos. *in utero*	6 mos.	12–16 mos.	2–2½ yrs.
		Second molar	6 mos. *in utero*	10–12 mos.	20–30 mos.	3 yrs.
Permanent dentition	Upper jaw	Central incisor	3–4 mos.	4– 5 yrs.	7– 8 yrs.	10 yrs.
		Lateral incisor	10 mos.	4– 5 yrs.	8– 9 yrs.	11 yrs.
		Canine	4–5 mos.	6– 7 yrs.	11–12 yrs.	13–15 yrs.
		First premolar	1½–1¾ yrs.	5– 6 yrs.	10–11 yrs.	12–13 yrs.
		Second premolar	2–2¼ yrs.	6– 7 yrs.	10–12 yrs.	12–14 yrs.
		First molar	At birth	2½– 3 yrs.	6– 7 yrs.	9–10 yrs.
		Second molar	2½–3 yrs.	7– 8 yrs.	12–13 yrs.	14–16 yrs.
		Third molar	7–9 yrs.	12–16 yrs.	17–21 yrs.	18–25 yrs.
	Lower jaw	Central incisor	3–4 mos.	4– 5 yrs.	6– 7 yrs.	9 yrs.
		Lateral incisor	3–4 mos.	4– 5 yrs.	7– 8 yrs.	10 yrs.
		Canine	4–5 mos.	6– 7 yrs.	9–10 yrs.	12–14 yrs.
		First premolar	1¾–2 yrs.	5– 6 yrs.	10–12 yrs.	12–13 yrs.
		Second premolar	2¼–2½ yrs.	6– 7 yrs.	11–12 yrs.	13–14 yrs.
		First molar	At birth	2½– 3 yrs.	6– 7 yrs.	9–10 yrs.
		Second molar	2½– 3 yrs.	7– 8 yrs.	11–13 yrs.	14–15 yrs.
		Third molar	8–10 yrs.	12–16 yrs.	17–21 yrs.	18–25 yrs.

failure of the deciduous root to resorb may bring about prolonged retention of the deciduous tooth (Figs. 2–10 and 2–11).

Mandibular lateral incisors erupt very soon after the central incisors, and often simultaneously. The *maxillary central incisors* erupt next in the chronological order, and the *maxillary lateral incisors* make their appearance about a year later (*cf.* "Chronology of Human Dentition," above and Figs. 2–2 and 2–3): The *first premolars* follow the maxillary laterals in sequence when the child is ten years old, approximately; the *mandibular canines* (cuspids) often appear at the same time. The *second premolars* follow during the next year and then the *maxillary canines*. Usually the second molars come in when the individual is about twelve; they are posterior to the first molars and are commonly called "twelve-year molars." The maxillary canines occasionally erupt along with the second molars, but in most instances of normal eruption the canines precede them somewhat.

The *third molars* do not come in until the age of seventeen years or later. Considerable jaw growth is required after the age of twelve to allow room for these teeth. Third molars are subject to many anomalies and variations of form. Insufficient jaw development for their accommodation complicates matters in the majority of cases. Individuals who have properly developed third molars in good alignment are very much in the minority. Third molar anomalies and variations with the complications brought about by malalignment and subnormal jaw development comprise a subject too vast to be covered here.

The usual order in which the permanent teeth appear is as follows:

1. First molars
2. Mandibular central and lateral incisors
3. Maxillary central incisors
4. Maxillary lateral incisors

5. Mandibular canines
6. First premolars
7. Second premolars
8. Maxillary canines
9. Second molars
10. Third molars

The "Chronology of the Human Dentition," which is a table of calcification and eruption of both deciduous and permanent teeth, was reported by Logan and Kronfeld in 1936 and modified later by McCall and Schour. The table has been recognized generally and has been utilized as an index of tooth development; in fact, this book uses the revised table as authority for all references to the chronology of tooth development.

Dr. Carmen Nolla at the University of Michigan reported the results of new research in 1952. The report covered radiographic studies of tooth development, separating the records of boys and girls, at the Elementary School, University of Michigan. This work progressed over a long period under scientific procedure. The results are most interesting and promise to modify further the original work on this problem by Logan and Kronfeld. Dr. Carmen Nolla refers continually to their original table as modified and makes direct comparisons with it where her research seemed to differ in detail.

Some of the comments of Dr. Nolla, with illustrations and tables follow:

"A method for appraising the development of permanent teeth in terms of the

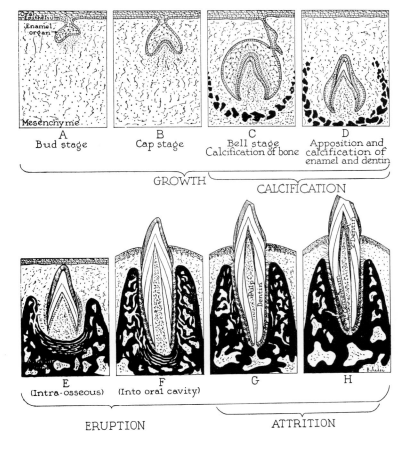

Figure 2–4. Diagram of life cycle of a human deciduous incisor. The normal resorption of the root is not indicated. Enamel and bone are drawn in black. (Slightly modified after Schour and Massler from Maximow and Bloom.) (Schour, *Oral Histology and Embryology,* 8th ed. Lea & Febiger.)

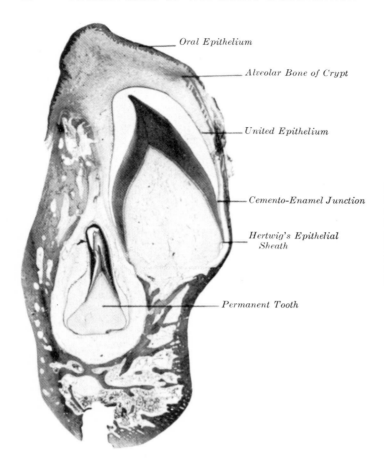

Oral Epithelium

Alveolar Bone of Crypt

United Epithelium

Cemento-Enamel Junction

Hertwig's Epithelial Sheath

Permanent Tooth

Figure 2–5. Section of mandible of 9-month-old infant cut through unerupted deciduous canine and its permanent successor which lies lingually and apically to it. The enamel of the deciduous canine crown is completed and lost because of decalcification. Root formation has begun. (After Schour, *Oral Histology and Embryology,* 8th Edition, Lea & Febiger).

Ages for Completion of Calcification of Permanent Teeth

Teeth Mand.		Crown Completed (Nolla)		Root Completed (Nolla)		Logan and Kronfeld, 1944 (Modified by Schour and Massler) Root Completed
		Boys	Girls	Boys	Girls	
1	1	3 yrs. 8 mo.	3 yrs. 6 mo.	10 yrs.	8 yrs. 6 mo.	9 yrs.
2	2	4 yrs. 4 mo.	4 yrs.	10 yrs. 6 mo.	9 yrs. 8 mo.	10 yrs.
3	3	6 yrs.	5 yrs. 8 mo.	13 yrs. 6 mo.	12 yrs.	12–14 yrs.
4	4	7 yrs.	6 yrs. 6 mo.	14 yrs.	12 yrs. 6 mo.	12–13 yrs.
5	5	7 yrs. 8 mo.	7 yrs. 2 mo.	15 yrs.	14 yrs. 6 mo.	13–14 yrs.
6	6	4 yrs.	3 yrs. 10 mo.	11 yrs. 6 mo.	10 yrs.	9–10 yrs.
7	7	8 yrs. 2 mo.	7 yrs.	16 yrs. 6 mo.	15 yrs. 6 mo.	14–15 yrs.
Max.						
1	1	4½ yrs.	4½ yrs.	11 yrs.	10 yrs.	10 yrs.
2	2	5½ yrs.	5 yrs. 2 mo.	12 yrs.	11 yrs.	11 yrs.
3	3	6½ yrs.	5 yrs. 10 mo.	15 yrs.	12½ to 13 yrs.	13–15 yrs.
4	4	7 yrs. 4 mo.	6 yrs. 4 mo.	14½ yrs.	12 yrs. 9 mo.	12–13 yrs.
5	5	8 yrs. 5 mo.	7 yrs. 3 mo.	15½ yrs.	14 yrs.	13–14 yrs.
6	6	4½ yrs.	4 yrs. 2 mo.	11½ yrs.	9½ yrs.	9–10 yrs.
7	7	8 yrs. 2 mo.	7 yrs. 6 mo.	16½ yrs.	15 yrs. 6 mo.	14–16 yrs.

Norms for the Maturation of Permanent Teeth for Boys (Nolla)

Dental Age (Yrs.)	Mandibular Teeth (Growth Stage)								Maxillary Teeth (Growth Stage)							
	1|1	2|2	3|3	4|4	5|5	6|6	7|7	8|8	1|1	2|2	3|3	4|4	5|5	6|6	7|7	8|8
3	5.2	4.5	3.2	2.6	1.1	5.0	0.7		4.3	3.4	3.0	2.0	1.0	4.2	1.0	
4	6.5	5.7	4.2	3.5	2.2	6.2	2.0		5.4	4.5	3.9	3.0	2.0	5.3	2.0	
5	7.5	6.8	5.1	4.4	3.3	7.0	3.0		6.4	5.5	4.8	4.0	3.0	6.4	3.0	
6	8.2	7.7	5.9	5.2	4.3	7.7	4.0		7.3	6.4	5.6	4.9	4.0	7.4	4.0	
7	8.8	8.5	6.7	6.0	5.3	8.4	5.0	0.8	8.2	7.2	6.3	5.7	4.9	8.2	5.0	
8	9.3	9.1	7.4	6.8	6.2	9.0	5.9	1.4	8.8	8.0	7.0	6.5	5.8	8.9	5.8	1.0
9	9.7	9.5	8.0	7.5	7.0	9.5	6.7	1.8	9.4	8.7	7.7	7.2	6.6	9.4	6.5	1.8
10	10.0	9.8	8.6	8.2	7.7	9.8	7.4	2.0	9.7	9.3	8.4	7.9	7.3	9.7	7.2	2.3
11			9.1	8.8	8.3	9.9	7.9	2.7	9.95	9.7	8.8	8.6	8.0	9.8	7.8	3.0
12			9.6	9.4	8.9		8.4	3.5	9.95		9.2	9.2	8.7		8.3	4.0
13			9.8	9.7	9.4		8.9	4.5			9.6	9.6	9.3		8.8	4.9
14			10.0	9.7			9.3	5.3			9.8	9.8	9.6		9.3	5.9
15				10.0			9.7	6.2			9.9	9.9	9.9		9.6	6.6
16½							10.0	7.3							10.0	7.7
17								7.6								8.0

Norms for the Maturation of Permanent Teeth for Girls (Nolla)

Dental Age (Yrs.)	Mandibular Teeth (Growth Stage)								Maxillary Teeth (Growth Stage)							
	1|1	2|2	3|3	4|4	5|5	6|6	7|7	8|8	1|1	2|2	3|3	4|4	5|5	6|6	7|7	8|8
3	5.3	4.7	3.4	2.9	1.7	5.0	1.6		4.3	3.7	3.3	2.6	2.0	4.5	1.8	
4	6.6	6.0	4.4	3.9	2.8	6.2	2.8		5.4	4.8	4.3	3.6	3.0	5.7	2.8	
5	7.6	7.2	5.4	4.9	3.8	7.3	3.9		6.5	5.8	5.3	4.6	4.0	6.9	3.8	
6	8.5	8.1	6.3	5.8	4.8	8.1	5.0		7.4	6.7	6.2	5.6	4.9	7.9	4.7	
7	9.3	8.9	7.2	6.7	5.7	8.7	5.9	1.8	8.3	7.6	7.0	6.5	5.8	8.7	5.6	
8	9.8	9.5	8.0	7.5	6.6	9.3	6.7	2.1	9.0	8.4	7.8	7.3	6.6	9.3	6.5	2.1
9	10.0	9.9	8.7	8.3	7.4	9.7	7.4	2.3	9.6	9.1	8.5	8.1	7.4	9.7	7.2	2.4
10		10.0	9.2	8.9	8.1	10.0	8.1	3.2	10.0	9.6	9.1	8.7	8.1	10.0	7.9	3.2
11			9.7	9.4	8.6		8.6	3.7		10.0	9.5	9.3	8.7		8.5	4.3
12			10.0	9.7	9.1		9.1	4.7			9.8	9.7	9.3		9.0	5.4
13				10.0	9.4		9.5	5.8			10.0	10.0	9.7		9.5	6.2
14					9.7		9.7	6.5					10.0		9.7	6.8
15					10.0		9.8	6.9							9.8	7.3
16							10.0	7.5							10.0	8.0
17								8.0								8.7

amount of maturation was developed (radiographic records). The data obtained by this procedure are used to provide dental age values presented in the tables. The observational method used to appraise the development of each tooth in the maxillary and the mandibular arch is illustrated in Figures 2–6 and 2–7, titled calcification of maxillary and mandibular teeth, respectively.

"In order to obtain an appraisal of the development of a particular tooth, the

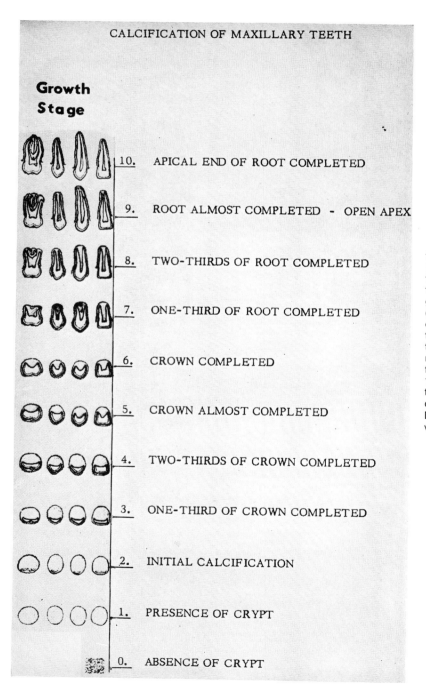

CALCIFICATION OF MAXILLARY TEETH

Growth Stage

10. APICAL END OF ROOT COMPLETED

9. ROOT ALMOST COMPLETED - OPEN APEX

8. TWO-THIRDS OF ROOT COMPLETED

7. ONE-THIRD OF ROOT COMPLETED

6. CROWN COMPLETED

5. CROWN ALMOST COMPLETED

4. TWO-THIRDS OF CROWN COMPLETED

3. ONE-THIRD OF CROWN COMPLETED

2. INITIAL CALCIFICATION

1. PRESENCE OF CRYPT

0. ABSENCE OF CRYPT

Figure 2–6 and 2–7. Under the column entitled growth stage is a set of drawings illustrating the ten stages of development of the teeth as observed radiographically. The first column (right) appraises the growth stage of the central and lateral incisors; the second the canine; the third the premolars and the fourth the molars. The drawings illustrate for each of the ten stages (1 to 10 inclusive) the appearance of the stage of tooth development as observed radiographically. (Child Development Laboratories, University of Michigan.)

radiograph is matched as closely as possible with the comparative figure. For example, if one-third of the crown is completed, the observation is given the value 3; if one-third of the root is completed the observation is graded 7.0. When the radiographic reading lies between two grades, this appraisal is indicated as the value of 0.5. For example, if the X-ray reading is between one-third and two-thirds of the root completed, it is given the value of 7.5. When the X-ray shows a reading that is slightly

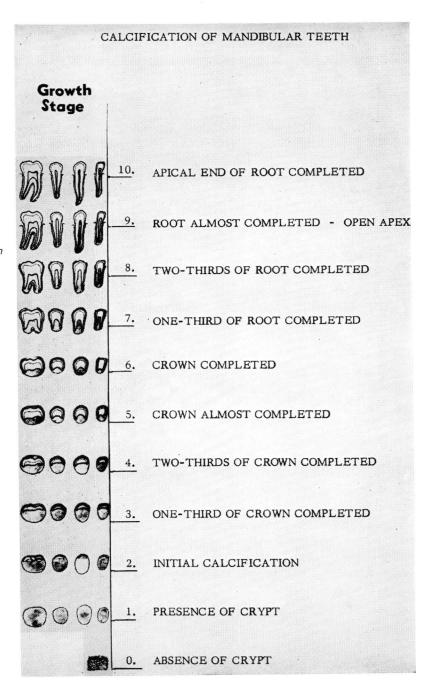

Figure 2–7.   *(See legend on opposite page.)*

CALCIFICATION OF MANDIBULAR TEETH

Growth Stage

10.   APICAL END OF ROOT COMPLETED

9.   ROOT ALMOST COMPLETED - OPEN APEX

8.   TWO-THIRDS OF ROOT COMPLETED

7.   ONE-THIRD OF ROOT COMPLETED

6.   CROWN COMPLETED

5.   CROWN ALMOST COMPLETED

4.   TWO-THIRDS OF CROWN COMPLETED

3.   ONE-THIRD OF CROWN COMPLETED

2.   INITIAL CALCIFICATION

1.   PRESENCE OF CRYPT

0.   ABSENCE OF CRYPT

greater than the illustrated grade, but not as much as halfway between that stage and the next, the value 0.2 is added. For example, if slightly more than two-thirds of the crown is completed, the grade will be 4.2, or if somewhat more than two-thirds of the root is completed it will be 7.2. If the development is slightly less than the grade indicated, the value 0.7 is added to the preceding grade. For example, if two-thirds of the crown is approximately completed, the grade will be 3.7, or if two-thirds of the root is almost completed, the grade will be 7.7.

"Thus, it is possible without too much difficulty to assign the observation value as seen on the growth level, above the growth level, halfway between the growth stage and close to the next level. Attempts to appraise radiographs more accurately than this do not seem feasible.

"In the succeeding annual radiographs, the quantitative increase in calcification easily is determined. The outline of the radiolucent pulp can be followed readily through the different stages of development. The completion of the apical end of the root is the final stage in the process of maturation to be observed radiographically.

"Maturation of teeth may, in this way, be used as a criterion of dental age and of the physiologic age of the patient. It provides an index of physiologic maturity of the permanent dentition."

In an article in the *Journal of Dentistry for Children*, Dr. Nolla stated:

"In the study of child growth and development it has been pointed out by various investigators that the development of the dentition has a close correlation to some other measures of growth. In the laboratory school of the University of Michigan, the nature of growth and development has been investigated by serial examination of the same children at yearly intervals, utilizing a set of objective measurements of various physical and mental attributes. It has been found by Olson and Hughes that there is an intimate relationship in the functioning of all the aspects of normal growth, as has been shown by the plotting of a number of measurements in the same graph. When this relationship is appreciated one thinks of the development of the teeth, not as an isolated process, but as one which relates to other developmental processes.

"So far, the only available measure of dental age has been secured by noting the eruption of teeth. Although the eruption of the teeth may differ greatly in the time of appearance in the mouths of different children, the majority of the children exhibit some pattern in the sequence of eruption. However, consideration of eruption alone makes one cognizant of only one phase of the development of the dentition. A measure of calcification (maturation) at different age levels will provide a more precise index for determining dental age and will contribute to the concept of the organism as a whole."

DEVELOPMENT OF THE TEETH

Apparently there are *four or more centers of formation* for each tooth. The formation of each center proceeds until there is a coalescence of all of them. Each of these centers (when one is speaking of the crown portion) is called a *lobe*.

Although no lines of demarcation are found in the dentin to show this development, there are signs to be found on the surfaces of the crowns and roots; these are called *developmental grooves* (Fig. 4–23).

After the *crown* of the tooth is formed, the *root portion* is begun. At the cervical border of the enamel, at the cervix of the crown, cementum starts to form as a root covering of the dentin. The *cementum* is hard tissue (similar in some ways to bone tissue) which covers the root of the tooth in a thin layer. The junction of enamel and cementum is called the *cementoenamel junction.* For descriptive purposes in dental anat-

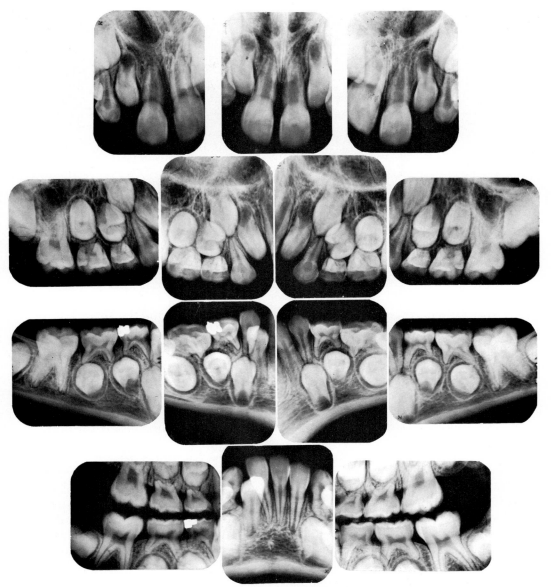

Figure 2–8. Radiographs of teeth of a child eight years old. Maxillary teeth have crowns pointed downward, whereas mandibular teeth have crowns pointed upward. Some of the permanent teeth have erupted, while others may be seen forming above or below deciduous predecessors. Note the resorption of the roots of deciduous teeth.

omy this is spoken of as the *cervical line*, forming a line of demarcation between the crown and root.

The development of the crown and root takes place within a bony crypt in the jaw bone.*

---

*A macroscopic approach will be made to the subject of jaw development and tooth eruption. A summary of what happens chronologically will assist in clinical evaluations. Information concerning the intricate biological processes by which gross anatomy is created must be looked for elsewhere under the title of histology and embryology.

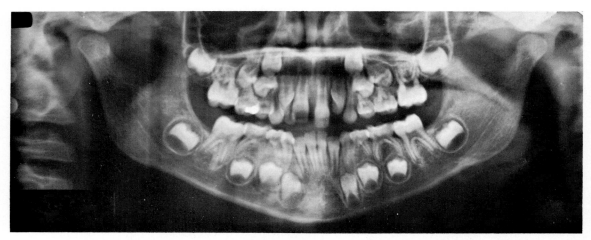

Figure 2–9. Panoramic radiograph of a child about seven years old. This type of examination is of great value in registering an overall record of development. (Dental Radiography and Photography, Eastman Kodak Company, Vol. 43, No. 2, 1970.)

Figures 2–10 to 2–14 are photographs of the skull of a child who was probably in his tenth year. The skull has been dissected to show the positions of the remaining deciduous teeth and their root resorption, as well as the positions and development of the permanent teeth.

After the crown and part of the root are formed, the tooth penetrates the mucous membrane and makes its entry into the mouth. Further formation of the root is supposed to be an active factor in pushing the crown toward its final position in the mouth. Eruption of the tooth is said to be completed when most of the crown is in evidence and when it has made contact with its antagonist or antagonists in the opposing jaw. Actually, eruption may and usually does continue after this; *i.e.,* more of the crown may become exposed, and the tooth may move farther occlusally to accommodate itself to new conditions.

Formation of root dentin and cementum continues after the tooth is in use. The *root* formation is about half finished when the tooth emerges. Ultimately the root is completed. Cementum covers the root. The pulp tissue continues to function with its blood and nerve supply after the tooth is formed. The pulp cavity within the tooth has by this time become small in comparison with the tooth size. Its outline is similar to

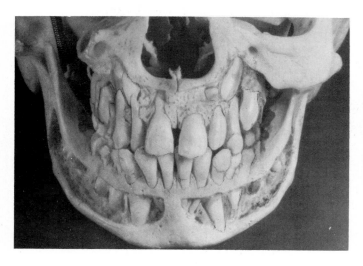

Figure 2–10. Front view of skull of child nine or ten years of age. Note the stages of development and eruption of the various teeth. The canines are lingual to the roots of predecessors. The relation and development of the teeth are normal except for the prolonged retention of the maxillary right lateral incisor, which is locked in a lingual relation to the mandibular teeth.

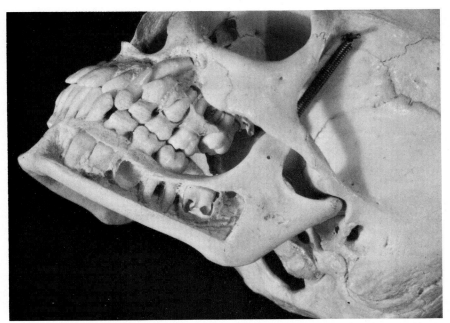

Figure 2–11.   Left side of the skull shown in Figure 2–10. Note the placement of the permanent maxillary canine and the second premolar; also observe the position and stage of development of the maxillary second permanent molar.

The bony crypt of the mandibular second permanent premolar is in full view, since the developing tooth was lost from the specimen.

Observe the large openings in the developing roots of the mandibular second permanent molar.

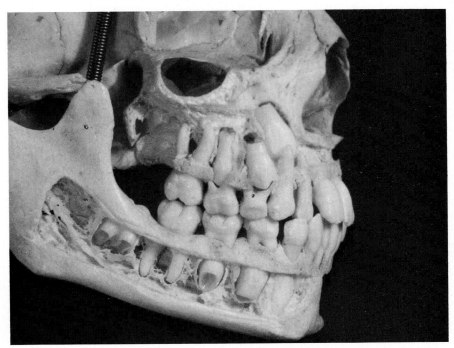

Figure 2–12.   View of the right side of the skull shown in Fig. 2–10. Note the amount of resorption of the roots of the deciduous upper molars which has taken place and the relation of the developing premolars above them. The roots of the first permanent molars have been completed. Note the open pulp chambers and the pulp canals in the developing mandibular teeth. The lingual inclination of the lower second premolar is common. The developing upper second molar has been lost from the specimen.

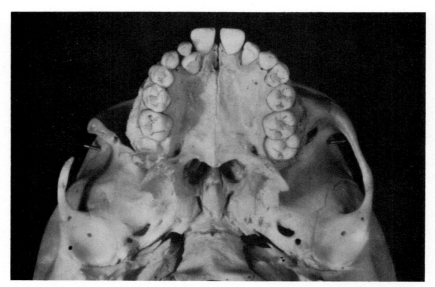

Figure 2–13. Occlusal view of the skull shown in the preceding illustrations. Both maxillary lateral incisors have erupted, but the right lateral has come in lingually to the deciduous tooth because of prolonged retention of the latter. (Compare with Fig. 2–10.) The deciduous canines and molars remain in position. The left maxillary second permanent molar is no longer covered by bone.

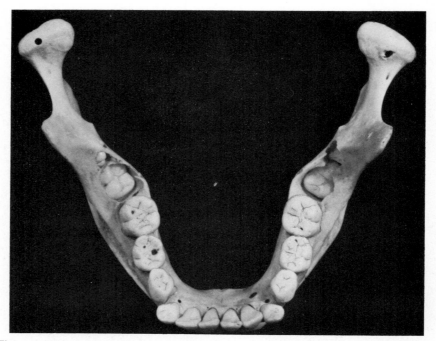

Figure 2–14. Occlusal view of the mandibular arch of the skull shown in Fig. 2–13. The development is typical, with a distal inclination of the lower lateral incisors (permanent) and a labial inclination of the canines (deciduous). Note the openings which have been started in the bone immediately lingual to the deciduous canines to facilitate the eruption of the permanent successors. Also note the developing second molars, typically located, and a tip of the developing third molar (right). The deciduous canines are approaching exfoliation. The deciduous molars remain in their normal positions with good contact relation.

the outline of the crown and root, and the opening of the pulp cavity at the apex is constricted. This opening is called the *apical foramen*. The pulp keeps its tissue-forming function, in that it may form *secondary dentin* on occasion as a protection to itself.

Formation of the tooth is said to be *completed* when the apex of the root is formed; as a matter of fact, however, this process continues slowly throughout the life of the tooth. The pulp cavity becomes smaller and more constricted with age. Sometimes the pulp chamber within the crown is entirely obliterated, and in rare instances the entire pulp cavity has been found filled with secondary deposit. This process is not so extensive in deciduous teeth, since the years of their usefulness are fewer; nevertheless, the same powers are inherent in the deciduous pulp. Deciduous teeth will show secondary dentin in their pulp chambers as a result of the irritation produced by caries or excessive wear.

The *dental pulp* is a connective-tissue organ containing a number of structures, among which are arteries, veins, a lymphatic system and nerves. Its primary function is to form the dentin of the tooth. When the tooth is newly erupted, the dental pulp is large; it becomes progressively smaller as the tooth is completed. The pulp is relatively large in deciduous teeth and also in young permanent teeth. For this reason the teeth of children and young people are more sensitive than teeth of older people to thermal change and dental operative procedure.

At the time of its eruption, the enamel of the crown of the tooth is covered by the *enamel cuticle*. This is a thin horny material called *keratin*, which may be worn off in exposed areas, but which remains in places that are not subject to friction, such as the deepest portions of developmental grooves, interproximal areas and the cervix of the crown, where it is protected by the gingival tissue with its epithelial attachment. The enamel cuticle has been called *Nasmyth's membrane*.

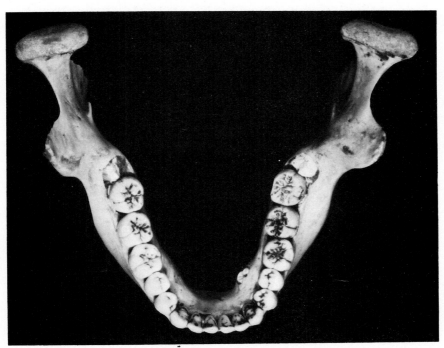

Figure 2–15. A mandible illustrating extra tooth development. A fourth molar is appearing on each side, and a supernumerary premolar is showing to the lingual side of the mandibular second premolars on the left side.

General References

Atkinson, S. R.: Changing Dynamics of the Growing Face. American Journal of Orthodontics, *35*:815–836, 1949.

Atkinson, S. R.: Growth and Development of Teeth and Jaws. Journal of Orthodontics & Oral Surgery. *26*:829–842, 1940.

Atkinson, S. R.: The Permanent Maxillary Lateral Incisor. Am. Journal of Orthodontics & Oral Surgery, *29*:685–698, 1943.

Broadbent, B. H.: The Face of the Normal Child. The Angle Orthodontist, Vol. 7., Oct., 1937.

Broomell, I. N., and Fischelis, P.: Anatomy and Histology of the Mouth and Teeth. 6th ed., Philadelphia, Blakiston, 1923.

Finn, S. B.: Clinical Pedodontics, 2nd ed., Philadelphia, W. B. Saunders Co., 1962.

Gregory and Hellman: Evolution of Dental Occlusion from Fish to Man. First International Orthodontic Congress. C. V. Mosby Co., 1927.

Logan, W. H. G., and Kronfeld, R.: Development of the human jaws and surrounding structures from birth to age fifteen. J.A.D.A., *20*:379–424, 1935.

Massler, M., Schour, I., and Poncher, H. G.: Development pattern of the child as reflected in the calcification pattern of the teeth. American Journal of Dentistry for Children, July, 1941.

McCall, J. O., and Wald, S. S.: Clinical Dental Roentgenology. 2nd ed., Philadelphia, W. B. Saunders Co., 1947.

Nolla, C. M.: Development of the permanent teeth. J. Den. Children, 27:254, 1960.

Nolla, C. M.: The Development of Permanent Teeth. Ann Arbor, Univ. of Michigan, 1962. Sixty page thesis.

Noyes, F. B., Schour, I., Noyes, H. J.: Dental Histology and Embryology, 5th ed., Philadelphia, Lea & Febiger, 1938.

Olson, W. C., and Hughes, B. O.: Growth of the Child as a Whole. *In* Barker, R. C., Kounin, J. S., and Wright, H. F.: Child Behavior and Development. New York, McGraw-Hill, 1943, pp. 199–208.

Schour, I., and Massler, M.: The development of the human dentition. J.A.D.A., 28:1153–60, 1941.

Schour, I., and McCall, J. O.: Chronology of the Human Dentition. *In* Orban, B.: Oral Histology and Embryology, St. Louis, C. V. Mosby, 1944, p.240.

Schour, I., and Noyes, H. J.: Oral Histology and Embryology. 8th ed., Philadelphia, Lea & Febiger, 1960.

Watson, E. H., and Lowrey, G. H.: Growth and Development of Children. 2nd ed., Chicago, Year Book Publishers, 1954.

3

The Deciduous
or Primary Teeth

IMPORTANCE OF THE DECIDUOUS TEETH*

In recent years the health of children has been given increasing thought and consideration by everyone. The medical profession, along with all of its allied groups, has conceded that no child health program is complete without the inclusion of dental health.

The deciduous teeth should be watched and cared for during the child's years of greatest physical development, approximately eleven years in all. Consequently, there is no need to "sell" the importance of the deciduous dentition today to anyone interested in dental care. The contemporary scene has changed. In the year 1940, when this work went to press for the first time, the situation was quite different. The average person, and even some dental personnel, regarded the deciduous dentition as temporary and perhaps of doubtful value when compared with the permanent dentition which was to take its place in due time. Today no one questions the value of delivering good treatment and comfort to a child during these very important years in his life.

Therefore, in this book the deciduous teeth will be described in advance of the permanent dentition, so that they may be given their proper sequence in the study of dental anatomy and physiology. Alignment and occlusion will be under discussion also.

As the term "deciduous" implies, these teeth are shed in order to make way for their permanent successors. The process of exfoliation takes place between the seventh and the twelfth years. This does not, however, indicate the period at which the root resorption of the deciduous tooth begins. For only a year or two after the root is completely formed and the apical foramen is established, resorption begins at the apical extremity and continues in the direction of the crown until resorption of the entire root has taken place and the crown is lost from lack of support. The subject of den-

---

*The term "primary dentition" has been accepted as preferable to the term "deciduous dentition" by the Terminology Committee of the American Society of Dentistry for Children. However, the term "deciduous dentition" will have to be given preference in this text because it is more acceptable to all groups interested in dental anatomy, human or comparative.

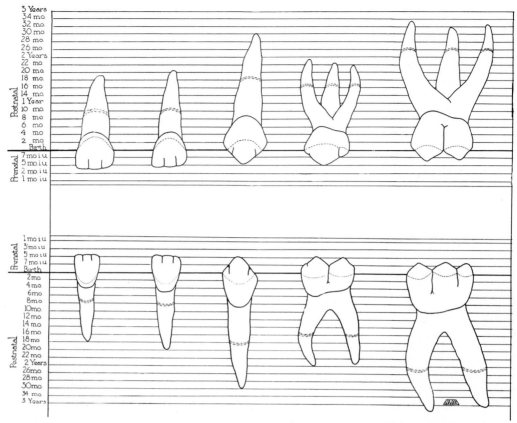

Figure 3–1.   Diagrammatic representation of the chronology of the deciduous teeth. Eruption is completed at the approximate time indicated by the dotted area on the roots of the teeth. (Modified after McBeath, from Noyes, Schour and Noyes, *Dental Histology and Embryology,* Lea & Febiger.)

tal histology and embryology should be consulted for more complete information in this area.

The deciduous teeth are *twenty* in number, ten in each jaw, and they are classified as follows: four *incisors,* two *canines* and four *molars* in each jaw. Beginning with the median line, the teeth are named in each jaw on each side of the mouth as follows: *central incisor, lateral incisor, canine, first molar,* and *second molar.*

The deciduous teeth have been called "temporary," "milk," and "baby" teeth. These terms are improper because they foster the implication that these teeth are useful for a short period only. It should be emphasized again that they are needed for many years of growth and physical development. Premature loss of deciduous teeth is to be avoided.

The first permanent molar, commonly called the *six-year molar,* makes its appearance in the mouth *before any of the deciduous teeth are lost.* It comes in immediately distal to the deciduous second molar.

The deciduous molars are replaced by *permanent premolars.* There are no premolars in the deciduous set, and there are no teeth in the deciduous set which resemble the permanent premolar. However, the crowns of the deciduous *maxillary* first molars resemble the crowns of the permanent premolars as much as they do any of the permanent molars. Nevertheless, they have three well-defined roots, which

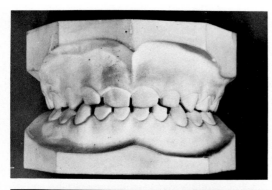

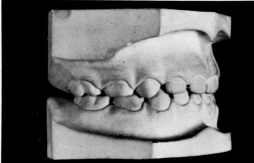

Figure 3–2. Casts of normally developed teeth of a child five years and six months old. Note the form and occlusion of the teeth and their even separation. *Top,* Labial aspect; *Bottom,* buccal aspect. Occlusal aspects of these casts are shown in Fig. 1, Chapter I. (Courtesy Columbia Dentoform Co., New York.)

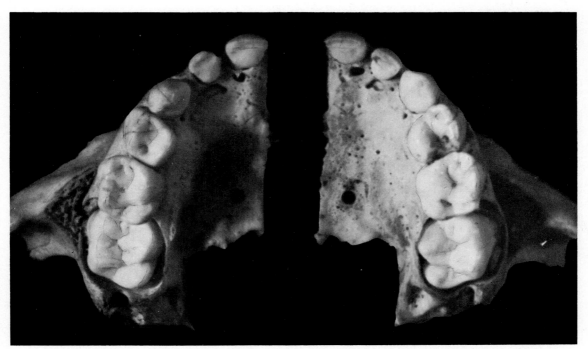

Figure 3–3. Occlusal aspect of maxillae of an individual approximately five and one-half years of age. The anterior teeth have separated considerably, and openings in the bone lingual to them have appeared in anticipation of the eruption of the permanent anterior teeth. The deciduous canines and molars remain in contact with each other. Well-formed permanent first molar crowns have lost their bone covering and are at the point of eruption distal to the second deciduous molars. The value of the deciduous second molar as a guide in influencing the future position of the permanent first molar is emphasized in this illustration.

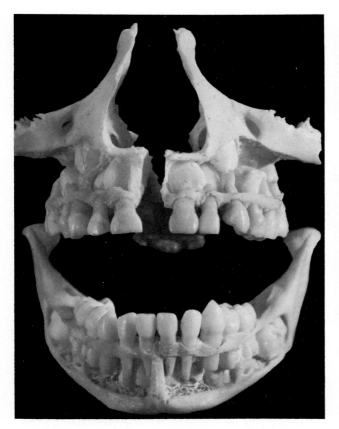

Figure 3–4. This is a picture of a remarkable specimen of a five- to six-year-old child. It was carefully prepared to show a full complement of deciduous teeth in place, the beginning of resorption of deciduous roots in some, and no apparent resorption in others. This straight front view shows the relative positions of the developing tooth crowns of the permanent anterior teeth. The maxillary central and lateral incisors and the canine are shown overlapped in a narrow space, waiting for future development of the maxilla that will allow them to develop roots and improve the alignment. See also Figures 3–5 and 3–6.

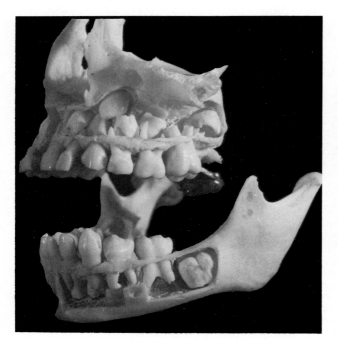

Figure 3–5. A view from the left of the specimen in Figure 3–4. Note the crowns of permanent maxillary premolars located between the roots of first and second deciduous molars, with their roots still intact. Another interesting observation is the well-developed first permanent maxillary molar entirely erupted with half its roots formed. Ordinarily, the mandibular first permanent molar comes in and takes its place first, the maxillary molar following. The specimen shows the mandibular molar still covered with bone and no roots in evidence.

The maxillary second molar crown is well developed and located in a place which is about level with the present root development of the permanent maxillary first molar.

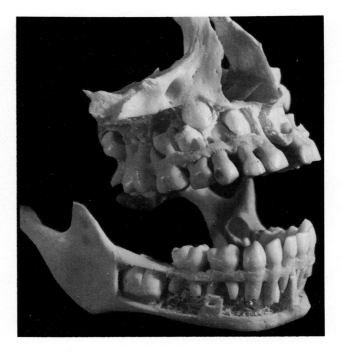

Figure 3–6. This picture of the specimen shown in Figure 3–4 was taken from the right side and slightly forward. It makes an interesting study from a different aspect. It does show the developing anterior maxillary crowns a little better. Unless they were lost in preparation, no development shows of mandibular permanent premolars. The tiny cusps formed at this age would be lost easily in preparation.

number matches that of the maxillary first permanent molar. The deciduous *mandibular* first molar is unique in that it has a crown form unlike that of any permanent tooth. It does, however, have two strong roots, one mesial and one distal—an arrangement similar to that of a mandibular permanent molar. These two deciduous teeth, the maxillary and mandibular first molars, differ from any teeth in the permanent set when comparing crown forms in particular. The deciduous first molars, maxillary and mandibular, will be described in detail later on.

SOME MAJOR CONTRASTS APPARENT WHEN DECIDUOUS TEETH ARE COMPARED WITH THEIR COUNTERPARTS IN THE PERMANENT DENTITION

A comparison of deciduous and permanent teeth will show the following major *differences* in form:

1. The crowns of deciduous anterior teeth are wider mesiodistally in comparison with their crown length than are the permanent teeth.

2. The roots of deciduous anterior teeth are narrower and longer comparatively. Narrow roots with wide crowns present an arrangement at the cervical third of crown and root that differs markedly from the permanent anterior teeth. From mesial and distal aspects the proportions are similar, except that the crown width is greater at the cervical third, contrasting a wide crown with a narrow root.

3. The roots of the deciduous molars accordingly are longer and *more slender* than the roots of the permanent teeth. They also flare more, extending out beyond projected outlines of the crowns. This flare allows more room between the roots for

A   B

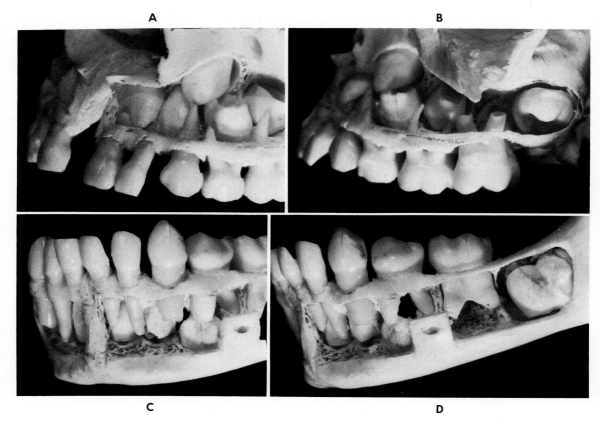

C   D

Figure 3–7. *A.* A sectional close-up of Figure 3–4. This section is somewhat anterior to the left side of the maxilla. The developing crowns of the central and lateral incisors, the canine and two premolars are clearly in view.

B. The left side of the maxilla of the specimen, taken from an angle posteriorly. The molar relationship, both deciduous and permanent, is accented here.

C. This angle of the specimen in Figure 3–4 presents a good view of the mandible anteriorly and to the left. Permanent central and lateral incisors and the canine may be seen. Notice that the permanent canine develops distally to the deciduous canine root.

D. Posteriorly, examination of the specimen mandible fails to find crown development of permanent premolars. However, the hollow spaces showing between the roots of deciduous molars may indicate a loss of material during the difficult process of dissection. The first permanent molar has progressed in crown formation but the maturation of the whole tooth with alignment is far behind its opposition in the maxilla above it. (See Figure 3–5.)

the development of permanent tooth crowns before it is time for deciduous molars to lose their anchorage. (Figs. 3–24 and 3–25.)

4. Again, when viewing the mesial or distal aspects of anterior deciduous teeth, it will be noted that the cervical ridges of enamel seen labially and lingually are quite prominent, showing more prominence by far than that displayed by permanent anterior teeth. These bulges must be considered seriously when they are involved in any operative procedure. (Fig. 3–17.)

5. When looking at the buccal aspect, the crowns and roots of deciduous molars at their cervical portions are more slender mesiodistally than are those of permanent molars. In short, they are narrower at the "necks."

6. The cervical ridges buccally on the deciduous molars are much more pronounced, especially on first molars, maxillary and mandibular. (Figs. 3–28, 3–29, 3–30, and 3–31.)

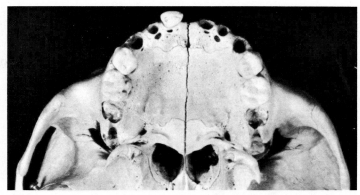

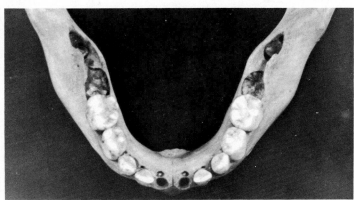

Figure 3–8. Maxillae and mandible of a five-year-old child. Some of the anterior deciduous teeth have been lost from the specimen, which shows the empty alveoli. Note the relative position of the developing permanent second molar in the left maxilla. Tips of the mandibular central incisors are making their appearance lingual to the alveoli of the deciduous central incisors. The mandibular canines and molars are still in contact with each other in this specimen.

7. The buccal and lingual surfaces of deciduous molars are flatter above the cervical curvatures than those of permanent molars, thereby narrowing the occlusal surfaces by their taper occlusally. (Fig. 3–26.)

8. The deciduous teeth are usually lighter in color than are the permanent teeth.

PULP CHAMBERS AND PULP CANALS IN DECIDUOUS TEETH

Cross sections of deciduous teeth will emphasize morphological details which are important when studying the shape and relative size of pulp chambers and canals (Fig. 3–9).

1. Crown widths in all directions are large in comparison with root trunks and cervices.

2. The enamel is relatively thin and has a consistent depth.

3. The dentin thickness between the pulp chambers and the enamel is limited, particularly in some areas (Fig. 3–10, lower second deciduous molar).

4. The pulpal horns are high and pulp chambers are large.

5. Deciduous roots are narrow and long when compared with crown width and length.

6. Molar roots of deciduous teeth flare markedly, and thin out rapidly as the apices are approached.

It is well, at all times, to study the comparisons between the deciduous and the

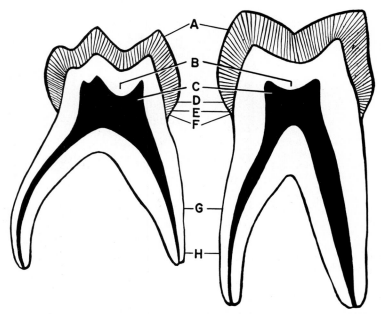

Figure 3–9. Comparison of maxillary, deciduous and permanent second molars, linguobuccal cross section. *A,* The enamel cap of deciduous molars is thinner and has a more consistent depth. *B,* There is a comparatively greater thickness of dentin over the pulpal wall at the occlusal fossa of deciduous molars. *C,* The pulpal horns are higher in deciduous molars, especially the mesial horns, and pulp chambers are proportionately larger. *D,* The cervical ridges are more pronounced, especially on the buccal aspect of the first deciduous molars. *E,* The enamel rods at the cervix slope occlusally instead of gingivally as in the permanent teeth. *F,* The deciduous molars have a markedly constricted neck compared to the permanent molars. *G,* The roots of the deciduous teeth are longer and more slender in comparison with crown size than those of the permanent teeth. *H,* The roots of the deciduous molars flare out nearer the cervix than do those of the permanent teeth. (From Finn, S. B.: *Clinical Pedodontics,* 2nd edition, W. B. Saunders Co.)

permanent dentitions (Figs. 3–11 and 3–12). Further variations between the macroscopic form of the deciduous and the permanent teeth will follow, with a detailed description of each deciduous tooth.

A DETAILED DESCRIPTION OF EACH DECIDUOUS TOOTH, THE ALIGNMENT OF DECIDUOUS TEETH AND OCCLUSION

MAXILLARY CENTRAL INCISOR

Labial Aspect (Fig. 3–13 and 3–14). In the crown of the deciduous central incisor the mesiodistal diameter is greater than the cervicoincisal length. (The opposite is true of permanent central incisors.) The labial surface is very smooth and the incisal edge is nearly straight. Developmental lines are usually not seen. The root is cone-shaped with even, tapered sides. The root length is greater in comparison with the crown length than that of the permanent central incisor. It is advisable when studying the deciduous teeth, and also the permanent teeth later on, to make direct compari-

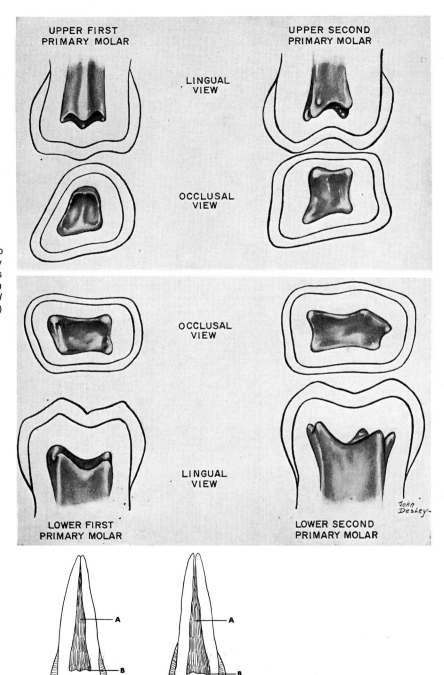

UPPER FIRST PRIMARY MOLAR

UPPER SECOND PRIMARY MOLAR

LINGUAL VIEW

OCCLUSAL VIEW

OCCLUSAL VIEW

LINGUAL VIEW

LOWER FIRST PRIMARY MOLAR

LOWER SECOND PRIMARY MOLAR

Figure 3–10. Pulp chambers in the primary molars. Note the contours of the pulp horns within them. (Finn, S. B.: *Clinical Pedodontics,* 2nd Edition.)

Figure 3–11   Figure 3–12

Figure 3–11. Permanent central incisor. This figure represents a sectioned central incisor of a young person. Although the pulp canal is rather large, it is smaller than the pulp canal shown in Figure 3–12 and it becomes more constricted apically. Note the dentin space between the pulp horns and the incisal edge of the crown. *A,* Pulp canal; *B,* pulp horn.

Figure 3–12. Deciduous central incisor. This figure represents a sectioned deciduous central incisor. It will be noted that the pulp chamber with its horns and the pulp canal are broader than those found in Fig. 3–11. The apical portion of the canal is much less constricted than that of the permanent tooth. Note the narrow dentin space incisally. A, Pulp canal; B, pulp horns.

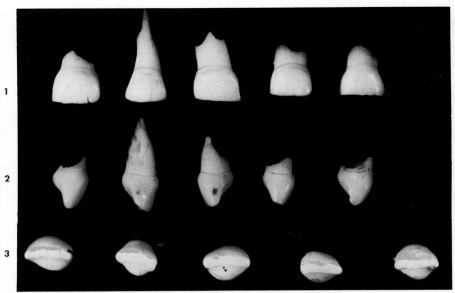

Figure 3-13. *Deciduous Maxillary Central Incisors (First Incisors).*

1. Labial aspect. Note the lack of character in the mold form. Also note the mesiodistal width when compared with the shorter crown length. A little of the crown length was lost through abrasion before the date of extraction.

2. Mesial aspect. The cervical ridges are quite prominent labially and lingually, with the bulge much greater than that found on permanent incisors. This characteristic is common to each deciduous tooth to a varied degree. Normally, these curvatures are covered by gum tissue with epithelial attachment. (See Chapter 5, Physiologic Tooth Form Protecting the Periodontium.)

3. Incisal aspect.

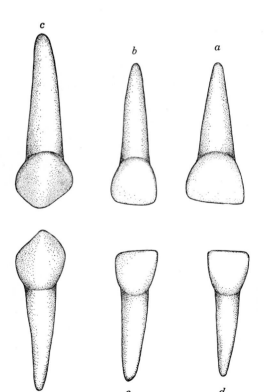

Figure 3-14. Deciduous right anterior teeth, labial aspect. *a,* Maxillary central incisor; *b,* maxillary lateral incisor; *c,* maxillary canine; *d,* mandibular central incisor; *e,* mandibular lateral incisor; *f,* mandibular canine.

sons between the table of measurements of the deciduous teeth (see below) and the table of measurements for the permanent teeth which was given in Chapter 1 (page 20).

Lingual Aspect (Figs. 3–3 and 3–13). The lingual aspect of the crown shows well-developed marginal ridges and a highly developed cingulum. The cingulum extends up toward the incisal ridge far enough to make a partial division of the concavity on the lingual surface below the incisal edge, practically dividing it into a mesial and distal fossa.

The root narrows lingually and presents a ridge for its full length in comparison with a flatter surface labially. A cross section through the root where it joins the crown shows an outline which is somewhat triangular in shape, with the labial surface making one side of the triangle and mesial and distal surfaces making up the other two sides.

Mesial and Distal Aspects (Figs 3–13 and 3–17). The mesial and distal aspects of the deciduous maxillary central incisors are similar. The measurement of the crown at the cervical third shows the crown from this aspect to be wide in relation to its total length. The average measurement will be only about 1 mm. less than the entire crown length cervicoincisally. Because of the short crown and its labiolingual measurement, the crown appears thick at the middle third and even down toward the incisal third. The *curvature of cervical line*, which represents the *cementoenamel junction*, is distinct, curving toward the incisal ridge. However, the curvature is not as great as that found on its permanent successor. The cervical curvature distally is less than the amount of curvature mesially, a design that compares favorably with the permanent central incisor.

Although the root from this aspect appears more blunt than it did from the labial and lingual aspects, still it is of an even taper and is the shape of a long cone. It is,

Table of Measurements of the Deciduous Teeth of Man (G. V. Black) (Averages Only)

Upper Teeth	Length Over All	Length of Crown	Length of Root	Mesio-distal Diameter of Crown	Mesio-distal Diameter at Cervix	Labio-lingual Diameter of Crown	Labio-lingual Diameter at Cervix
Central Incisor	16.0°	6.0	10.0	6.5	4.5	5.0	4.0
Lateral Incisor	15.8	5.6	11.4	5.1	3.7	4.0	3.7
Canine	19.0	6.5	13.5	7.0	5.1	7.0	5.5
First Molar	15.2	5.1	10.0	7.3	5.2	8.5	6.9
Second Molar	17.5	5.7	11.7	8.2	6.4	10.0	8.3
Lower Teeth							
Central Incisor	14.0	5.0	9.0	4.2	3.0	4.0	3.5
Lateral Incisor	15.0	5.2	10.0	4.1†	3.0	4.0	3.5
Canine	17.0	6.0	11.5	5.0	3.7	4.8	4.0
First Molar	15.8	6.0	9.8	7.7	6.5	7.0	5.3
Second Molar	18.8	5.5	11.3	9.9	7.2	8.7	6.4

° Millimeters.

however, blunt at the apex. Usually the mesial side of the root will have a developmental groove or concavity, whereas distally the surface is generally convex.

Note the development of the cervical ridges of enamel at the cervical third of the crown labially and lingually.

Incisal Aspect (Figs. 3–3 and 3–13). An important feature to note from the incisal aspect is the measurement mesiodistally as compared with the measurement labiolingually. The incisal edge is centered over the main bulk of the crown and is relatively straight. Looking down on the incisal edge, one sees that the labial surface is much broader and also smoother than the lingual surface. The lingual surface tapers toward the cingulum.

The mesial and the distal surfaces of this tooth are relatively broad. The mesial and distal surfaces toward the incisal ridge or at the incisal third are generous enough to make good contact areas with the adjoining teeth, although this facility is used for a short period only because of rapid changes which take place in the jaws of children.

MAXILLARY LATERAL INCISOR (Figs. 3–14, 3–15, 3–16, 3–17 and 3–18)

In general, the maxillary lateral incisor is similar to the central incisor from all aspects, but its dimensions differ. Its crown is smaller in all directions. The cervicoincisal length of the lateral crown is greater than its mesiodistal width. The distoincisal angles of the crown are more rounded than is the central incisor. Although the root has a similar shape, it is much longer in proportion to its crown than the central ratio indicates when a comparison is made.

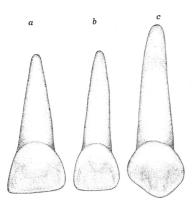

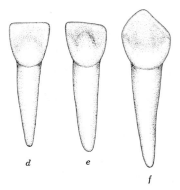

Figure 3–15. Deciduous right anterior teeth, lingual aspect. *a,* Maxillary central incisor; *b,* maxillary lateral incisor; *c,* maxillary canine; *d,* mandibular central incisor; *e,* mandibular lateral incisor; *f,* mandibular canine.

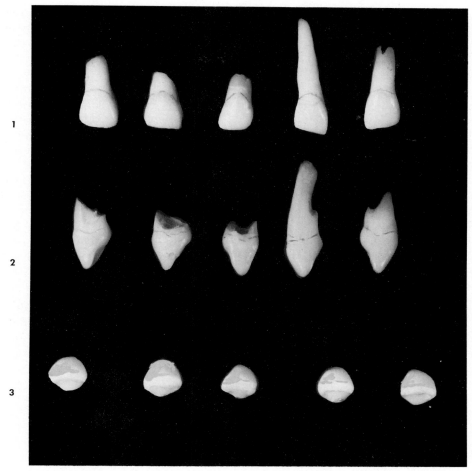

Figure 3–16. Deciduous maxillary lateral incisors. (Second incisors.) 1, Labial aspect; 2, mesial aspect; 3, incisal aspect.

MAXILLARY CANINE

Labial Aspect (Fig. 3–14, C). Except for the root form, the labial aspect of the maxillary canine does not resemble either the central or the lateral incisors. The crown is more constricted at the cervix in relation to its mesiodistal width, and the mesial and distal surfaces are more convex. Instead of an incisal edge, relatively straight, it has a long, well-developed and sharp cusp.

Compared with that of the permanent maxillary canine, the cusp on the deciduous canine is much longer and sharper, and the crest of contour mesially is not so far down toward the incisal portion. A line drawn through the contact areas of the deciduous canine would bisect a line drawn from the cervix to the tip of the cusp. In the *permanent* canine the contact areas are not at the same level. When the cusp is intact the mesial slope of the cusp will be longer than the distal slope.

The root of the deciduous canine is long, slender and tapering and is more than twice the crown length.

Lingual Aspect (Fig. 3–15, C). The lingual aspect shows pronounced enamel ridges which merge with each other. They are the cingulum, mesial and distal marginal ridges, and incisal ridges, besides a tubercle at the cusp tip which is a continuation of the lingual ridge connecting the cingulum and the cusp tip. This lingual ridge divides the lingual surface into shallow mesiolingual and distolingual fossae.

The root of this tooth tapers lingually. It is usually inclined distally also above the middle third (Figs. 3–14, C, 3–17, C.)

Mesial Aspect (Fig. 3–17, C).   From the mesial aspect, the outline form is similar to that of the lateral and central incisors. However, there is a difference in proportion. The measurement labiolingually at the cervical third is much greater. This increase in crown dimension, in conjunction with the root width and length, permits resistance against forces the tooth must withstand during function. The function of this tooth is to punch, tear and apprehend food material.

Distal Aspect.   The distal outline of this tooth is the reverse of the mesial aspect. No outstanding differences may be noted except that the curvature of the cervical line toward the cusp ridge is less than on the mesial surface.

Incisal Aspect (Fig. 3–18, C).   From the incisal aspect one observes that the crown is essentially diamond-shaped. The angles which are found at the contact areas mesially and distally, at the cingulum on the lingual surface and at the cervical third, or enamel ridge, on the labial surface are more pronounced and less rounded in effect than are those found on the permanent canines. The tip of the cusp is distal to the center of the crown, and the mesial cusp slope is longer than the distal cusp slope. This allows for intercuspation with the lower, or mandibular, canine, which has its longest slope distally (Fig. 3–14).

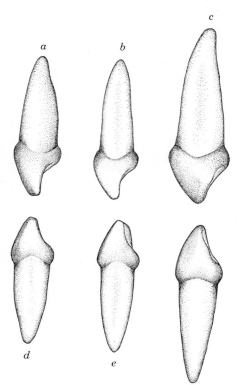

Figure 3–17. Deciduous right anterior teeth, mesial aspect. *a*, Maxillary central incisor; *b*, maxillary lateral incisor; *c*, maxillary canine; *d*, mandibular central incisor; *e*, mandibular lateral incisor; *f*, mandibular canine.

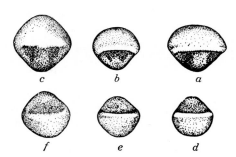

Figure 3–18. Deciduous right anterior teeth, incisal aspect. *a,* Maxillary central incisor; *b,* maxillary lateral incisor; *c,* maxillary canine; *d,* mandibular central incisor; *e,* mandibular lateral incisor; *f,* mandibular canine.

MANDIBULAR CENTRAL INCISOR

Labial Aspect (Fig. 3–14, D).   The labial aspect of this crown has a flat face with no developmental grooves. The mesial and distal sides of the crown are tapered evenly from the contact areas, the measurement being less at the cervix. This crown is wide in proportion to its length in comparison with that of its permanent successor. The heavy look at the root trunk makes this small tooth resemble the permanent maxillary lateral incisor.

The root of the deciduous central incisor is long, and evenly tapered down to the apex, which is pointed. The root is almost twice the length of the crown.

Lingual Aspect (Fig. 3–15, D).   On the lingual surface of the crown the marginal ridges and the cingulum may be located easily. The lingual surface of the crown at the middle third and the incisal third may have a flattened surface level with the marginal ridges, or it may present a slight concavity, called the *lingual fossa.* The lingual portion of the crown and root converges so that it is narrower toward the lingual than toward the labial surface.

Mesial Aspect (Fig. 3–17, D).   The mesial aspect shows the typical outline of an incisor tooth even though the measurements are small. The incisal ridge is centered over the center of the root and between the crest of curvature of the crown, labially and lingually. The convexity of the cervical contours labially and lingually at the cervical third is just as pronounced as in any of the other deciduous incisors and more pronounced by far than the prominences found at the same locations on a permanent mandibular central incisor. As mentioned before, these cervical bulges are important.

Although this tooth is small, its labiolingual measurement is only about a millimeter less than that of the deciduous maxillary central incisor. The deciduous incisors seem to be built for strenuous service.

The mesial surface of the root is nearly flat and is evenly tapered; the apex presents a more blunt appearance than is found when one observes the lingual or labial aspects.

Distal Aspect.   The outline of this tooth from the distal aspect is the reverse of that found from the mesial aspect. There is little difference to be noted between these aspects except that the cervical line of the crown is less curved toward the incisal ridge than that found on the mesial surface. Often there is a developmental depression on the distal side of the root.

Incisal Aspect (Fig. 3–18, D).   The incisal ridge is straight and bisects the crown labiolingually. The outline of the crown from the incisal aspect emphasizes the crests of contour at the cervical third labially and lingually. There is a definite taper toward the cingulum on the lingual side.

The labial surface from this view presents a flat surface slightly convex, whereas the lingual surface presents a flattened surface slightly concave.

MANDIBULAR LATERAL INCISOR (FIGS. 3-14, 3-15, 3-17, 3-18)

The fundamental outlines of the deciduous mandibular lateral incisor are similar to those of the deciduous central incisor. These two teeth supplement each other in function. The lateral incisor is somewhat larger in all measurements except the labiolingual, where the two teeth are practically identical. The cingulum of the lateral incisor may be a little more generous than that of the central incisor, and the lingual surface of the crown between the marginal ridges may be more concave. In addition, there is a tendency for the incisal ridge to slope downward distally. This design lowers the distal contact area apically in order that proper contact may be made with the mesial surface of the deciduous mandibular canine.

MANDIBULAR CANINE (FIGS. 3-14, 3-15, 3-17, 3-18)

There is very little difference in functional form between this tooth and the maxillary canine. The difference is mainly in the dimensions. The crown is perhaps 0.5 mm. shorter, and the root is at least 2 mm. shorter; the mesiodistal measurement of

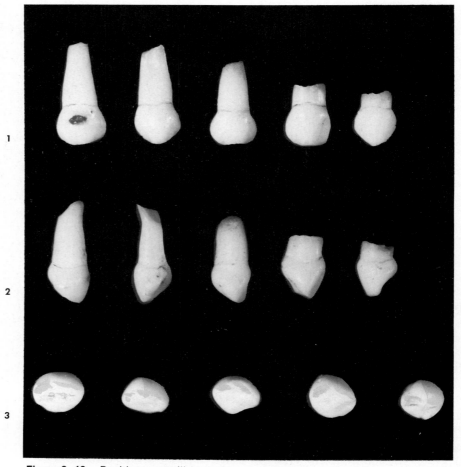

Figure 3-19. Deciduous maxillary canines. 1, Labial aspect; 2, mesial aspect; 3, incisal aspect.

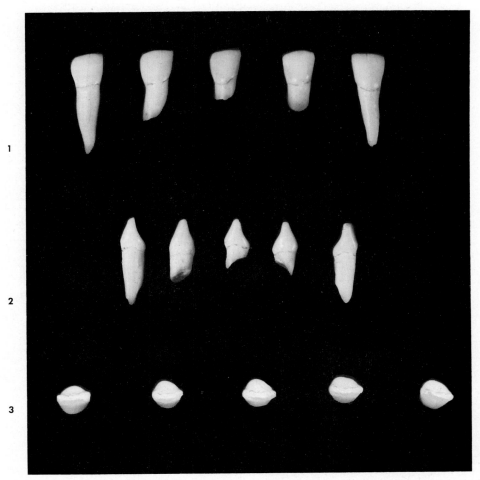

Figure 3–20. Deciduous mandibular central incisors. 1. Labial aspect; 2, mesial aspect; 3, incisal aspect.

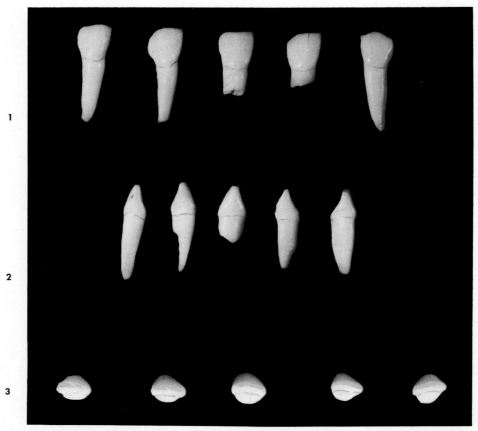

Figure 3–21. Deciduous mandibular lateral incisors. 1. Labial aspect; 2, mesial aspect; 3, incisal aspect.

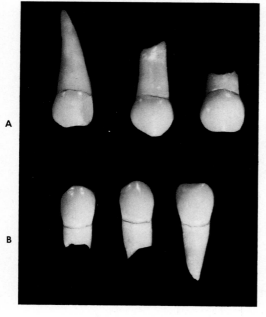

Figure 3–22. A comparison of deciduous canines, both in the size and shape of the crowns. Two of them have their roots intact and showing no dissolution. *A*, Maxillary canines; *B*, mandibular canines. Compare Figures 3–19 and 3–23.

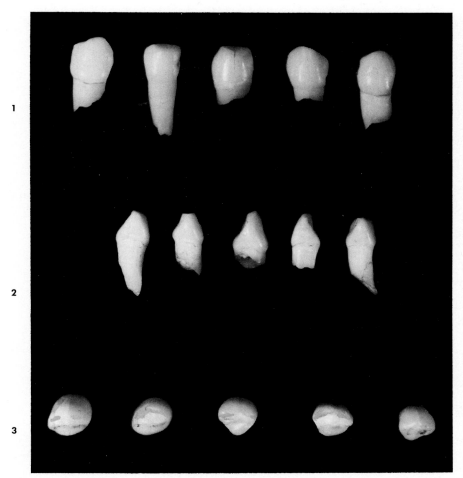

Figure 3–23.   Deciduous mandibular canines. 1, Labial aspect; 2, mesial aspect; 3, incisal aspect.

the mandibular canine at the root trunk is greater when compared with its mesio-distal measurement at the contact areas than is the maxillary canine (Fig. 3–22). It is "thicker" accordingly at the "neck" of the tooth. The outstanding variation in size between the two deciduous canines is shown by the labiolingual calibration. The deciduous maxillary canine is much larger labiolingually (Fig. 3–17).

The cervical ridges labially and lingually are not quite as pronounced as those found on the maxillary canine. The greatest variation in outline form when one compares the two teeth is seen from the labial and lingual aspects; the distal cusp slope is longer than the mesial slope. The opposite arrangement is true of the maxillary canine. This makes for proper intercuspation of these teeth during mastication.

MAXILLARY FIRST MOLAR

Buccal Aspect (Fig. 3–24).   The widest measurement of the crown of the maxillary first molar is at the contact areas mesially and distally. From these points the crown converges toward the cervix, the measurement at the cervix being fully 2 mm.

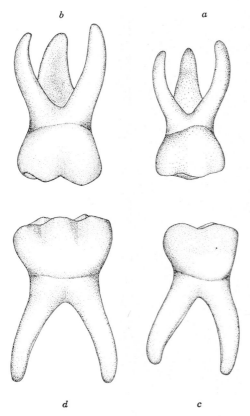

Figure 3–24. Deciduous right molars, buccal aspect, a, Maxillary first molar; b, maxillary second molar; c, mandibular first molar; d, mandibular second molar.

less than the measurement at the contact areas. This dimensional arrangement furnishes a narrower look to the cervical portion of crown and root of the deciduous maxillary first molar than that of the same portion of the permanent maxillary first molar. The occlusal line is slightly scalloped but with no definite cusp form. The buccal surface is smooth, and there is little evidence of developmental grooves. It is from this aspect that one may judge the relative size of the deciduous maxillary first molar when it is compared with the second molar. It is much smaller in all measurements than the second molar. Its relative shape and size suggest that it was designed to be the "premolar section" of the deciduous dentition. In function it acts as a compromise between the size and shape of the anterior deciduous teeth and the molar area; this area being held temporarily by the larger deciduous second molar. At six years of age, the large first permanent molar is expected to take its place distal to the second deciduous molar, which will complete a more extensive molar area for masticating efficiency.

The *roots* of the maxillary first molar are slender and long, and they spread widely. All three roots may be seen from this aspect. The distal root is considerably shorter than the mesial one. The bifurcation of the roots begins almost immediately at the site of the cervical line (cementoenamel junction). Actually, this arrangement is in effect for the entire root trunk, which includes a "trifurcation," and this is a characteristic of all deciduous molars, maxillary and mandibular.

This characteristic is not possessed by permanent molars. The root trunk on all permanent molars is much heavier, with a greater calibration between the cervical line and the points of bifurcation (Figs. 11–7, 11–8).

Lingual Aspect (Fig. 3–25). The general outline of the lingual aspect of the

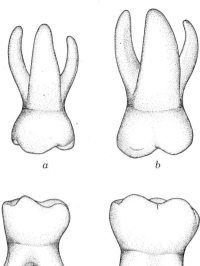

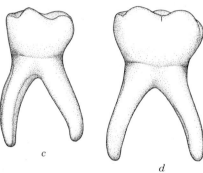

Figure 3–25. Deciduous right molars, lingual aspect. *a*, Maxillary first molar; *b*, maxillary second molar; *c*, mandibular first molar; *d*, mandibular second molar.

crown is similar to the buccal aspect. The crown converges considerably in a lingual direction, making the lingual portion calibrate less mesiodistally than the buccal portion.

The mesiolingual cusp is the most prominent cusp on this tooth. It is the longest and sharpest cusp. The distolingual cusp is poorly defined: it is small and rounded when it exists at all. From the lingual aspect the distobuccal cusp may be seen, since it is longer and better developed than the distolingual cusp. There is a type of deciduous maxillary first molar which is not uncommon and which presents one large lingual cusp with no developmental groove in evidence lingually. This type is apparently a three-cusped molar (Fig. 3–28, division 4, second from left).

All three roots may be seen from this aspect also. The lingual root is larger than the others.

Mesial Aspect (Fig. 3–26).   From the mesial aspect the dimension at the cervical third is greater than the dimension at the occlusal third. This is true of all molar forms, but it is more pronounced on deciduous teeth than on permanent teeth. The mesiolingual cusp is longer and sharper than the mesiobuccal cusp. There is a pronounced convexity on the buccal outline in the cervical third. This convexity is an outstanding characteristic of this tooth. Actually, it gives the impression of over-development in this area when comparisons are made with any other tooth, deciduous or permanent, the mandibular first deciduous molar being a close contender. The cervical line mesially shows some curvature in the direction of the occlusal surface.

The mesiobuccal and lingual roots only are visible when one looks at the mesial side of this tooth from a point directly opposite the contact area. The distobuccal root is hidden behind the mesiobuccal root. The lingual root from this aspect looks long and slender and extends lingually to a marked degree. It curves sharply in a buccal direction above the middle third.

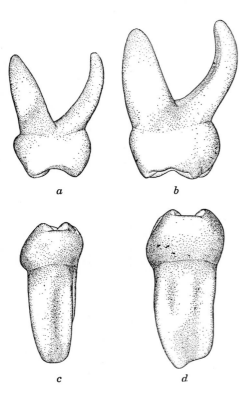

a   *b*

Figure 3–26. Deciduous right molars, mesial aspect. *a*, Maxillary first molar; *b*, maxillary second molar; *c*, mandibular first molar; *d*, mandibular second molar.

c   *d*

Distal Aspect.   From the distal aspect the crown is narrower distally than mesially; it tapers markedly toward the distal (Fig. 3–27). The distobuccal cusp is long and sharp, and the distolingual cusp is poorly developed. The prominent bulge seen from the mesial aspect at the cervical third does not continue distally. The cervical line may curve occlusally, or it may extend straight across from the buccal surface to the lingual surface. All three roots may be seen from this angle, but the distobuccal root is superimposed on the mesiobuccal root so that only the buccal surface and the apex of the latter may be seen. The point of bifurcation of the distobuccal root and the lingual root is near the cementoenamel junction as described heretofore as being typical.

Occlusal Aspect (Fig. 3–27, A).   The calibration of the distance between the mesiobuccal line angle and the distobuccal line angle is definitely greater than the calibration between the mesiolingual line angle and the distolingual line angle. Therefore, the crown outline converges lingually. Also, the calibration from the mesiobuccal line angle to the mesiolingual line angle is definitely greater than that found at the distal line angles. Therefore, the crown converges distally also. Nevertheless, these convergencies are not reflected entirely in the working occlusal surface, because it is more nearly rectangular with the shortest sides of the rectangle represented by the marginal ridges. The occlusal surface is more nearly rectangular, with the shortest side of the rectangle represented by the marginal ridges.

The occlusal surface has a *central fossa*. There is a *mesial triangular fossa*, just inside the mesial marginal ridge, with a mesial pit in this fossa and a sulcus with its central groove connecting the two fossae. There is also a well-defined *buccal develop-*

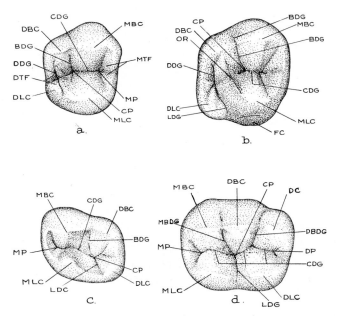

Figure 3–27. *a,* Maxillary first molar. *MBC,* mesiobuccal cusp; *MTF,* mesial triangular fossa; *MP,* mesial pit; *CP,* central pit; *MLC,* mesiolingual cusp; *DLC,* distolingual cusp; *DTF,* distal triangular fossa; *DDG,* distal developmental groove; *BDG,* buccal developmental groove; *DBC,* distobuccal cusp; *CDG,* central developmental groove.

  b, Maxillary second molar. *BDG,* buccal developmental groove; *MBC,* mesiobuccal cusp; *CDG,* central developmental groove; *MLC,* mesiolingual cusp; *FC,* fifth cusp; *LDG,* lingual developmental groove; *DLC,* distolingual cusp; *DDG,* distal developmental groove; *OR,* oblique ridge; *DBC,* distobuccal cusp; *CP,* central pit.

  c, Mandibular first molar. *CDG,* central developmental groove; *DBC,* distobuccal cusp; *BDG,* buccal developmental groove; *CP,* central pit; *DLC,* distolingual cusp; *LDG,* lingual developmental groove; *MLC,* mesiolingual cusp; *MP,* mesial pit; *MBC,* mesiobuccal cusp.

  d, Mandibular second molar. *DBC,* distobuccal cusp; *CP,* central pit; *DC,* distal cusp; *DBDG,* distobuccal developmental groove; *DP,* distal pit; *CDG,* central developmental groove; *DLC,* distolingual cusp; *LDG,* lingual developmental groove; *MLC,* mesiolingual cusp; *MP,* mesial pit; *MBDG,* mesiobuccal developmental groove; *MBC,* mesiobuccal cusp.

mental groove dividing the mesiobuccal cusp and the distobuccal cusp occlusally. There are supplemental grooves radiating from the pit in the mesial triangular fossa. These grooves radiate as follows: one buccally, one lingually and one toward the marginal ridge, the last sometimes extending over the marginal ridge mesially.

  Sometimes the deciduous maxillary first molar has a well-defined triangular ridge connecting the mesiolingual cusp with the distobuccal cusp. When well developed, it is called the *oblique ridge.* In some of these teeth the ridge will be very indefinite and the central developmental groove will extend from the mesial pit to the *distal developmental groove.* This disto-occlusal groove is always seen and may or may not extend through to the lingual surface, outlining a distolingual cusp. The distal marginal ridge is thin and poorly developed in comparison with the mesial marginal ridge.

  Summary of the Occlusal Aspect of This Tooth.   The form of the maxillary first deciduous molar varies from that of any tooth in the permanent dentition. Although there are no premolars in the deciduous set, in some respects the crown of this deciduous molar resembles a permanent maxillary premolar. Nevertheless, the divisions of the occlusal surface and the root form with its efficient anchorage make it a molar, both in type and function.

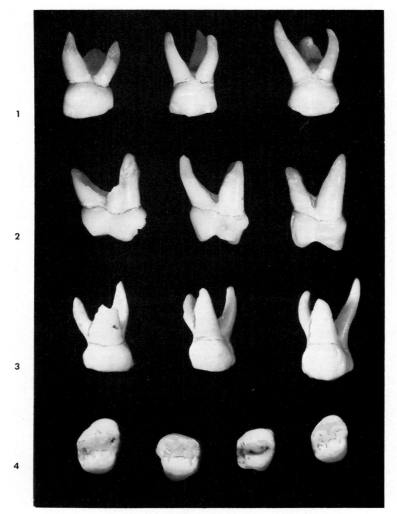

Figure 3–28.   Deciduous Maxillary First Molars.

1, Buccal aspect; note the flare of roots. 2, Mesial aspect; the cervical ridge on the buccal surface is curved to the extreme. Also note the flat or concave buccal surface above this bulge as it approaches the occlusal surface. 3, Lingual aspect. 4, Occlusal aspect. This aspect emphasizes the extensive width of the mesial portion of deciduous first molars. The four specimens show size differentials even in deciduous teeth. See Figure 3–27.

MAXILLARY SECOND MOLAR

Buccal Aspect (Figs. 3–24, B; 3–29, I).   The deciduous maxillary second molar has characteristics resembling the *permanent* maxillary first molar but it is smaller (Fig. 3–3).

The buccal view of this tooth shows two well-defined buccal cusps with a buccal developmental groove between them. In line with all deciduous molars, the crown is narrow at the cervix in comparison with its mesiodistal measurement at the contact areas. This crown is much larger than that of the first deciduous molar. Although the roots, from this aspect, appear slender, they are much longer and heavier than those that are a part of the maxillary first molar. The point of bifurcation between the buccal

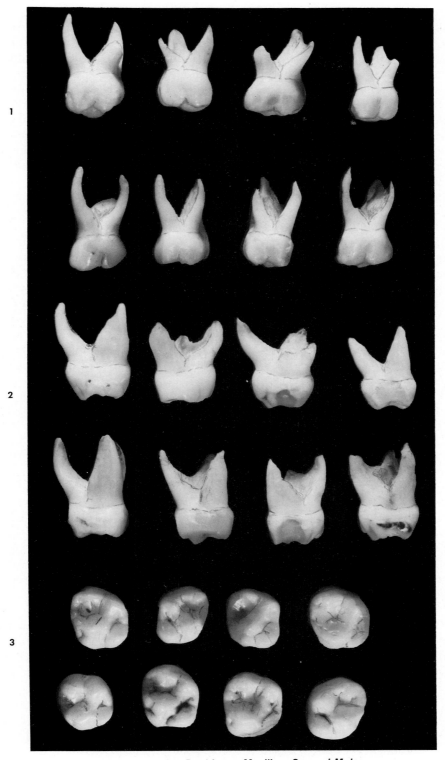

Figure 3–29. *Deciduous Maxillary Second Molars.*

1. Buccal aspect; 2, mesial aspect; 3, occlusal aspect.

roots is close to the cervical line of the crown. The two buccal cusps are more nearly equal in size and development than those of the deciduous maxillary first molar.

Lingual Aspect (Fig. 3–25, B).   Lingually, the crown shows three cusps: (1) the mesiolingual cusp, which is large and well developed; (2) the distolingual cusp, which is well developed (more so than that of the deciduous first molar), and (3) a third supplemental cusp, which is apical to the mesiolingual cusp and which is sometimes called the *tubercle of Carabelli* or the fifth cusp. This cusp is poorly developed and merely acts as a buttress or supplement to the bulk of the mesiolingual cusp. If the tubercle of Carabelli seems to be missing, some traces of developmental lines or "dimples" will remain. (Fig. 3–29, division 3). A well-defined developmental groove separates the mesiolingual cusp from the distolingual cusp and connects with the developmental groove which outlines the fifth cusp.

All three roots are visible from this aspect; the lingual root is large and thick in comparison with the other two roots. It is approximately the same length as the mesiobuccal root. If it should differ, it will be on the short side.

Mesial Aspect (Fig. 3–26, B).   From the mesial aspect the crown has a typical molar outline which resembles that of the permanent molars very much. The crown appears short because of its width buccolingually in comparison with its length. The crown of this tooth is usually only about 0.5 mm. longer than the crown of the first deciduous molar, but the buccolingual measurement is 1.5 to 2 mm. greater. In addition, the roots are 1.5 to 2 mm. longer. The mesiolingual cusp of the crown with its supplementary fifth cusp appears large in comparison with the mesiobuccal cusp. The mesiobuccal cusp from this angle is relatively short and sharp. There is very little curvature to the cervical line. Usually it is almost straight across from buccal surface to lingual surface.

The mesiobuccal root from this aspect is broad and flat. The lingual root has somewhat the same curvature as the lingual root of the maxillary first deciduous molar.

It extends lingually far out beyond the crown outline. The point of bifurcation between the mesiobuccal root and the lingual root is 2 or 3 mm. apical to the cervical line of the crown; this differs in depth on the root trunk from comparisons of this area in the recent discussion of deciduous molars. The mesiobuccal root presents itself as being quite wide from the mesial aspect. It will measure approximately two thirds the width of the root trunk, leaving one third for the lingual root. The mesiolingual cusp is directly below their bifurcation. Although the curvature lingually on the crown from this aspect is strong at the cervical portion, as on most deciduous teeth, the crest of curvature buccally at the cervical third is nominal and resembles the curvature found at this point on the permanent maxillary first molar. In this it differs entirely from the prominent curvature found on the deciduous maxillary first molars at the cervical third buccally.

Distal Aspect.   From the distal aspect it is apparent that the distal calibration of the crown is less than the mesial measurement, but there is not the variation found on the crown of the deciduous maxillary first molar. From both the distal and the mesial aspects the outline of the crown lingually creates a smooth rounded line, whereas a line describing the buccal surface is almost straight from the crest of curvature to the tip of the buccal cusp. The distobuccal cusp and the distolingual cusp are about the same in length. The cervical line is approximately straight, as was found mesially.

All three roots are seen from this aspect, although only a part of the outline of the mesiobuccal root may be seen, since the distobuccal root is superimposed over it. The distobuccal root is shorter and narrower than the other roots. The point of bifurcation between the distobuccal root and the lingual root is more apical in location than any of the other points of bifurcation. The point of bifurcation between these two roots on the distal is more nearly centered above the crown than that on the mesial between the mesiobuccal and lingual roots.

Occlusal Aspect (Fig. 3–27, B).   From the occlusal aspect this tooth resembles the permanent first molar. It is somewhat rhomboidal and has four well-developed cusps and one supplemental cusp: mesiobuccal, distobuccal, mesiolingual, distolingual and fifth cusps. The buccal surface is rather flat, with the developmental groove between the cusps less marked than that found on the first permanent molar. Developmental grooves, pits, oblique ridge, etc., are almost identical. The character of the "mold" is constant.

The occlusal surface has a *central fossa* with a *central pit*, a well-defined *mesial triangular fossa*, just distal to the *mesial marginal ridge*, with a mesial pit at its center. There is, too, a well-defined developmental groove called the *central groove* at the bottom of a sulcus connecting the mesial triangular fossa with the central fossa. The *buccal developmental groove* extends buccally from the central pit, separating the triangular ridges which are occlusal continuations of the mesio- and distobuccal cusps. Supplemental grooves often radiate from these developmental grooves.

The *oblique ridge* is prominent and connects the mesiolingual cusp with the distobuccal cusp. Distal to the oblique ridge one finds the *distal fossa*, which harbors the *distal developmental groove*. The distal groove has branches of supplemental grooves within the *distal triangular fossa* which is rather indefinitely outlined just mesial to the distal marginal ridge.

The distal groove acts as a line of demarcation between the mesiolingual and distolingual cusps and continues on to the lingual surface as the *lingual developmental groove*. The *distal marginal ridge* is as well developed as the *mesial marginal ridge*. It will be remembered that the marginal ridges are not developed equally on the deciduous maxillary first molar.

MANDIBULAR FIRST MOLAR

This tooth does not resemble any of the other teeth, deciduous or permanent. Because it varies so much from all others, it appears strange and primitive.

Buccal Aspect (Figs. 3–24, C and 3–31, A).   From the buccal aspect the mesial outline of the crown of the deciduous mandibular first molar is almost straight from the contact area to the cervix, constricting the crown very little at the cervix. The outline describing the distal portion, however, converges toward the cervix more than usual, making the contact area extend distally to a marked degree.

The distal portion of the crown is shorter than the mesial portion, the cervical line dipping apically where it joins the mesial root.

The two buccal cusps are rather distinct, although there is no developmental groove between them. The mesial cusp is larger than the distal cusp. There is a developmental depression dividing them (not a groove), which extends over to the buccal surface.

The roots are long and slender, and they spread greatly at the apical third beyond the outline of the crown.

The strange primitive look of this tooth is emphasized by the *buccal aspect*. The deciduous first mandibular molar from this angle impresses one with the thought of the possibility that at some time in the dim past there was a fusion of two teeth that ended in a strange single combination.

That thought seems particularly apropos when one is able to find a well-formed specimen of the tooth in question—one with its roots intact, showing no evidences of decalcification.

Viewing the buccal aspect, if a line is drawn from the bifurcation of the roots to the occlusal surface, the tooth will be evenly divided mesiodistally. However, the mesial portion will represent a tooth with a crown almost twice as tall as the distal half, and the root will be a third again as long as the distal one. Two complete teeth will be represented, but their dimensions will differ considerably (Figs. 3–25, 3–28).

Lingual Aspect (Fig. 3–30). The *crown and root* converge lingually to a marked degree on the mesial surface. Distally the opposite arrangement is true of both crown and root. The distolingual cusp is rounded and suggests a developmental groove between this cusp and the mesiolingual cusp. The mesiolingual cusp is long and sharp at the tip, more so than any of the other cusps. The sharp and prominent mesiolingual cusp (almost centered lingually but in line with the mesial root) is an outstanding characteristic found occlusally on the deciduous first mandibular molar. It will be noted that the mesial marginal ridge is so well developed that it might almost be considered another small cusp lingually. Part of the two buccal cusps may be seen from this angle.

From the lingual aspect the crown length mesially and distally is more uniform than it is from the buccal aspect. The cervical line is straighter.

Mesial Aspect (Fig. 3–31, B). The most noticeable detail from the mesial aspect is the extreme curvature buccally at the cervical third. Except for this detail, the crown outline of this tooth from this aspect resembles the mesial aspect of the deciduous second molar and that aspect of the permanent mandibular molars. In this comparison, the buccal cusps are placed over the root base, and the lingual outline of the crown extends out lingually beyond the confines of the root base.

Both the mesiobuccal cusp and the mesiolingual cusp are in view from this aspect, as is the well-developed mesial marginal ridge. Since the mesiobuccal crown length is greater than the mesiolingual crown length, the cervical line slants upward buccolingually. Note the flat appearance of the buccal outline of the crown from the crest of curvature of the buccal surface at the cervical third to the tip of the mesiobuccal cusp. All of the deciduous molars have flattened buccal surfaces above this cervical ridge.

The outline of the mesial root from the mesial aspect does not resemble the outline of *any other deciduous tooth root*. The buccal and lingual outlines of the root drop straight down from the crown and are approximately parallel for over half their length, tapering only slightly at the apical third. The root end is flat and almost square. A developmental depression usually extends almost the full length of the root on the mesial side.

Distal Aspect. The distal aspect of the mandibular first molar differs from the mesial aspect in the following points: The cervical line does not drop buccally. The length of crown buccally and lingually is more uniform, and the cervical line extends almost straight across buccolingually. The distobuccal cusp and the distolingual cusp are not as long or as sharp as the two mesial cusps. The distal marginal ridge is not as straight and well-defined as the mesial marginal ridge. The distal root is rounder and shorter and tapers more apically.

Occlusal Aspect (Fig. 3–30, 3). The general outline of this tooth from the occlusal aspect is rhomboidal. The prominence mesiobuccally is noticeable from this aspect, a fact which accents the mesiobuccal line angle of the crown in comparison with the distobuccal line angle, thereby accenting the rhomboidal form.

The mesiolingual cusp may be seen as the largest and the best developed of all the cusps, and it has a broad flattened surface lingually. The *buccal developmental*

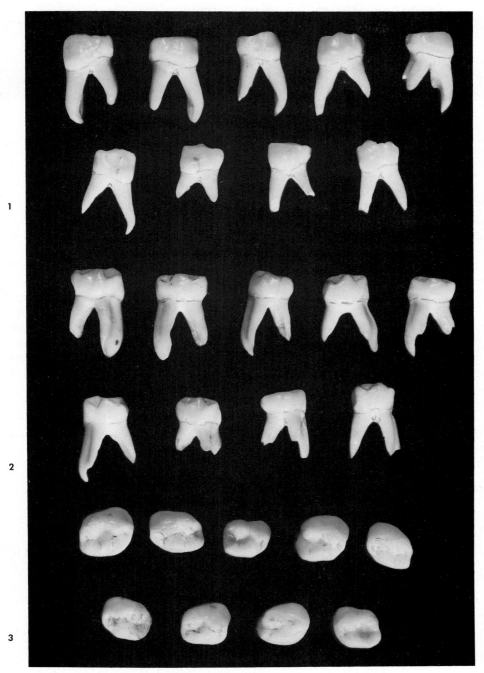

Figure 3–30. *Deciduous Mandibular First Molars.*

This tooth has characteristics unlike any other tooth in the mouth, deciduous or permanent. See text. 1. Buccal aspect; 2, lingual aspect; 3, occlusal aspect.

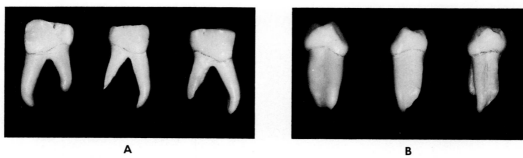

A   **B**

Figure 3–31. Three rare specimens of the deciduous mandibular first molars. *A.,* buccal aspect; *B.,* mesial aspect.

These three specimens have their roots intact with little or no resorption showing. They enable the viewer to observe the actual shape and size of the mesial and distal roots. The mesial root is very broad, curved and long, with fluting down the center. This makes for tremendous anchorage. The distal root is much shorter, but it is heavy and also curved. It does its share in bracing the crown, being in partnership with the mesial root during the process.

groove of the occlusal surface divides the two buccal cusps evenly. This developmental groove is short, extending from between the buccal cusp ridges to a point approximately in the center of the crown outline at a *central pit.* The *central developmental groove* joins it at this point and extends mesially, separating the mesiobuccal cusp and the mesiolingual cusp. The central groove ends in a *mesial pit* in the *mesial triangular fossa* which is immediately distal to the *mesial marginal ridge.* Two supplemental grooves join the developmental groove in the center of the mesial triangular fossa; one supplemental groove extends buccally and the other extends lingually.

The mesiobuccal cusp exhibits a well-defined triangular ridge on the occlusal surface which terminates in the center of the occlusal surface buccolingually at the *central developmental groove.* The *lingual developmental groove* extends lingually from this point, separating the mesiolingual cusp and the distolingual cusp. Usually the lingual developmental groove does not extend through to the lingual surface but stops at the junction of lingual cusp ridges. There are some supplemental grooves immediately mesial to the *distal marginal ridge* in the *distal triangular fossa* which join with the central developmental groove.

MANDIBULAR SECOND MOLAR

The *deciduous* mandibular *second* molar has characteristics which resemble those of the *permanent* mandibular *first* molar, although its dimensions differ.

Buccal Aspect (Figs. 3–24, D; 3–32, 1).   From the buccal aspect the deciduous mandibular second molar has a narrow mesiodistal calibration at the cervical portion of the crown when compared with the calibration mesiodistally on the crown at contact level. The mandibular first *permanent* molar, accordingly, is wider at the cervical portion.

From this aspect also, it will be noted that mesiobuccal and distobuccal developmental grooves divide the buccal surface of the crown occlusally into three cuspal portions almost equal in size. This arrangement forms a straight buccal surface presenting three cusps; a mesiobuccal, a buccal and a distobuccal cusp. It differs, therefore, from the mandibular *first permanent* molar, which has an uneven distribution buccally, presenting two buccal cusps and one distal cusp.

The roots of the deciduous second molar from this angle are slender and long. They have a characteristic flare mesiodistally at the middle and apical thirds. The roots of this tooth may be twice as long as the crown.

The point of bifurcation of the roots starts immediately below the cemento-enamel junction of crown and root.

Lingual Aspect (Figs. 3–25, D; 3–32, 2).   From the lingual aspect one sees two cusps of almost equal dimensions. Between them is a short lingual groove. The two lingual cusps are not quite as wide as the three buccal cusps; this arrangement narrows the crown lingually. The cervical line is relatively straight, and the crown extends out over the root more distally than it does mesially. The mesial portion of the crown seems to be a little higher than the distal portion of the crown when viewed from the lingual aspect. It gives the impression of being tipped distally. A portion of each of the three buccal cusps may be seen from this aspect.

The roots from this aspect give somewhat the same appearance as from the buccal aspect. Note the length of the roots.

Mesial Aspect (Figs 3–26, D; 3–32, 3).   From the mesial aspect the outline of the crown resembles the permanent mandibular first molar. The variations are: The crest of contour buccally is more prominent on the deciduous molar, and the tooth seems to be more constricted occlusally because of the flattened buccal surface above this cervical ridge.

The crown is poised over the root of this tooth in the same manner as all mandibular posteriors; its buccal cusp is over the root and the lingual outline of the crown extending out beyond the root line. The marginal ridge is high, a characteristic which makes the mesiobuccal cusp and the mesiolingual cusp appear rather short. The lingual cusp is longer, or extends higher at any rate, than the buccal cusp. The cervical line is regular, although it extends upward buccolingually, making up for the difference in length between the buccal and lingual cusps.

The mesial root is unusually broad and flat with a blunt apex which is sometimes serrated.

Distal Aspect.   The crown is not as wide distally as it is mesially; therefore it is possible to see the mesiobuccal cusp as well as the distobuccal cusp from the distal aspect. The distolingual cusp appears well developed, and the triangular ridge from the tip of this cusp extending down into the occlusal surface is seen over the distal marginal ridge.

The distal marginal ridge dips down more sharply and is shorter buccolingually than the mesial marginal ridge. The cervical line of the crown is regular, although it has the same upward incline buccolingually on the distal as on the mesial.

The distal root is almost as broad as the mesial root, and it is flattened on the distal surface. The distal root tapers more at the apical end than does the mesial root.

Occlusal Aspect (Figs. 3–27, D; 3–32, 4).   The occlusal aspect of the deciduous mandibular second molar is somewhat rectangular. The three buccal cusps are similar in size. The two lingual cusps are also equally matched. However, the total mesiodistal width of the lingual cusps is less than the total mesiodistal width of the three buccal cusps.

There are well-defined triangular ridges extending occlusally from each one of these cusp tips. The triangular ridges end in the center of the crown buccolingually in a *central developmental groove* which follows a staggered course from the *mesial triangular fossa*, just inside the *mesial marginal ridge*, to the *distal triangular fossa*, just mesial to the *distal marginal ridge*. The distal triangular fossa is not so well defined as the mesial triangular fossa. Developmental grooves branch off from the central groove both buccally and lingually, dividing the cusps. The two *buccal grooves* are confluent with the buccal developmental grooves of the buccal surface, one *mesial* and one *distal*, and the single *lingual developmental groove* is confluent with the *lingual groove* on the lingual surface of the crown.

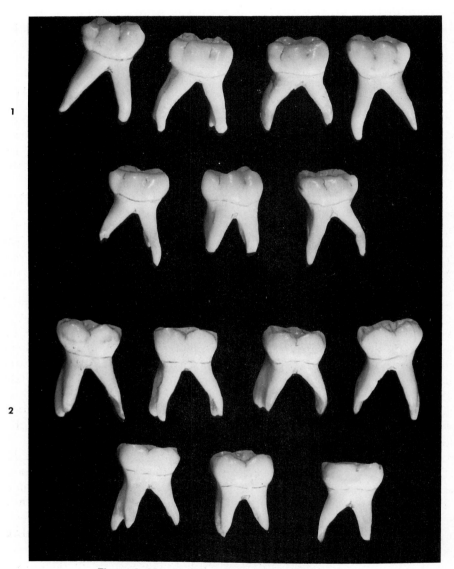

Figure 3–32.   *Deciduous Mandibular Second Molars.*

1. Buccal aspect; 2, lingual aspect.

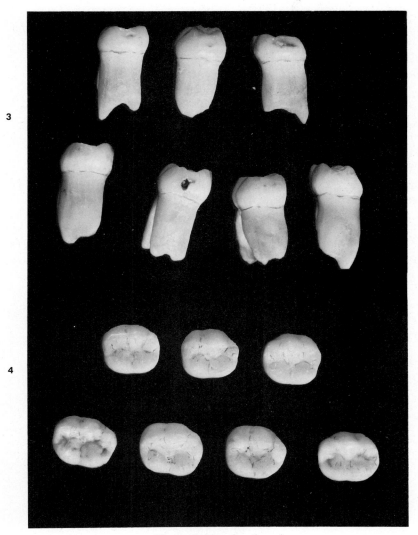

Figure 3–32. *Continued*

3, mesial aspect; 4, occlusal aspect.

Scattered over the occlusal surface are supplemental grooves on the slopes of triangular ridges and in the mesial and distal triangular fossae. The mesial marginal ridge is better developed and more pronounced than the distal marginal ridge. The outline of the crown converges distally. An outline following the tips of the cusps and the marginal ridges conforms to the outline of a rectangle more closely than does the gross outline of the crown in its entirety.

A comparison occlusally between the deciduous mandibular second molar and the permanent mandibular first molar brings out the following points of difference: The deciduous molar has its mesiobuccal, distobuccal and distal cusps almost equal in size and development. The distal cusp of the permanent molar is smaller than the other two. Because of the small buccal cusps, the deciduous tooth crown is narrower buccolingually in comparison with its mesiodistal measurement, than is the permanent tooth.

THE OCCLUSION OF THE DECIDUOUS TEETH

The deciduous teeth are arranged in the jaws in the form of two arches: a maxillary and a mandibular. An outline following the labial and buccal surfaces of the maxillary teeth describes the segment of an ellipse, an outline which is larger than the segment following the same surfaces on the mandibular teeth (see Fig. 1–1, A, Chapter 1).

The relation between the maxillary and mandibular deciduous teeth when in occlusion is such that each tooth, with the exception of the mandibular central incisor and the maxillary second molar, occludes with two teeth of the opposing jaw. The

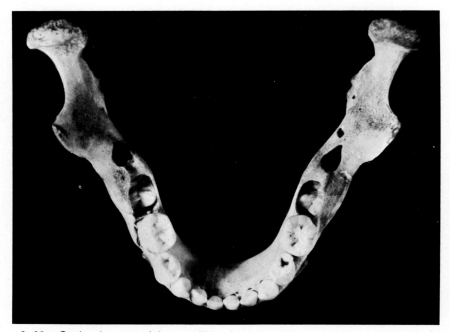

Figure 3–33.   Occlusal aspect of the mandible of specimen shown in Fig. 3–3. Permanent first molar crowns are well developed, and openings in the bone have appeared over the developing permanent second molars. Note the extent of development of the mandible between the distal surface of the second deciduous molar and the anterior border of the ramus.

deciduous teeth should be in normal alignment and occlusion shortly after the age of two, with all the roots fully formed by the time the child is three years old. A year or so after the teeth have fully erupted and have assumed their respective positions in the arches, the rapid development of the jaws is sufficient to create a slight space, or *diastema*, between some of them.

The anterior teeth separate and usually show greater separation as time goes on — a process which is caused by the growth of the jaws and the approach of the permanent teeth from the lingual side. This separation usually begins between the ages of four and five years. The canines and molars are supposed to keep their positive contact relation during all the jaw growth. However, some shifting and separation is seen quite often. Since the teeth do not hold their relative positions for long, they are worn off rapidly on incisal ridges and occlusal surfaces. As an example, when a deciduous canine is lost eight years or more after its eruption, its long, sharp cusp has in most instances been worn down. If the deciduous teeth are in good alignment, the occlusion is most efficient during the time that these teeth are in their original positions (see Figs. 3–34 and 3–35). This situation exists for only a relatively short time.

After normal jaw growth has resulted in considerable separation, the occlusion is supported and made more efficient by the eruption and occlusion of the *first permanent molars* immediately *distal* to the *deciduous second molars*. The child is now approximately *six years* of age, and he will use some of his deciduous teeth for *six more years*.

DETAILS OF OCCLUSION (FIGS. 3–34 AND 3–35)

The occlusion of deciduous teeth, in a three-year-old child, will be described. After separation has begun, the migration of the teeth changes the occlusion. Nevertheless, if development is normal, the spacing of the teeth is rather uniform (Fig. 3–2). This biological change opens up contacts in the arch between teeth and increases occlusal wear. Nature seems to have anticipated the child's needs, however, because

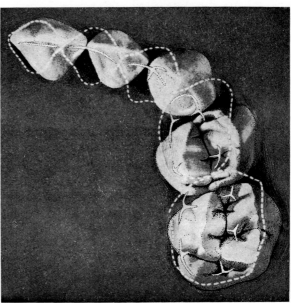

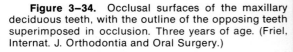

Figure 3–34. Occlusal surfaces of the maxillary deciduous teeth, with the outline of the opposing teeth superimposed in occlusion. Three years of age. (Friel, Internat. J. Orthodontia and Oral Surgery.)

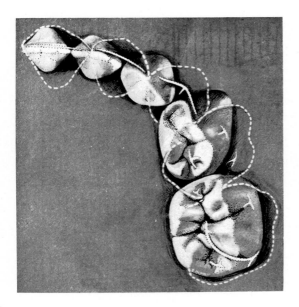

Figure 3–35. Occlusal surface of the mandibular deciduous teeth, with the outlines of the opposing teeth superimposed in occlusion. Three years of age. (Friel, Internat. J. Orthodontia and Oral Surgery.)

if normal healthy reactions are in effect the child seldom suffers from mechanical irritations during this severe adjustment period.

Normal occlusion of deciduous teeth at the age of three years is as follows:

1. Mesial surfaces of maxillary and mandibular central incisors are in line with each other at the median line.

2. The maxillary central incisor occludes with the mandibular central incisor and the mesial third of the mandibular lateral incisor. The mandibular anterior teeth strike the maxillary anterior teeth lingually above the level of the incisal ridges.

3. The maxillary lateral incisor occludes with the distal two-thirds of the mandibular lateral incisor and that portion of the mandibular canine which is mesial to the point of its cusp.

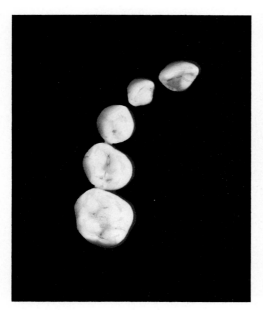

Figure 3–36. *Deciduous Dentition, Upper Right.*

These maxillary deciduous teeth belonged to one person. They were set up in wax approximately in their original arrangement. Normally the anterior contacts open up as the jaw develops. The contact distal to the canine and the contact between the molars should remain functional. This is due to the static character of this section of both jaws. Apparently it is a way of preserving space for the succedaneous premolars.

This figure is a good one to study when making comparisons of the size and shape of deciduous teeth.

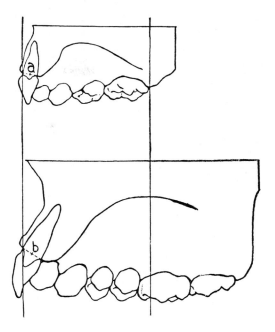

Figure 3–37. *Drawing of a Sagittal Section Through the Permanent and Deciduous Maxillary Incisors.*

The labial surface at the cervical margin is oriented in the same plane. Note that the midalveolar point of the permanent incisors, *b*, is more lingual than the midalveolar point of the deciduous incisor, *a*, but that the incisal edge of the permanent incisors is more labial than that of the deciduous incisors. (Friel, Internat. J. Orthodontia and Oral Surgery.)

4. The maxillary canine occludes with that portion of the mandibular canine distal to its cusp tip and the mesial third of the mandibular first molar (that portion mesial to the tip of the mesiobuccal cusp).

5. The maxillary first molar occludes with the distal two-thirds of the mandibular first molar and the mesial portion of the mandibular second molar, which portion is represented by the mesial marginal ridge and the mesial triangular fossa.

6. The maxillary second molar occludes with the remainder of the mandibular second molar, the distal surface of the maxillary molar projecting slightly over the distal portion of the mandibular second molar.

The interrelation of cusps and incisal ridges of the opposing arches of deciduous teeth may be studied in the illustrations by Sheldon Friel. The relation in size of deciduous and permanent arches is also illustrated by him in Figure 3–37. (See also Fig. 1–1, Chapter 1).

4

General Considerations
in the Physiology
of the Permanent Dentition

FORM AND FUNCTION

The teeth are regarded as instruments — instruments to be used for the comminution of food during the digestive process. Because they need to be kept sound and firmly attached in the jaws, presumably for a lifetime, the tissues that support the teeth must be preserved also. Normal tooth form, plus proper alignment in the jaws, promotes efficiency during mastication, but in addition the *major portion* of the form operates to insure the life of the tooth through stabilization. Proper root form for anchorage, and certain intricate crown contours combine to protect vulnerable soft tissues; all facilities combined serve to preserve the *periodontium*.

Since the design of the individual tooth helps protect its investing tissues — its form having another important function besides that of reducing food material — we come to the important observation, *form and function*. To illustrate: surgical instruments, mechanic's tools and the like are designed for certain purposes. The better each tool or instrument obeys fundamental physical laws in design, the more efficient it will be. Its form governs its function, and its function in turn requires a positive design.

Human teeth are no exception to this rule: Their anatomy is such that they are enabled to perform two major functions during life: (1) *they incise and reduce food material during mastication*, and (2) *they help sustain themselves in the dental arches by assisting in the development and protection of the tissues that support them.*

Protection of the investing tissues and stabilization of alignment are provided by the normal form of the individual teeth, by their proper alignment with others in the same jaw, by normal development of the jaws, and by the proper relation of one jaw to the other during functional movements.

The relation of one jaw to the other has an effect upon the forces brought to bear on the teeth. A normal jaw relation applies the forces equally in directions which the teeth, in normal alignment, are designed to withstand.

The function of the dental apparatus is primarily the mastication of food. However, it has other important values.

Good teeth make one physically more attractive. Socially, good diction is an asset, and correct speech is made possible by the normal development of teeth and jaws.

Psychologically, physical and mental concentration are aided by clenching the teeth firmly together during almost any activity. Strong teeth with good occlusion add in this manner to one's assets and capabilities.

ALIGNMENT, CONTACTS AND OCCLUSION

When the teeth in the mandibular arch come into contact with those in the maxillary arch in any *functional relation*, they are said to be *in occlusion*. There is therefore a central relation of one arch to the other, which is called *centric* or *central occlusion*. When the occlusion of the teeth of one jaw with those in the opposing jaw is abnormal, the teeth are said to be in *malocclusion*.

In proper alignment the teeth are arranged in arches in each jaw and placed in strong contact with their neighbors (Fig. 4–1). If, in addition, each tooth in the arch is placed at its most advantageous angle to withstand forces brought to bear upon it, each tooth is more efficient and the arches are stabilized by the collective action of the teeth in supporting each other (Figs. 4–2 and 4–3). Compare the plaster casts in Figure 4–4, for example, with those in Figure 4–5. It is readily seen that irregularly arranged teeth are less likely to stabilize themselves or to help in stabilizing the others.

Contact of each tooth with its fellows in the arch protects the *gingiva* between them in the *interproximal spaces*. Figures 4–6 and 4–7 are given as examples. The gingiva is the soft tissue in the mouth which covers the alveolar bone and surrounds the teeth.

INTERPROXIMAL FORM

The interproximal space between the teeth is a triangular region, normally filled with gingival tissue, which is bounded by the two proximal surfaces of contacting teeth and the alveolar bone between the teeth, which acts as the base of the triangle.

The gingiva within this space is called the *gingival or interdental papilla* (Fig. 5–35). Normally, the gingiva covers part of the cervical third of the tooth crowns and fills the interproximal spaces (Figs. 4–6 and 5–17). The *gingival line* follows the curvature, but not necessarily the level of the cervical line. The cervical line is defined as the "cementoenamel junction of crown and root." The gingival line and the cervical line must not be thought of as being identical; although they normally follow a similar curvature, they are seldom at the same level on the tooth. The cervical line is a stable anatomic demarcation, whereas the gingival line merely represents the gingival level on the tooth at any one period in the individual's life, and this level is variable. Malalignment of the teeth will change the gingival line – something not conducive to the health of the tissue (Fig. 4–8).

Even though the teeth are in good alignment, unless the proper relation is kept between the *width* of each tooth *at the cervix* and the width *at the point of contact* with neighboring teeth, the spacing interdentally will be changed. This is an important point to observe in clinical examinations.

When considering the tooth form from the mesial and distal aspects, we find cur-

A

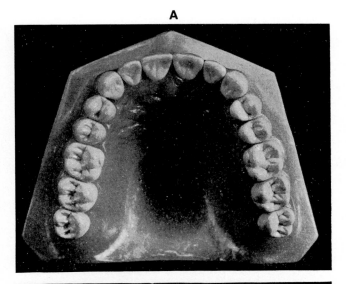

B

Figure 4–1.   Model teeth placed in "ideal" alignment and contact relation. A, Maxillary arch; B, mandibular arch.

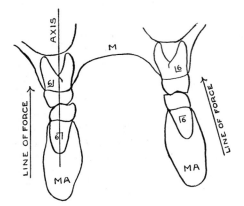

Figure 4–2.   Outline of a cross section through the maxilla and mandible at the site of the first molars. The line of force exerted when the teeth come into contact should be parallel to the long axis of the teeth. If the teeth are in the proper position to withstand this force their positions will be stable.

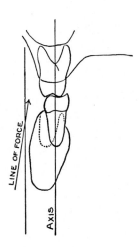

Figure 4–3. A drawing showing the first mandibular molar out of normal position. Its axis is not parallel with the line of force, and consequently the act of mastication would tend to change the position and angulation of the teeth, making them unstable.

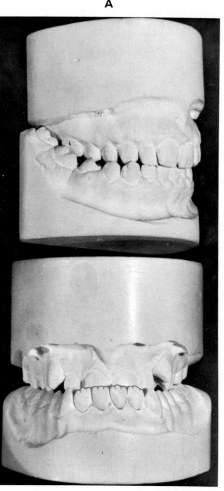

A

Figure 4–4. Plaster casts of two sets of jaws, each demonstrating malocclusion. *A,* Fair occlusion of maxillary central and lateral incisors with those of the mandible, but gross malocclusion of the right canines and posterior teeth. *B,* Extensive malocclusion with improper relationship of the maxillary and mandibular arches. Note the *mamelons,* which are still intact on the incisal portion of the mandibular central and lateral incisors.

B

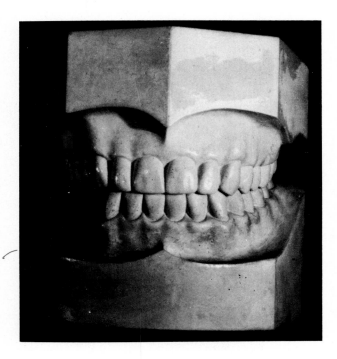

Figure 4–5. This cast demonstrates normal occlusion. The teeth in each arch are in proper alignment, the jaw relationship is normal, and therefore the relationship of each mandibular tooth to its antagonist in the maxilla is normal. These teeth will support each other in keeping normal arch relationship.

vature on the crowns at the cervical third above the cervical line, labially or buccally and lingually—a factor which must be treated with respect. This prominence holds the gingiva under proper tension and serves to protect the investing tissues of the teeth during mastication. It is called the cervicoenamel ridge (Figs. 1–15 and 1–16), or merely cervical ridge, with the location added (buccocervical ridge, and so forth).

IMPORTANT PHYSIOLOGIC RELATIONS

The *length* and *shape of the root* (or roots) of each tooth must be considered important: the canine, for instance, because of its position and the work required of it, would be torn out of its socket, or at least displaced, by forces brought to bear upon it, if the root were not of extra size and length (Fig. 4–9). Fracture would be imminent if the root were not larger than that of other single-rooted teeth. The root form therefore is associated with the *over-all form* of the tooth and the *work* it has to do.

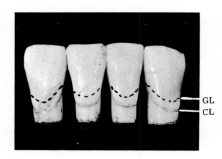

Figure 4–6. The mandibular centrals and laterals contact each other at the incisal third. The form of each tooth, plus the location of the contact areas, creates narrow pointed spaces between the teeth which differ from other interproximal spaces in other segments of the arches. *CL*, cervical line as established by the cementoenamel junction. *GL*, the variable gingival line which represents the gingival level.

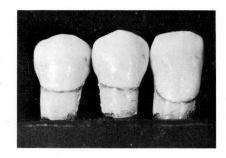

Figure 4–7. Contact design and interproximal (sometimes called interdental) spaces illustrated by the mandibular canine and first and second premolars. Note the variation in contact areas in relation to crown length.

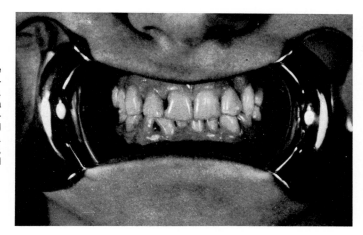

Figure 4–8. The maxillary teeth are surrounded by normal gingival tissue, because these teeth are in good alignment. Observe the irregular outline of the gingiva around the mandibular teeth and the destruction apparent in this young individual between the right lateral incisor and canine. The alignment is especially bad at this point, and therefore the contact and interproximal spacing are abnormal.

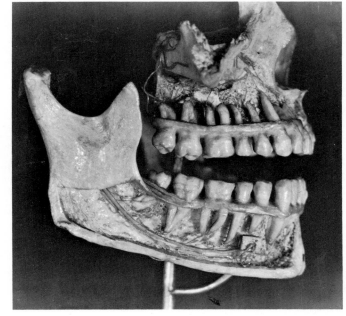

Figure 4–9. A view of a specimen from a point opposite the first molar. Note that the teeth are placed at different angulations. The position of the tooth in the jaw and the relation between its axis and the lines of force brought to bear upon it are very important.

The *angle* at which the incisal and occlusal surfaces of the tooth crowns are placed with respect to the root bases is also important. The mesial view of an anterior tooth will show that the incisal ridge or cusp is centered over the root (Fig. 1–15, Chapter 1). The mesial view of an upper first molar, which is a multi-cusped tooth, demonstrates the same principle. The points on the occlusal surface that are contacted by opposing teeth will prove to be well within the confines of the root base of the crown. The measurement from cusp tip to cusp tip buccolingually is much less than the buccolingual diameter of the root base. (Figure 1–16, Chapter 1. Note the flare of roots for stabilization.)

COMPENSATING OCCLUSAL CURVATURE

Close observation indicates that the occlusal and incisal surfaces of all the crowns taken together in either arch would not contact a flat plane. Looking at the teeth from a point opposite the first molars buccally, one sees that a line following the occlusal and incisal surfaces describes a curve.

This arrangement was described originally in the German literature in 1890 by F. Graf von Spee, and it is called the *Curve of Spee* (Fig. 4–10). The occlusal curvature of tooth alignment was described as conforming to arcs of circles. Today we prefer to think of the composite arrangement of the occlusal surfaces of all of the teeth in each dental arch and of their approximate conformation to a segment of a sphere, which gives the curvature three-dimensional quality (Figs. 4–11 and 16–15). This curvature is called the *compensating occlusal curvature.* We say that the compensating occlusal curvature of the mandibular teeth is *concave* and that of the maxillary teeth *convex* (Fig. 4–11). Actually, the compensating occlusal curvature adaptability of any tooth in the jaws is reflected in its own makeup. The occlusal surface of a maxillary molar, as an example, shows very plainly an acute angulation mesially with the long axis of its roots (Fig. 4–12).

The length and shape of the roots, the angle at which the incisal and occlusal surfaces are placed with respect to the roots, sufficient dimensions for strength, and an efficient design for thorough work with resistance against lines of force; all these play a part in a magnificent scheme to stabilize the dental arches and to resist physiologic change.

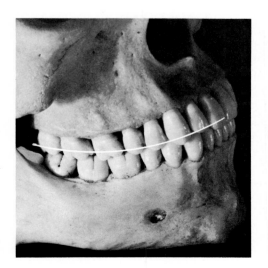

Figure 4–10. Centric occlusion. The occlusion of natural teeth is seldom if ever "ideal." This illustration shows normal occlusion. Note the "Curve of Spee." Also note the margin of the alveolar bone in its relation to the cervical line of the teeth. (Observe fourth mandibular molar, an anomaly.)

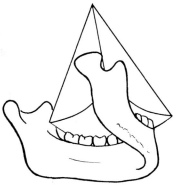

Figure 4–11. A segment of a sphere placed on the occluding surfaces of the mandibular teeth, showing their compensating occlusal curvature.

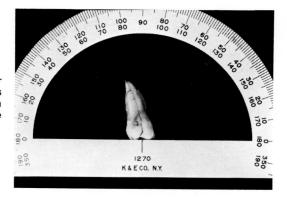

Figure 4–12. Molar tooth placed within a protractor to show axial inclinations. When the teeth are set in the jaws in proper alignment, the occlusal surfaces will combine in a manner producing compensating occlusal curvature (see Fig. 4–11).

COMPARATIVE DENTAL ANATOMY

The fundamentals of tooth form in the human subject will be better understood by making comparisons with other dentitions in comparative dental anatomy. The physiologic significance of anatomical details means more after a study of evolutionary concepts, development of form and function and so forth; a detailed description of the form of individual teeth will have more meaning after a comparison is made.

The study of the evolutionary concepts of tooth development leading to the higher forms is a fascinating one. Anyone interested in dental anatomy should take every opportunity to pursue the subject in depth, thereby enhancing his knowledge of the fundamentals of tooth form.

A superficial summary of the topic is presented here. It includes an outline of development in the vertebrates only, starting with the primordial form of tooth, the single cone or lobe which was the forerunner of combinations of lobes forming the more complicated teeth found in highly developed animals and in the human being today.

Figure 4–13 graphically illustrates with a schematic drawing the four stages of tooth development:

    a. The Reptilian stage (Haplodont)
    b. Early Mammalian stage (Triconodont)
    c. Triangular stage (Tritubercular molar)
    d. Quadritubercular molar

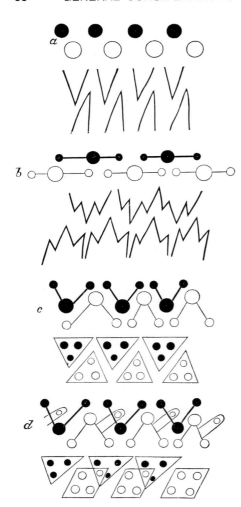

Figure 4–13. Phyletic history of the molar cusps. (After Osborn.)

    a. The Reptilian stage. (Haplodont.)
    b. Early Mammalian stage. (Triconodont.)
    c. Triangular stage. (Tritubercular molar.)
    d. Quadritubercular molar.

(From Dewey and Thompson, *Comparative Dental Anatomy,* The C. V. Mosby Company, 2nd Edition.)

The *Reptilian* or *Haplodont* stage is represented by the simplest form of tooth, the single cone (Fig. 4–14). This type of dentition usually includes many teeth in both jaws that limit jaw movement. There is no occlusion of the teeth in this class, the teeth being used mainly for prehension or combat. Their main function is the procurement of food. The limitation of jaw relation is confined to that of a simple hinge movement. Jaw movements are related to and governed by tooth form in all cases.

The *Early Mammalian* or *Triconodont* stage exhibits three cusps in line in the development of posterior teeth. The largest, or anthropologically, the original cusp, is centered with a smaller cusp located anteriorly and another posteriorly. Today examples are not seen with a purely triconodont dentition. Some of the teeth in some breeds of dogs and other carnivori have some teeth that certainly indicate a triconodont background (Fig. 4–15). Nevertheless, the dog and other animals carnivorous by nature are considered to be in the third category, namely, the *Tritubercular* class (Figs. 4–16 and 4–17).

According to the recognized theories explaining evolutionary tooth development, the triconodont line of three changed to a three-cornered shape, with the teeth still bypassing each other more or less when the jaw opened or closed. The next stage of

Figure 4–14. *The Mississippi Alligator.*

(Kronfeld, Dental Histology and Comparative Dental Anatomy. Lea & Febiger.) An interesting commentary on the anatomy of the alligator: because of the alligator's physical problems, the upper jaw is the mobile one. The lower jaw, closer to the ground, is static.

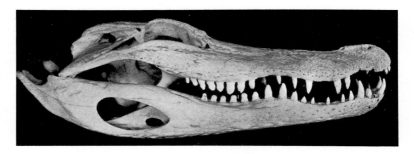

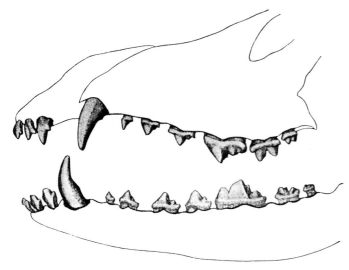

Figure 4–15. Permanent dentition of Canis familiaris. (After Marett Tims.)

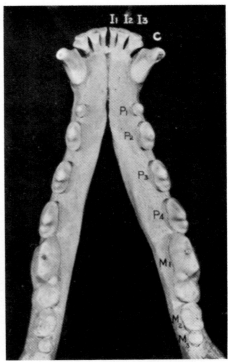

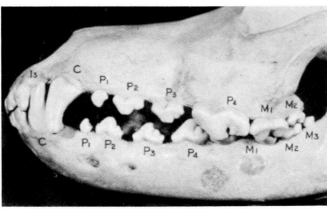

Figure 4–16. Jaws of a dog (collie). The premolars are tritubercular and widely spaced; the upper carnassial (fourth premolar, P_4) articulates with the lower carnassial (first molar, M_1). (From Kronfeld, *Dental Histology and Comparative Anatomy*, Lea & Febiger, 1937.)

Figure 4–17. Occlusal view of the mandible of a dog (collie). The mandible is long and slender. The cutting edges of the four premolars and three molars are arranged in a sagittal plane. (From Kronfeld, *Dental Histology and Comparative Anatomy*, Lea & Febiger, 1937.)

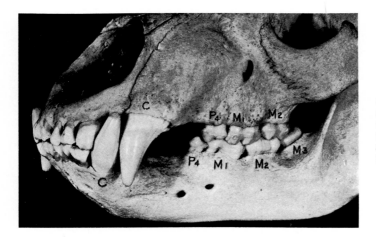

Figure 4–18. The bear. The extent of development of teeth and jaws and occlusion is often used to rate animal forms. A comparison of this figure with Fig. 4–19 is interesting. (Kronfeld, *Dental Histology and Comparative Dental Anatomy*, Lea & Febiger.)

development created projections on the triangular form that finally occluded with an antagonist in the opposing jaw. As this development progressed, occlusion was established and the *Quadritubercular stage* had arrived. During these eons of time, and as an accommodation to the changes in tooth form, the anatomy and articulation of the jaws changed accordingly.

The *herbivorous* animal possesses the greatest range in jaw movement; the *omnivorous* is next in line; Man (*homo sapiens*) joins this group. The *carnivorous* animals have a limited range of jaw movement, partly because of the extreme over development of canines that locks the jaws when fully closed.

The animals with a dentition similar to that of Man are anthropoid apes. This group of animals includes the chimpanzee, gibbon, gorilla and orangutan (Fig. 4–19).

The shapes of individual teeth in these animals are amazingly close to their counterparts in the human mouth. Nevertheless, the development of the canines, the arch form and the jaw development are quite different.

As mentioned earlier, a serious student of dentistry should pursue his interest in comparative dental anatomy. Many men in the profession with a scientific bent have

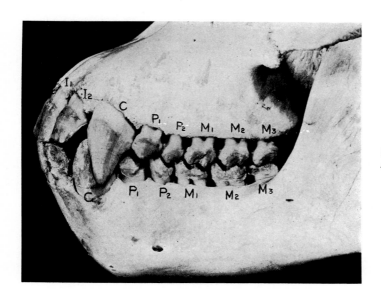

Figure 4–19. The ape. (Kronfeld, *Dental Histology and Comparative Dental Anatomy*, Lea & Febiger.)

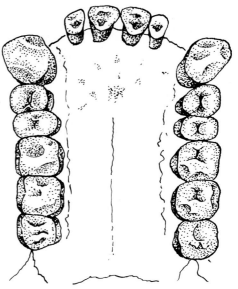

Figure 4–20. Occlusal view of the upper jaw of an orangutan. The arch is square, and the canines, premolars, and molars stand in a straight sagittal line. Note the diastema between lateral incisor and canine. (After Kronfeld, *Dental Histology and Comparative Dental Anatomy*. Lea & Febiger.)

made the study a "collateral hobby," much to their pleasure and enlightenment. The proper approach, of course, would be to consult specialized literature on the subject.

The multiplication and fusion of lobes during tooth development are demonstrated graphically when human teeth are viewed from the mesial or distal aspects. Anterior teeth which are used for incising or apprehending food reflect the single cone, whereas the posterior or multicusp teeth, which are used for grinding food in addition to a shearing action, appear to be two or more cones fused (Fig. 4–21). Although the schematic form of the teeth from the mesial or distal aspects is that of a single cone in anteriors, or what seems to be an indication of a fusion of two or more cones in posteriors, close observation causes one to come to the conclusion that each tooth crown, regardless of location, will appear to be a combination of four or more lobes. Each lobe represents a primary center of formation.

Figure 4–21. The functional form of the teeth when outlined schematically from the mesial or distal aspects is that of the fusion of two or three cones. *a*, Maxillary incisor; *b*, maxillary premolar; *c*, maxillary first molar. Note that the major portion of the incisor in view is made up of one cone or lobe.

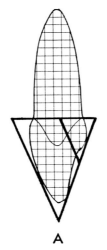

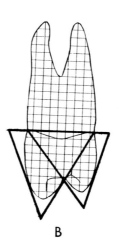

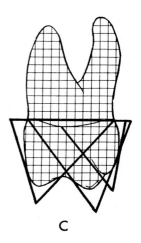

A   B   C

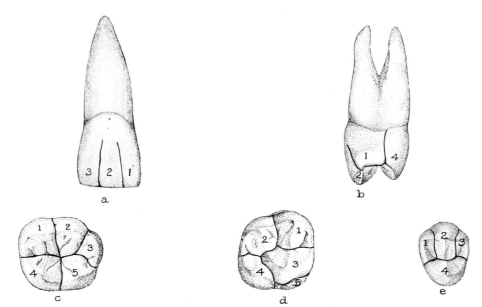

Figure 4–22. This illustration shows the general outlines of some of the lobes.

a, Labial aspect of maxillary central incisor, showing the labial grooves marking the division of the lobes. 1, Mesial lobe; 2, labial lobe; 3, distal lobe. (Lingual lobe or cingulum not in view.) (See Fig. 4–23, A-4.)

b and *e,* Mesial and occlusal aspects of maxillary first premolar. 1, Mesial lobe; 2, buccal lobe; 3, distal lobe; 4, lingual lobe.

c, Occlusal aspect of mandibular first molar. 1, Mesiobuccal lobe; 2, distobuccal lobe; 3, distal lobe; 4, mesiolingual lobe; 5, distolingual lobe. (Lobes on molars are named the same as cusps.)

d, Occlusal aspect of maxillary first molar. 1, Mesiobuccal lobe; 2, distobuccal lobe; 3, mesiolingual lobe; 4, distolingual lobe; 5, fifth lobe (fifth cusp).

All anterior teeth show traces of four lobes, three labially and one lingually, the lingual lobe being represented by the cingulum. Each labial lobe of the incisor terminates incisally in rounded eminences known as *mamelons.* These mamelons are prominent in newly erupted incisors (Fig. 4–4). Soon after eruption they are worn down by use unless through malalignment they escape incisal wear. Maxillary central incisors often show traces of the fusion of three lobes on the labial face by visible markings in the enamel called *labial grooves* (Fig. 4–22, A).

In the anterior teeth the four lobes are called the *mesial, labial, distal* and *lingual lobes.* In *premolars* they are called *mesial, buccal, distal* and *lingual lobes;* or, as in the case of the mandibular second premolar, which often has two lingual cusps, the *mesial, buccal, distal, mesiolingual* and *distolingual lobes,* making five in all (Fig. 10–17).

The *molar lobes* are named the same as the cusps: *mesiobuccal lobe,* etc. The tip of each cusp represents the primary center of formation of each lobe.[*]

It is possible, of course, to find a variation in the number of lobes in molars. Tubercles of enamel may be found in addition to the primary lobes. When present, they are usually smaller than, and supplementary to, the major lobes.

[*]Tables of development of the teeth will be given under the complete description of each tooth. The description of the formation of the teeth histologically, however, will not be included. For this refer to a work on dental histology and embryology. See also, the color charts on pages 28–29.

A GEOMETRIC CONCEPT OF CROWN OUTLINES

In a general way, all aspects of each tooth crown except the incisal or occlusal aspects may be outlined schematically within three gometric figures: a *triangle*, a *trapezoid* and a *rhomboid.* To one unfamiliar with dental anatomy it may seem an exaggeration to say that curved outlines of tooth crowns can be included within geometric figures. Nevertheless, to one who realizes the problems involved in crown design it seems very plausible to consider fundamental outlines schematically to assist in visualization.

In freehand drawing, the outlines of a subject are sketched roughly at first in order to get proportion and outline form. In sculpture the subject is "blocked in," a method which follows the same plan as sketching in drawing except that three dimensions are involved. Therefore, since it is possible to reduce the fundamental outline of tooth crowns to three generalizations (except, as has been pointed out, for the incisal or occlusal aspects), this method of approach may be used.

FACIAL AND LINGUAL ASPECTS OF ALL TEETH

The outlines of the facial and lingual aspects of all the teeth may be represented by *trapezoids* of various dimensions. The shortest of the uneven sides represent the bases of the crowns at the cervices, and the longest of the uneven sides represent the working surfaces, or the incisal and occlusal surfaces, the line made through the points of contact of neighboring teeth in the same arch (Fig. 4–25). Disregarding the overlap of anterior teeth and the cusp forms of the cusped teeth in the schematic drawing, one can easily see the fundamental plan governing the form and arrangement of the teeth from this aspect.

Figure 4–23. *A,* Lingual aspect of maxillary canine, with primary centers marked. 1, Mesial lobe; 2, central lobe (cusp); 3, distal lobe; 4, lingual lobe (cingulum).

B, Incomplete formation demonstrated by a developmental groove distolingually on a maxillary lateral incisor. This groove will sometimes harbor fissures at various points along its length, especially in the coronal portion. A tooth with this handicap is more subject to caries and gum infections.

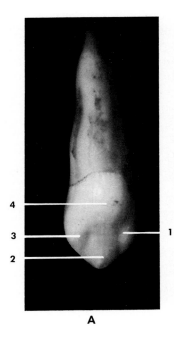
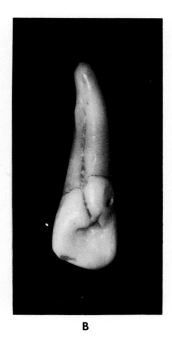

A   B

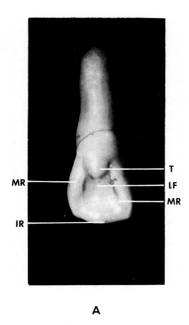
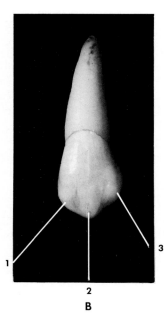

Figure 4–24. *A,* Maxillary lateral incisor which shows prominences at the centers of calcification. *T,* Tubercle, prominence equal to a small cusp at the cingulum; *LF,* lingual fossa; *MR,* marginal ridges; *IR,* incisal ridge with a prominent enamel rise.

B, Maxillary canine showing evidences of lobe formation. 1, Mesial lobe; 2, labial lobe; 3, distal lobe.

A   B

The occlusal line which forms the longest uneven side of each of the trapezoids represents the approximate point at which the opposing teeth come together when the jaw is closed. The viewer must not become confused at this point and think that the teeth actually occlude level with their points of contact. The illustration is made to help in visualizing the fundamental shape of the teeth from the labial and buccal aspects. (See Fig. 4–26.)

This arrangement brings out the following *fundamentals* of form:

1. Interproximal spaces may accommodate interproximal tissue.

2. Spacing between the roots of one tooth and those of another allows sufficient bone tissue for investment for the teeth and a supporting structure required to hold up gingival tissue to a normal level. Sufficient circulation of blood to the parts would be impossible without this spacing.

3. Each tooth crown in the dental arches must be in contact at some point with its neighbor, or neighbors, to help protect the interproximal gingival tissue from trauma

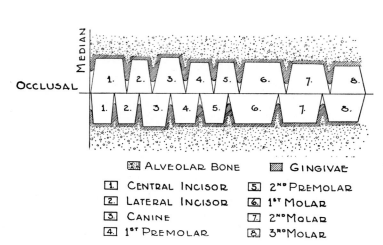

Figure 4–25. Schematic drawing of facial (labial and buccal) aspects of the teeth only, illustrating the teeth as trapezoids of various dimensions. Note the relations of each tooth to its opposing tooth or teeth in the opposite arch. Each tooth has two antagonists except number 1 below and number 8 above.

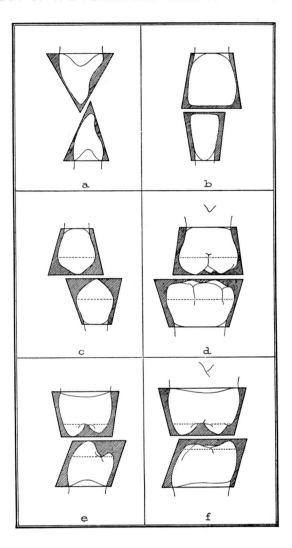

Figure 4–26. Outlines of crown forms within geometric outlines—triangles, trapezoids and rhomboids. The upper figure in each square represents a maxillary tooth, the lower figure a mandibular tooth. Note that the trapezoid outline will not include the cusp form of posteriors actually. It does include the crowns from cervix to contact point or cervix to marginal ridge, however. Remember that this is a schematic drawing to emphasize certain fundamentals. *a,* Anterior teeth, mesial or distal; *b,* anterior teeth, labial or lingual; *c,* premolars, buccal or lingual; *d,* molars, buccal or lingual; *e,* premolars, mesial or distal; *f,* molars, mesial or distal.

during mastication. The contact of one tooth with another in the arch tends to insure their respective positions by mutual support.

4. Each tooth in each dental arch has two antagonists in the opposing arch excepting the mandibular central incisor and the maxillary third molar. In the event of loss of any tooth, this arrangement tends to prevent elongation of antagonists and helps stabilize the remaining teeth over a longer period than would be likely if each tooth had but a single antagonist.

MESIAL AND DISTAL ASPECTS OF THE ANTERIOR TEETH

The mesial and distal aspects of the anterior teeth, central incisors, lateral incisors and canines, maxillary and mandibular, may be included within *triangles*. The base of the triangle is represented by the cervical portion of the crown, and the apex by the incisal ridge (Fig. 4–26, A).

The fundamentals protrayed here are:

1. A wide base to the crown for strength.

2. A tapered outline labially and lingually, narrowing down to a relatively thin ridge which facilitates the penetration of food material.

MESIAL AND DISTAL ASPECTS OF MAXILLARY POSTERIOR TEETH

The outlines of the mesial and distal aspects of all maxillary posterior teeth (premolars and molars) can be included within *trapezoidal* figures. Naturally, the uneven sides of the premolar figures are shorter than those of the molars (Fig. 4–26, *E* and *F*). Notice that in this instance the trapezoidal figures show the longest uneven side representing the *base* of the crown instead of the *occlusal line,* as was the case in showing the same teeth from the buccal or lingual view. In other words, the schematic outline used to represent the buccal aspect of premolars or molars is turned upside down to represent the mesial or distal aspects of the same teeth. (In Fig. 4–26, compare maxillary figures *C* and *D* with *E* and *F*.)

The fundamental considerations to be observed when reviewing the mesial or distal aspects of maxillary posterior teeth are:

1. Because the occlusal surface is constricted the tooth can be forced into food material more easily.

2. If the occlusal surface were as wide as the base of the crown the additional chewing surface would multiply the forces of mastication; then, too, the tooth would be less "self cleansing" during the process.

It has been found necessary to emphasize the fundamental outlines of these aspects through the medium of schematic drawings because the correct anatomy is overlooked so often. The tendency is to take for granted that the tooth crowns are narrowest at the cervix *from all angles,* which is not true. The measurement of the cervical portion of a posterior tooth is smaller than that of the occlusal portion when viewed from buccal or lingual aspects only; when it is observed from the mesial or distal aspects, the comparison is just the reverse; the occlusal surface tapers from the wide root base. (Compare *E* and *F*, Fig. 4–26, with *C* and *D*.)

MESIAL AND DISTAL ASPECTS OF MANDIBULAR POSTERIOR TEETH

Finally, the mandibular posterior teeth, when approached from the mesial or distal aspects, are somewhat *rhomboidal* in outline (Fig. 4–26, *E* and *F*). The occlusal surfaces are constricted in comparison with the bases—similar to the maxillary posterior teeth. The rhomboidal outline inclines the crowns lingual to the root bases, bringing the cusps into proper occlusion with the cusps of their maxillary opponents. At the same time, the axes of crowns and roots of the teeth of both jaws are kept parallel (Fig. 4–2 and 4–3). If the mandibular posterior crowns were to be set on their roots in the same relation of crown to root as that of the maxillary posterior teeth, the cusps would clash with one another. This would not allow the intercusp relations necessary for proper function.

SUMMARY OF SCHEMATIC OUTLINES

Outlines of the tooth crowns, when viewed from the labial or buccal, lingual, mesial and distal aspects, are described in a general way by triangles, trapezoids or rhomboids (Fig. 4–26, *A* to *F*).

Triangles
    Six anterior teeth, maxillary and mandibular
        1. Mesial aspect
        2. Distal aspect
Trapezoids
    A. Trapezoid with longest uneven side toward occlusal or incisal surface
        1. *All anterior teeth,* maxillary and mandibular
            a. Labial aspect
            b. Lingual aspect
        2. *All posterior teeth*
            a. Buccal aspect
            b. Lingual aspect
    B. Trapezoid with shortest uneven side toward occlusal surface
        1. *All maxillary posterior teeth*
            a. Mesial aspect
            b. Distal aspect
Rhomboids
    All mandibular posterior teeth
        1. Mesial aspect
        2. Distal aspect

5

Physiologic Tooth Form Protecting the Periodontium; Tooth Form and Dental Maintenance

FUNDAMENTAL CURVATURES

The teeth possess certain fundamental curvatures that serve to give the proper degree of protection to the *periodontium*. Some of these protective curvatures are so finely drawn that an increase or decrease in dimensions at vulnerable areas would affect seriously the future of a tooth. In short, these protective contours are physiologic.

Research on the physiologic significance of tooth forms has been very limited. Authorities are, nevertheless, agreed on this; that certain fundamental outlines of the individual teeth have functional significance which is important to them singly and collectively in improving or decreasing their efficiency. The term efficiency implies, of course, that each tooth must help insure its own position, thereby doing its share toward the stability of the entire dental arch. It does this by contributing toward the protection of investing tissues in addition to its efficiency in mastication. This chapter will concern itself with the subject of *tooth form and dental maintenance*.

Without sound tissues supporting it, a tooth cannot last long. Teeth are subject to *abnormal development* and *anomalies of form*, as are other parts of the body. Undoubtedly many teeth are lost prematurely because certain functional outlines fail to develop properly or because *malalignment of well-formed teeth in the dental arches made the important protective contours inoperative*. Naturally, a good diagnosis for subsequent dental treatment of any sort must take into serious consideration all that is known of physiologic tooth form, alignment and occlusion.

Briefly, the study of the protective functional form of the tooth crowns must include, among other things, the following:

1. Proximal contact areas.

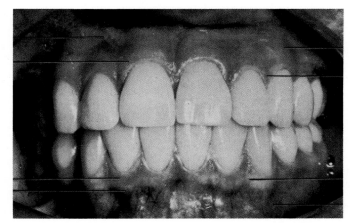

Alveolar
mucosa

Attached
gingiva

Mucogingival
junction

Interdental
papilla

Free gingival
groove

Mucogingival
junction

Attached
gingiva

Alveolar
mucosa

Figure 5–1.   Surface appearance of the clinically normal gingiva. This picture serves as an excellent example to illustrate the "self-cleansing" potential in nearly-perfect teeth in good alignment with healthy gingival tissue. Note the smooth interdental embrasures, both labially and incisally, and the slick labial faces of the anterior teeth. This figure demonstrates contact levels and contact designs as they are evidently intended to be. (Courtesy of Dr. Alfred L. Ogilvie. From Orban et al., *Periodontics,* C. V. Mosby Co., 1958, p. 17.)

2. Interproximal spaces (formed by proximal surfaces in contact).

3. Embrasures (spillways).

4. Labial and buccal contours at the cervical thirds (cervical ridges) and lingual contours at the middle thirds of crowns. (Both are protective contours.)

5. Curvatures of the cervical lines on mesial and distal surfaces (cementoenamel junction).

6. The role of tooth form in promoting sanitation in the mouth; the tooth is largely self cleansing, and it joins with all the others in the mouth to form an efficient combination promoting oral hygiene.

The above headings include the form which has a direct or primary bearing on the protection of the periodontium. Many other details of tooth form have an indirect bearing on the stability of the teeth through their contribution to the maintenance of efficiency during function. Some of these details are cusp forms, the proportions of various measurements of the crowns and roots, root form and anchorage and angles at which teeth are set in the jaws.

Further observation of the details of tooth form soon establishes another important fact: from all aspects, when well formed teeth are in normal alignment with normal gingival attachment (Fig. 5–1) they are remarkably "self cleansing." The smooth rounded form of the teeth contributes toward proper *dental hygiene* when assisted by the brushing activity of tongue and cheeks, the flushing action of saliva and the intake of fluids, plus the friction of food material during the functional activity of mastication. Needless to say, this form contributes to the efficient use of the tooth brush during home care of the teeth.

1. PROXIMAL CONTACT AREAS

Soon after the alignment of all of the teeth in their respective positions in the jaws takes place, there should be a positive contact relation mesially and distally of one tooth with another in each arch. Excepting the last molars (third molars, if present), each tooth has *two* contacting members adjoining it. The last molar is in contact only

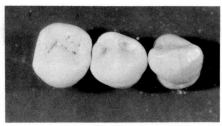

Figure 5–2. This is a photograph of three mandibular teeth removed from the same individual. This person was evidently well past middle age, but it so happened that the canine had never been in contact with the first premolar. The premolars had been in strong contact relation, as evidenced by their adaptation to each other at the contact areas.

The teeth were set up in their proper alignment to show the contrast between the "marble" contact of the canine and first premolar, a contrast which represents the contact design in extreme youth, since there had been no wear at the contact areas in this case, and the adaptation of one premolar to the other at the point of contact after many years of functional use.

with the tooth mesial to it. Although the areas of contact are still very circumscribed, especially on anterior teeth, these are *areas* and not mere *points* of contact. Actually the term "contact point," which term is often used to designate the contact of teeth in the same arch, is a misnomer. When the individual is quite young and the teeth are newly erupted, some of the teeth come close to having point contacts only when the contacting surfaces are nearly perfect curvatures (Fig. 5–2). Examples of the few contacts made by such rounded surfaces are located distally on canines and mesially on first premolars maxillary and mandibular.

The proper contact relation between neighboring teeth in each arch is important for the following reasons: (1) it serves to keep food from packing between the teeth, and (2) it helps to stabilize the dental arches by the combined anchorage of all the teeth in either arch in positive contact with each other (Figs. 5–3 and 5–4). Excepting the third molars, each tooth in the arch is supported in part by its contact with two neighboring teeth, one mesial and one distal. The third molars (and the second molars as well if there is no third molar) are prevented from drifting distally where there is no contacting tooth by the angulation of their occlusal surfaces with their roots and by the angle of the direction of the occlusal forces in their favor. This will be explained more fully in later chapters.

If for any reason food is allowed to escape between the teeth past the contact areas, the result may be pathologic. The gingival tissue which normally fills the interdental spaces may become inflamed so that *gingivitis* ensues. This inflammation may be followed by further degenerative processes unless it is checked. The final result may be a complete breakdown of the tissues, including destruction of the alveolar

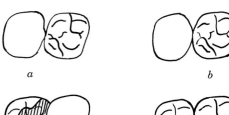

a

b

c

d

Figure 5–3. *a,* The projection of a point contact, as in a faulty restoration. This arrangement would not reproduce normal contact form or embrasure form. *b,* The contact is better than in *a,* but the supplementary embrasure form is faulty. *c,* Contact area is too great, with insufficient embrasure opening, buccal and lingual. *d,* Normal contact and embrasure form. The lingual escapement or embrasure form is more open than the buccal embrasure form.

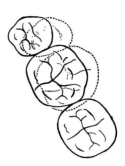

Figure 5–4.   Outline drawings from the occlusal aspect of the mandibular second premolar, first molar and second molar. Shadow drawings of occluding teeth show the adaptation of the contact and embrasure design to the occlusal relation.

bone and the possible loss of one or more teeth. Separation of the teeth through loss of contact causes a change in tooth alignment, which in turn brings about a shifting of the forces brought to bear upon the tooth or teeth in question during mastication.

When a tooth is subjected to occlusal forces at an angle that it is not designed to withstand, or if it must absorb more than its share of those forces through lack of support by its neighbors, it suffers from *occlusal trauma.* Prolonged occlusal trauma may also cause destruction of the supporting tissues.

Contact areas must be observed from *two aspects* in order to obtain the proper perspective for locating them: (1) the labial or buccal aspect, and (2) the incisal or occlusal aspect.

The *labial* or *buccal* view will demonstrate the relative positions of the contact areas cervicoincisally or cervico-occlusally. The center of the area from this aspect is gauged by its relation to the length of the crown portion of the tooth (Figs. 5–5 through 5–10).

The *incisal* or *occlusal* view will show the relative position of the contact areas labiolingually or buccolingually. In this instance the center of the area may be located in its relation to the labiolingual or buccolingual measurement of the crown (Figs. 5–11, 5–12, 5–14 and 5–15). The point at which the contact area is bisected will also depend upon the outline of the form of the crown from the incisal or occlusal aspect. This outline is governed by the *alignment* of the tooth in the arch and also by the *occlusal relation* with its antagonists in the opposing arch. The mandibular first molar is an excellent example (Figs. 5–4 and 5–14). The contact and embrasure design for this tooth will be explained later when the incisal and occlusal aspects of the teeth are considered.

2. INTERPROXIMAL SPACES (FORMED BY PROXIMAL SURFACES IN CONTACT)

The interproximal spaces between the teeth are triangularly shaped spaces normally filled by *gingival tissue (gingival papillae).* The base of the triangle is the alveolar process; the sides of the triangle are the proximal surfaces of the contacting teeth, and the apex of the triangle is in the area of contact. The form of the interproximal space will vary with the form of the teeth in contact and will depend also upon the relative position of the contact areas (compare Figs. 5–7, A and D).

Proper contact and alignment of adjoining teeth will allow proper spacing between them for the normal bulk of gingival tissue attached to the bone and teeth. This gingival tissue, which is a continuation of the gingiva covering all of the alveolar process, is a valuable aid in mouth hygiene. Assisted by the saliva and the friction of

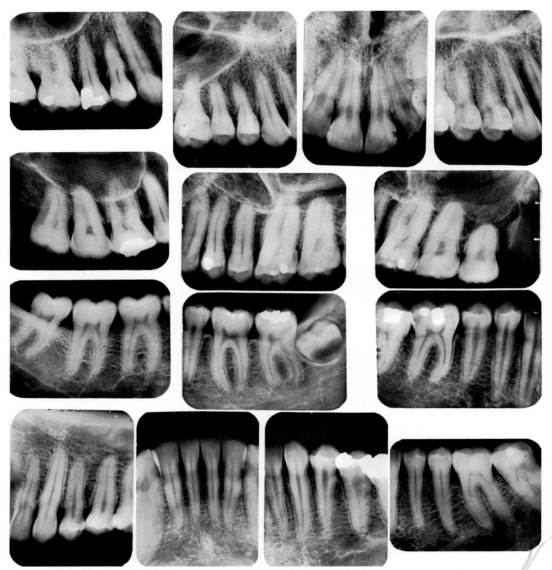

Figure 5–5. Radiographs of various groups of the permanent dentition. The radiographs demonstrate contact areas, occlusal embrasures, interproximal spacing, root forms, pulp cavities, root spacing, bone levels between the teeth, a carious cavity distal to a mandibular first molar, a developing unerupted tooth (right lower third molar), and so forth.

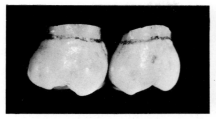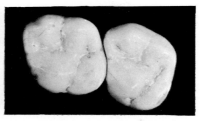

Figure 5–6. Photographs of maxillary first and second molars, taken from an elderly individual, showing considerable wear at their contact areas.

food during mastication, and aided somewhat by the fluid intake, the gingiva serves to prevent the stasis of food about and between the teeth by its elasticity and smoothness.

Since the teeth are narrower at the cervix mesiodistally than they are toward the occlusal surfaces and the outline of the root continues to taper from that point to the apices of the roots, considerable spacing is created between the roots of one tooth and the root of adjoining teeth. This arrangement allows sufficient bone tissue between one tooth and another, anchoring the teeth securely in the jaws. It also simplifies the problem of space for the blood and nerve supply to the surrounding alveolar process and other investing tissues of the teeth (Fig. 5–5).

The *type of tooth* also has a bearing upon the interproximal space. Some individuals have teeth which are wide at the cervices, constricting the space at the base. Others have teeth which are more slender at the cervices than usual; this type of tooth widens the space. Teeth which are oversize or unusually small will likewise affect the interproximal spacing. Nevertheless, this spacing will conform to a plan which is fairly uniform, provided the anatomic form is normal and the teeth are in good alignment.

3. EMBRASURES (SPILLWAYS)

When two teeth in the same arch are in contact, their curvatures adjacent to the contact areas form spillway spaces called *embrasures*. The spaces that widen out from the area of contact labially or buccally and lingually are called *labial* or *buccal* and *lingual interproximal embrasures*. These embrasures are continuous with the interproximal spaces between the teeth (Fig. 5–11). Above the contact areas incisally and occlusally, the spaces, which are bounded by the marginal ridges as they join the cusps and incisal ridges, are called the *incisal* or *occlusal embrasures*. These embrasures, and the labial or buccal and lingual embrasures, are continuous (Figs. 5–8 and 5–12). The curved proximal surfaces of the contacting teeth roll away from the contact area at all points, occlusally, labially or buccally, and lingually and cervically, and the embrasures and interproximal spaces are continuous, as they surround the areas of contact.

This embrasure form *serves two purposes*: (1) it makes a spillway for the escape of food during mastication, a physiologic form which reduces forces brought to bear upon the teeth during the reduction of any material which offers resistance; and (2) it makes the teeth more self cleansing because the rounded smooth surfaces of the enamel of the crowns are more exposed to the cleansing action of foods, fluids and the friction of the tongue, lips and cheeks. If the spaces did not widen out so freely, or if the surfaces of the teeth presented angles or corners for the lodgment of food, the situation would not promote proper dental hygiene.

The embrasure and contact form, when normal, protects the gingival tissue from undue frictional trauma, and paradoxically it allows just enough stimulation to permit the proper degree of frictional massage of tissue during mastication. Proper form provides *protection* or *stimulation* as needed, whereas improper contact and embrasure form will encourage pathologic change in the supporting tissues (Fig. 5–3).

The design of contact areas, interproximal spaces and embrasures varies with the form and alignment of the various teeth; each section of the two arches will show similarity of form. In other words, the contact form, the interproximal spacing and the embrasure form seem rather constant in sectional areas of the dental arches. These sections are named as follows: the maxillary anterior section, the mandibular anterior section, the maxillary posterior and the mandibular posterior sections. All embrasure spaces are reflections of the form of the teeth involved. Maxillary central and lateral incisors will exhibit one embrasure form, the mandibular incisors another and so on.

Maxillary posteriors and mandibular posteriors apparently require an embrasure design geared for their sections. In some cases the constancy has to be attained by a toothform adaptation (Fig. 5–13). The canines, for instance, are shaped so that they act

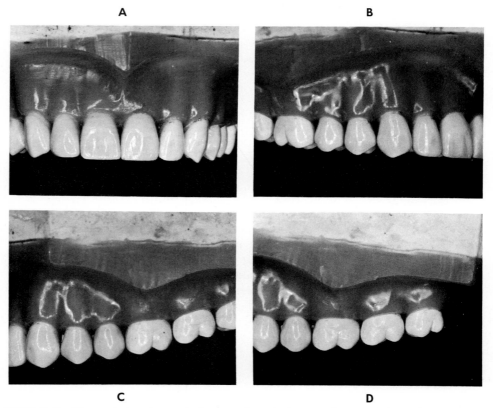

Figure 5–7. These photos demonstrate normal contact and embrasure form of the maxillary teeth from the labial and buccal aspects. (See Fig. 5–8.) Some of the interproximal spacing is visible. The interproximal, or interdental, space is normally filled by gingival tissue. *A,* Central and lateral incisors. *B,* Lateral incisor, canine and first premolar. *C,* Canine, first and second premolars and first molar. *D,* Second premolar, first, second and third molars.

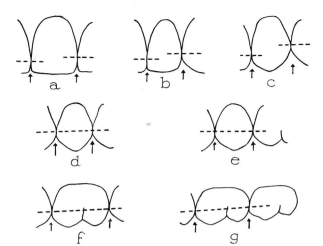

Figure 5–8. Outline drawings of the maxillary teeth in contact, with dotted lines bisecting the contact areas at the various levels as found normally. Arrows point to embrasure spaces.
a, Central and lateral incisors. *b,* Central and lateral incisors and canine. *c,* Lateral incisor, canine and first premolar. *d,* Canine, first and second premolars. *e,* First and second premolars and first molar. *f,* Second premolar, first molar and second molar. *g,* First, second and third molars.

as a catalyst in these matters between anterior and posterior teeth. A line bisecting the labial portion of either canine seems to create an anterior half mesially that resembles half of an anterior tooth, and a posterior half which resembles a posterior tooth. The mesial contact is at one level for contact with the lateral incisor, but the distal contact form must be at a level consistent with the contact form of the first premolar whether maxillary or mandibular (Fig. 5–8, *C*).

CONTACT AREAS AND INCISAL AND OCCLUSAL EMBRASURES FROM THE LABIAL AND BUCCAL ASPECTS

It is advisable to refer continually to the illustrations of contacts and embrasures during the reading of the descriptions which follow.

Figures 5–7 and 5–9 are close-ups of the labial and buccal surfaces of the teeth taken from several angles for the purpose of showing normal contacts and incisal or occlusal embrasures. Some of the interproximal spacing may be seen also. Dental radiographs will demonstrate interproximal spacing best (Fig. 5–5). Outline drawings of the tooth crowns in contact supplement the photographs (Figs. 5–8, 5–10, 5–12 and 5–15). These outlines emphasize the crests of curvature on the crowns mesially and distally that locate the contact areas. Dotted lines have been used to show the approximate points at which the contact areas may be bisected.

Locate the illustration of interest (i.e., Fig. 5–8, A) while reading the details concerning contact area levels in the following paragraphs. Often it will be of help to consult dental radiographs (Fig. 5–5).

Maxillary Teeth

Central Incisors.   The contact areas mesially on both central incisors are located at the incisal third of the crowns. Since the mesioincisal third of these teeth approaches a right angle, the incisal embrasure is very slight.

Central and Lateral Incisors.   The distal outline of the central incisor crown is rounded. The lateral incisor has a shorter crown and has a more rounded mesioincisal angle than the central incisor. The form of these two teeth coming into contact with each other therefore opens up an embrasure space distal to the central larger than the small one mesial to central incisors. A line bisecting the contact areas distal to the central incisor and mesial to the lateral approaches the junction of the middle and incisal thirds of each crown.

Lateral Incisor and Canine.   The distal contact area on the lateral incisor is approximately at the middle third. The mesial contact on the canine is at the junction of the incisal and middle thirds. The form of these teeth creates an embrasure which is more open than the two previously described.

Canine and First Premolar.   The canine has a long distal slope to its cusp, which puts the distal crest of curvature at the center of the middle third of the crown. The contact area is, therefore, at that point. This is a very important observation to be made clinically. As recently mentioned, it is at this point in the dental arch that the canine, situated between the anterior and posterior segments, becomes a part of both (Fig. 5–8, B and C).

The first premolar has a long cusp form also, which puts its mesial contact area rather high up on the crown. Usually it is just cervical to the junction of the occlusal and middle thirds. The embrasure between these teeth has a wide angle.

First and Second Premolars.   The contact areas of these teeth are similar to those just mentioned — usually a little cervical to the junction of the occlusal and middle thirds of the crowns. The form of these teeth creates a wide occlusal embrasure.

It should be noted that the design of the interproximal spaces changes also with the form and dimensions of the teeth in contact.

Second Premolar and First Molar.   The position of the contact areas cervico-occlusally is about the same as that found between the premolars.

The embrasure form changes somewhat because the mesiobuccal cusp of the molar is shorter than the cusp of the second premolar.

First and Second and Second and Third Molars.   These two contact and embrasure forms may be described together, since they are similar. The distal outline of the first molar is round — a fact that puts the contact area approximately at the center of the middle third of the crown. Here again it must be emphasized that contact levels on maxillary molars (and even on premolars to some extent) tend to be centered in the middle third of the anatomical crown.

The mesial contact area of the second molar also approaches the middle third of the crown. The occlusal embrasure is generous as a consequence, even though the cusps are not long.

The contact and embrasure design of the second and third molars is similar to those of the first and second molars. The molars become progressively shorter from the first through the third. Again, the dimensions of the tooth crowns will affect the contact and embrasure design.

Mandibular Teeth

Central Incisors.   The mesial contact areas on the mandibular central incisors are located at the incisal third of the crowns. At the time of the eruption of these teeth, the mesial and distal incisal angles are slightly rounded and the mamelons are noticeable on the incisal ridges. Soon, however, incisal wear reduces the incisal ridge to a straight surface, and the mesial and distal angles approach right angles in sharpness. This is due partly to wear at the contact areas (Fig. 5–9, A and 5–10). In many instances the contact areas extend to the mesioincisal angle. There will, therefore, be a

A B

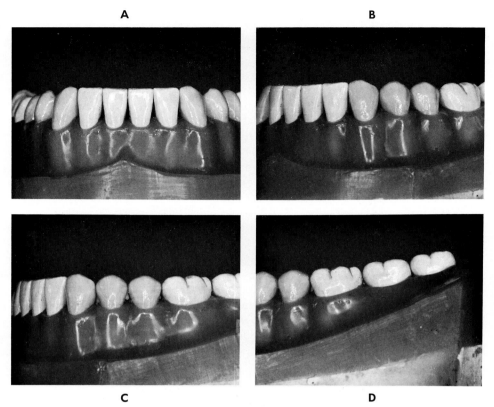

C D

Figure 5–9. Normal contact and embrasure form of the mandibular teeth from the labial and buccal aspects. *A,* Central and lateral incisors. *B,* Lateral incisor, canine and first premolar. *C,* Canine, first and second premolars and first molar. *D,* Second premolar, first, second and third molars.

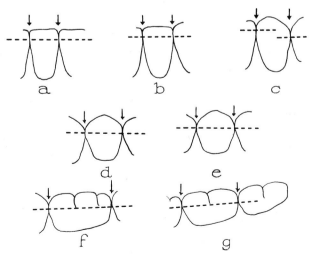

Figure 5–10. Contact levels found normally on mandibular teeth. Arrows point to embrasure spaces. *a,* Central and lateral incisors. *b,* Central and lateral incisors and canine. *c,* Lateral incisor, canine and first premolar. *d,* Canine, first and second premolars. *e,* First and second premolars and first molar. *f,* Second premolar, first and second molars. *g,* First, second and third molars.

small incisal embrasure mesially between the mandibular central incisors unless wear through usage obliterates it.

Central and Lateral Incisors.   The distal contact areas and the incisal embrasures on the central incisors and the mesial contact areas and incisal embrasures on the lateral incisors are similar to those just described. Since the mandibular central and lateral incisors are small mesiodistally and supplement each other in function, the design of their crowns brings about similar contact and embrasure forms.

Note the slender gothic arch-like spaces which circumscribe the interproximal spaces between the mandibular anterior teeth.

Lateral Incisor and Canine.   The positions of the contact areas distally on the lateral incisor and mesially on the canine are approximately the same, cervicoincisally, as the other two just described. The teeth are in contact at the incisal third close to the incisal ridges. However, the mesioincisal angle of the canine is more rounded than the others, which form opens up a small incisal embrasure at this point.

The interproximal spacing between lateral and canine is very similar in outline to the two interproximal spaces just described.

Canine and First Premolar.   The distal slope of the cusp of the mandibular canine is pronounced and long, which places the distal contact area on this tooth somewhat cervical to the junction of its incisal and middle thirds.

The first premolar has a long buccal cusp, and although its crown is shorter than the canine, the mesial contact area has about the same relation cervico-occlusally as that found distally on the canine—just cervical to the junction of the occlusal and middle thirds. Thus the whole arrangement places these contact areas level with each other.

The occlusal embrasure is quite wide and pronounced because of the cusp forms of the two teeth. The interproximal space has been reduced by the lowering of the contact areas cervically, comparing favorably to the design for posterior mandibular teeth.

First and Second Premolars.   From the buccal aspect the crowns of these two teeth are similar. The buccal cusp of the second premolar is not quite as long as that of the first premolar. The contact of these teeth is nearly level with that of the canine and first premolar. The slope of the cusps creates a large occlusal embrasure. The interproximal space is a little smaller than that between the canine and first premolar.

Second Premolar and First Molar.   The contact and embrasure design for these teeth is similar to that just described for the premolars. The mesiobuccal cusp of the first molar is shorter and more rounded than the cusp of the second premolar, which varies the embrasure somewhat, and since the crown of the molar is a little shorter, it reduces the interproximal space to that extent.

First and Second and Second and Third Molars.   These two contact and embrasure designs may be described together, since they are similar.

The proximal surfaces are quite round; that is, the distal surface of the first molar, mesial surface of the second molar, distal surface of the second molar and mesial surface of the third molar. The occlusal embrasures are, therefore, generous above the points of contact even though the cusps are short and rounded.

Because the molars become progressively shorter from the first to the third, the centers of the contact areas drop cervically also. A line bisecting the contact areas of the second and third molars is located approximately at the center of the middle thirds of the crowns.

The interproximal spaces have been reduced considerably because of their shortened form.

CONTACT AREAS, AND LABIAL, BUCCAL AND LINGUAL EMBRASURES FROM THE INCISAL AND OCCLUSAL ASPECTS *

In order to study the relative positions of contact areas and the related labial, buccal and lingual embrasures, and in order also to get proper perspective, the eye must be directed at the incisal surfaces of anterior teeth and directly above the surface of each tooth being examined in series. Posterior teeth are examined in the same manner. Look down on each tooth or group of teeth by facing the occlusal surfaces on a line with the long axis.

The problem at this point is to discover the relative positions of contacts in a labio- or buccolingual direction, and to observe the embrasure form facially and lingually created by the tooth forms and their contact relations (Fig. 5–11, A, B, C, D).

A generalization may be established in locating contact areas faciolingually. Anterior teeth will have their contacts centered labiolingually, whereas posterior teeth

---

*Refer to Figs. 5–11, 5–12, 5–14, and 5–15.

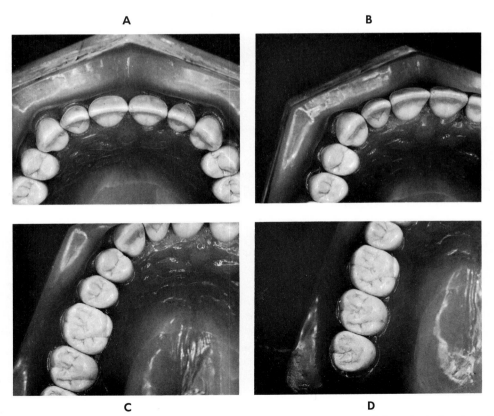

A   B

C   D

Figure 5–11.   Normal contact and embrasure form of the maxillary teeth from incisal and occlusal aspects. *A*, Central and lateral incisors. *B*, Lateral incisor, canine and first premolar. *C*, Canine, first and second premolars and first molar. *D*, First, second and third molars.

will have contact areas slightly buccal to the center buccolingually. This buccal inclination must be carefully studied and must not be overemphasized.

Except for the maxillary first molar, all crowns converge more lingually than facially from contact areas. The maxillary first molar is the only tooth wider lingually than buccally. Its formation makes a necessary adjustment of the mesiolingual embrasure when the tooth form of maxillary posteriors changes from the maxillary premolar form to the purely rhomboidal form of maxillary second and third molars. This situation will be discussed more fully later on (Fig. 5–13).

The narrower measurement lingually rather than facially causes wider embrasures lingually compared to facial embrasures. Compare the two types of embrasures displayed by maxillary central and lateral incisors (Fig. 5–11, B).

Maxillary Teeth (Figs. 5–11 and 5–12)

Central Incisors.   The contact areas of these teeth are centered labiolingually. The labial embrasure is a V-shaped space created by the labial form of these crowns. The lingual embrasure widens out more than the labial embrasure because of the lingual convergence of the crowns (Fig. 5–11, A). Note the centering of the labioincisal edge in respect to the crown outline of these teeth, and the narrowness of the lingual surfaces in comparison with the broad labial faces.

Central and Lateral Incisors.   The contact areas of these teeth are centered labiolingually also.

Lateral Incisor and Canine.   The contact area is centered labiolingually on both canine and lateral incisors. The lingual embrasure is similar to that of the central and lateral incisors, but the labial embrasure is changed somewhat by a definite convexity at the mesiolabial line angle of the canine.

Canine and First Premolar.   The contact area is centered on the distal surface of the canine, but is a little buccal to center on the mesial surface of the first premolar. The embrasure design lingually is marked by a concavity in the region of the distolingual line angle of the canine and by a developmental groove crossing the mesial marginal ridge of the first premolar.

First and Second Premolars.   The contact areas are nearly centered buccolingually. The embrasures buccally and lingually are regular in outline although slightly different in design.

The prominence of the mesio- and distobuccal line angles of the premolars is in direct contrast to the even taper of these teeth lingually, as viewed from the occlusal aspect. This form demonstrates a slight variation between buccal and lingual embrasures.

Second Premolar and First Molar.   As usual a line bisecting the contact areas of these teeth will be nearly centered on the distal surface of the second premolar. The area on the mesial surface of the first molar will be located farther buccally than other contact areas on the maxillary posterior teeth. The contact areas are wider on molars because of the greater width buccolingually of the molar teeth.

The buccal embrasure between these teeth and the location of the mesial contact area of the first molar are influenced by the prominence of the mesiobuccal line angle of the maxillary first molar and the matching prominence of the distobuccal line angle of the maxillary second premolar. The lingual embrasure is kept standard for the molar area by the enlargement of the mesiolingual cusp of the first molar. Occasionally this cusp will carry a small conformation lingually as part of the change in form.

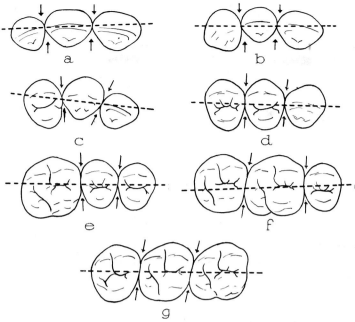

Figure 5–12.   Outline drawings of the maxillary teeth from the incisal and occlusal aspects with broken lines bisecting the contact areas. These illustrations show the relative positions of the contact areas labiolingually and buccolingually. Arrows point to embrasure spaces. *a,* Central incisors and lateral incisor. *b,* Central and lateral incisor and canine. *c,* Lateral incisor, canine and first premolar. *d,* Canine, first premolar and second premolar. *e,* First molar, second premolar and first molar. *f,* Second premolar, first molar and second molar. *g,* First, second and third molars.

(Fifth cusp, or cusp of Carabelli.) Usually, the mesiolingual cusp of the maxillary first molar will be rounded out, with no more than a developmental groove showing that an extra cusp formation may have been intended.

The mesiolingual lobe of this tooth is always large, however, causing the tooth to be wider lingually from its mesiolingual line angle to its distolingual line angle than it is from the mesiobuccal line angle to the distobuccal line angle. If it were not for this fact, the rhomboid form of the first molar in contact with the tapered form of the second premolar would open up a lingual embrasure of extremely large proportions. The large mesiolingual lobe makes up for the change in occlusal outline from premolar form to molar form, keeping the conformity of the lingual embrasures (Fig. 5–13).

First and Second and Second and Third Molars.   These contact and embrasure forms may be described together, since they are similar.

Although the mesiobuccal line angles of the second and third molars are not as sharp as that of the first molar, they are prominent nevertheless.

The distobuccal line angles of all the maxillary molars are indistinct and rounded, so that the buccal embrasure forms are shaped and characterized mainly by the prominent mesiobuccal line angle.

The mesiolingual line angles of the second and third molars are rounded and in conjunction with the rounded distolingual line angles; the lingual embrasures between first, second and third molars present a regular and open form (Fig. 5–12, *F* and *G*).

The contact areas are broad and centered buccolingually. The embrasures are uniform. Note the generous proportions of the buccal embrasures.

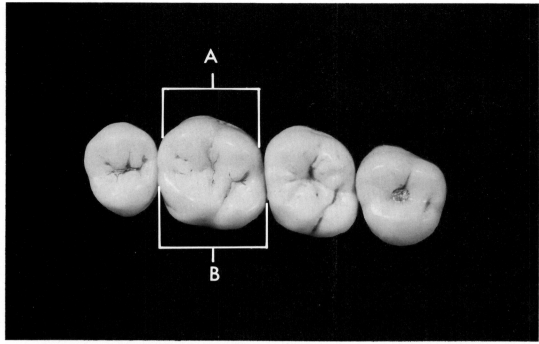

Figure 5–13. *Calibration of Maxillary First Molar.*

A, Calibration at prominent buccal line angles that functions by deflecting food material during mastication. *B,* Calibration of lingual contour from contact area mesially to contact area distally. There are no prominent line angles but the development of the mesiolingual cusp has widened the rounded lingual form. Thus, the two lingual embrasures are kept similar in size, even though the tooth makes contact with two teeth that are dissimilar lingually. This way the lingual gingival tissue interproximally is properly protected by the equalization of lingual embrasures.

Mandibular Teeth (Figs. 5–14 and 5–15)

Central Incisors and Central and Lateral Incisors. These contact areas and embrasures may be described together, since they are similar.

Although these teeth are narrow mesiodistally, their labiolingual measurements are not much less than those of the maxillary central and lateral incisors. The mandibular central incisors will come within a millimeter or so of having the same labiolingual diameter as that of the maxillary central incisors; the *mandibular* lateral incisors will have a labiolingual diameter as great if not greater than that of the *maxillary* lateral incisors.

The contact areas are centered labiolingually and the embrasures are uniform. Although the mesiodistal dimensions are less, the outline form of the incisal aspects of the mandibular central and lateral incisors is similar to that of the maxillary central and lateral incisors in that the lingual outlines have a rounded taper in comparison with broader, flattened labial faces.

Lateral Incisor and Canine. The contact areas are centered, and the lingual embrasure is similar to those just described. The labial embrasure is influenced by the prominence of the mesiolabial line angle of the canine. It will be remembered that the maxillary canine presents the same characteristic.

Canine and First Premolar. The contact areas are approximately centered, and the buccal embrasure is smooth and uniform in outline. The lingual embrasure is opened up somewhat by a slight concavity on the canine distolingually and by a char-

A

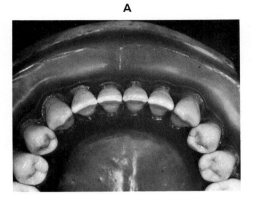

B

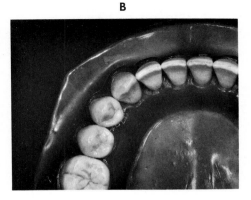

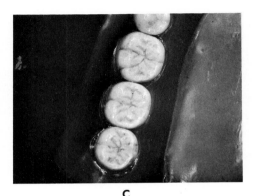

C

Figure 5–14. Normal contact and embrasure form of the mandibular teeth from the incisal and occlusal aspects. *A,* Central and lateral incisors. *B,* Lateral incisor, canine and first and second premolars. *C,* Second premolar, first, second and third molars.

acteristic developmental groove across the marginal ridge of the first premolar mesiolingually.

First and Second Premolars. The contact areas are nearly centered buccolingually; but are broader than those found mesial to them because the distal curvature of the first premolar describes a larger arc than the mesial curvature, and the mesial contacting surface of the second premolar is relatively broad and describes a shallower curved surface than that of the distal surface of the first premolar.

Because of the lingual convergence of the first premolar and the narrow lingual cusp form, the lingual embrasure is as wide as the one mesial to it.

Second Premolar and First Molar. The contact areas are wide and almost centered. The extent of the contact areas is sometimes increased by a slight concavity in the outline of the mesial surface of the first molar below the marginal ridge. The mesial contact area of the first molar is located farther buccally than any of the other contact areas on mandibular posterior teeth. It must be remembered that the same situation holds true in the upper dental arch when describing the contacts of maxillary first molars and second premolars.

The prominence of the first molar at the mesiobuccal line angle is readily apparent. The mesial outline of the crown tapers to the lingual, forming a generous lingual embrasure in conjunction with the smooth curvature of the second premolar distolingually.

First and Second Molar. The contact areas are nearly centered buccolingually, although they are not so broad as the contact just described. This variation is brought about by the design of the first molar distally. The distal contact area of the first molar

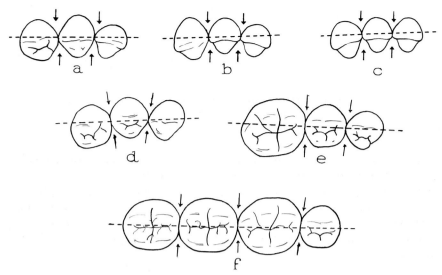

Figure 5–15. Contact relation of mandibular teeth labiolingually and buccolingually when surveyed from the incisal and occlusal aspects. Arrows point to embrasure spaces. *a*, Central incisors and lateral incisor. *b*, Central and lateral incisor and canine. *c*, Lateral incisor, canine and first premolar. *d*, Canine, first premolar and second premolar. *e*, First premolar, second premolar and first molar. *f*, Second premolar, first, second and third molars.

is confined to the distal cusp, which does not present the broad surface for contact with the second molar that was found mesially in contact with the second premolar. This form, along with the rounded outline at the distobuccal line angle, opens up both embrasures wider than those found immediately mesial.

The outline of the first molar crown just lingual to the distal contact area presents a straight line and occasionally a concavity.

The second molar outline buccally and lingually on both sides of the mesial contact area is uniformly rounded.

Second and Third Molars. The contact areas are broad, and they are nearly centered buccolingually. When the third molar is normally developed, it is similar in outline to the second molar from the occlusal aspect.

The buccal and lingual embrasures between these teeth are almost alike in form and extent.

A straight line may be drawn through the contact areas of the second premolar and the three molars, and it will come very near to bisecting all of the contact areas. These four mandibular teeth are set in a line that is almost straight (Figs. 5–14, *C*, 5–15 *F*).

4. FACIAL AND LINGUAL CONTOURS AT THE CERVICAL THIRDS (CERVICAL RIDGES) AND LINGUAL CONTOURS AT THE MIDDLE THIRDS OF CROWNS*

It might be well, at this point, to emphasize again the relation of tooth form to dental maintenance.

---

*All are protective contours. See Fig. 5–17 and Figs. 5–21 through 5–24.

The maintenance of the tooth in the dental arch is largely autogenetic in a state of health. The teeth are unique in that their static outside form is physiological. Even the maxillary teeth, which are firmly set in their alveoli, when moving through food material activated by mandibular movement change their functional crown form from a static to a dynamic form.

All details of tooth form will have some effect upon the stabilization of the tooth in the arch; therefore, *autogenous dental hygiene* is a most important feature.

All that is known of physiological tooth form should be utilized in the prevention and treatment of periodontal disease, or for that matter, in meeting any requirement of preservation or restoration.

Examinations will show that all tooth crowns, when viewed from mesial or distal aspects, have rather uniform curvatures at the cervical thirds and at the middle thirds labially or buccally or lingually, depending upon the teeth being examined (Fig. 5–16, *A*, *D*, and *E*). These contours must be recognized as having considerable physiologic importance. Apparently, the curvatures hold the gingiva under *definite tension* and also protect the gingival margins by *deflecting food* material away from the margins during mastication (Fig. 5–16, *A*). The proper degree of curvature will deflect food over the gingival margin, thereby preventing undue frictional irritation. Paradoxically, just the right amount of curvature, made operative by good alignment, will allow proper stimulation for periodontal health. Alignment is most important; if the tooth is malaligned, some phase of its functional form will be inoperative.

If the curvature is absent or too slight, the gingival tissue may be driven apically, and this would result in a recession of gum tissue and possible pathologic changes (Fig. 5–16, *B*). If the curvature is too great, another complication may arise: The gingiva is protected too much and loses tissue "tone." Food material and debris pack around the gingival area under this exaggerated contour and a veritable "backwater" results; this may be accompanied by stagnation of foreign material and chronic inflammation of the gingiva (Fig. 5–16, *C*).

The cervical third formation of the crowns is the area of soft tissue attachment. The *epithelial attachment* of soft tissue to the teeth, soon to be described more fully, is entirely within the area of the cervical third of the crowns. The cervical curvatures are often spoken of as *cervical ridges.* However, cervical *curvatures* is a more descrip-

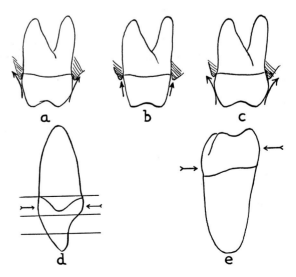

Figure 5–16. Schematic drawings of curvatures labially, buccally and lingually. *a,* Normal curvatures as found on maxillary molar. Arrow shows path of food material as it is avalanched over these curvatures during mastication. *b,* Molar with little or no curvature. The gingiva is apt to be stripped or pushed apically through lack of protection and consequent overstimulation. *c,* Molar with curvature in excess of the normal. The gingiva will be protected too much and will suffer from lack of proper stimulation. Food material and bacterial cultures may lodge under these curvatures, promoting pathological disturbance. *d,* Normal cervical curvatures as found on maxillary incisors. The crests of curvature are opposite each other labiolingually. *e,* Curvatures as found on mandibular posterior teeth. The protective curvature is located at the cervical third to the buccal and at the middle third to the lingual.

tive term, because few of these areas are pronounced enough to be called "ridges," and yet rarely will a normal tooth be seen with no curvature at all.

The *average cervical contour* labially or buccally and lingually for each group of teeth in the maxillary and mandibular arches will be described. This phase of tooth form has seldom been emphasized in dental literature, although it is most valuable in preserving the gingival outline and the investment tissues in the teeth. The contour under consideration is the curvature possessed by all tooth crowns above the cementoenamel junction, labially or buccally and lingually, which is usually found at the cervical third, or less often at the middle third when one observes the teeth from the mesial and distal aspects.

The curvatures above the cementoenamel junction seem to describe rather constant arcs, depending upon the location in the mouth; *i.e.,* the maxillary anterior teeth, maxillary posteriors, mandibular anteriors and mandibular posteriors. Each group exhibits an arc of curvature that is characteristic of that group, both as to location of the curvatures and as to the extent of the curvatures.

Variations are always possible, and therefore no hard and fast rule can be made. But after observing many teeth one may strike an *average* for that particular feature. Values that are "averages" or "norms" must be established in order properly to judge requirements in diagnosis or in restoration. Variations from the average are then better understood. Cervical contours may vary in individuals. If curvatures in any given case are found to be greater or less than average, it has been the author's observation that the variation will be uniform in that individual. Since there are variations, therefore, and since it is extremely difficult to restore the cervical curvature once it is

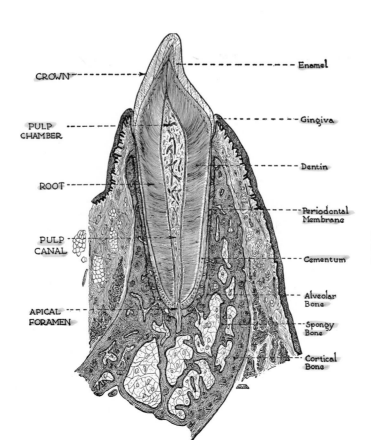

CROWN

PULP
CHAMBER

ROOT

PULP
CANAL

APICAL
FORAMEN

Enamel

Gingiva

Dentin

Periodontal
Membrane

Cementum

Alveolar
Bone

Spongy
Bone

Cortical
Bone

Figure 5–17. Diagrammatic representation of the dental tissues. (From Noyes, Schour and Noyes, *Dental Histology and Embryology,* Lea & Febiger.)

removed during operative procedures, these curvatures or "cervical ridges" *should be treated with respect and should be allowed to remain as they are whenever practicable.*

In young people, and some older ones, most of the curvature lies beneath the gingival crest (Fig. 5–17). In older persons, the cementoenamel line may be visible or may be just under the gingival crest, with most of the prominent curvature exposed.

Gradual recession of the gingivae throughout life may be a normal procedure, with no pathologic change in evidence. This process varies in different persons. If the recession occurs early with no apparent pathologic evidence, it may be found that the individual has "flat-faced" tooth crowns with little or no curvature, labially or lingually or buccally, to act as a protector of the gingiva. At least, such teeth are not favored by normal cervical curvature. By the same token, teeth having an excess of curvature over the average may be predestined to premature loss through their contribution to unhygienic conditions about the gingival sulci of their own periodontium.

All protective curvatures are most functional when the teeth are in proper alignment. *It should be quite plain that when teeth are malposed their curvatures are displaced and ineffective.*

The curvatures are rather uniform at the cervical third or lingual third of all of the maxillary teeth and on the buccal portion of mandibular posterior teeth (Figs. 5–21, 5–22 and 5–23).

The normal curvature from the cementoenamel junction to the crest of contour is approximately 0.5 mm. in extent. When the long axis of the tooth is placed vertically, it is found that this curvature is fairly constant and may be recognized as average or normal for the maxillary teeth, labially or buccally and lingually, and for the mandibular posterior teeth on the buccal surfaces. The curvature lingually of mandibular posterior teeth extends about a millimeter beyond the cervical line. Here, however, the extreme curvature does not contribute to the stasis of food material at the cervix because of the activity of the tongue in keeping the lingual surfaces of these teeth clean.

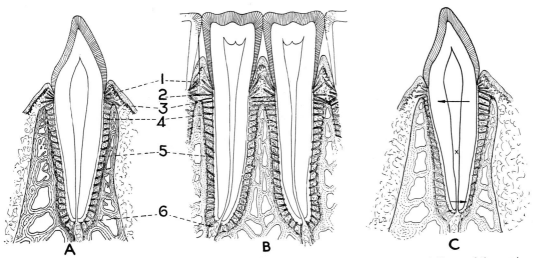

Figure 5–18. Diagrammatic representation of the arrangement of the principal fibers of the periodontal ligament. *A,* Labiolingual, and *B,* mesiodistal section through lower central incisors. 1, Free gingival group; 2, transseptal group; 3, alveolar crest group; 4, horizontal group; 5, oblique group; 6, apical group. *C,* Shows the tipping of the tooth lingually and the changes in the periodontal membrane under incisal stress. X indicates approximate fulcrum point. The periodontal ligament is shown disproportionately wide for clarity. (From Schour, I.: Noyes' *Oral Histology and Embryology,* 8th Edition, 1960, Lea & Febiger.)

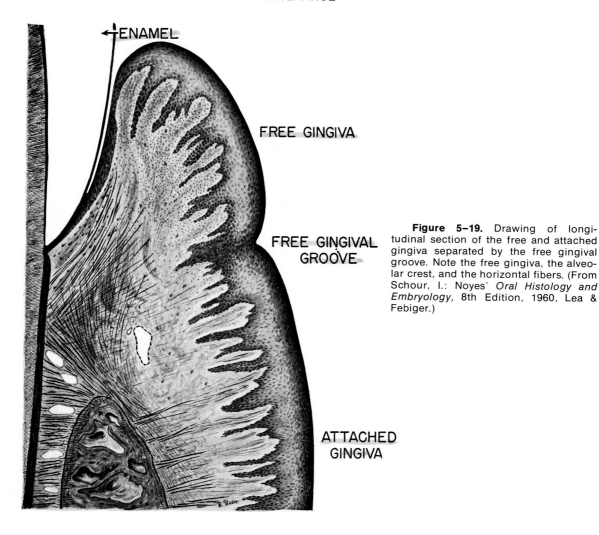

ENAMEL

FREE GINGIVA

FREE GINGIVAL
GROOVE

ATTACHED
GINGIVA

Figure 5–19. Drawing of longitudinal section of the free and attached gingiva separated by the free gingival groove. Note the free gingiva, the alveolar crest, and the horizontal fibers. (From Schour, I.: Noyes' *Oral Histology and Embryology,* 8th Edition, 1960, Lea & Febiger.)

Figure 5–21 shows that the maxillary central incisor and canine have curvatures labially and lingually which are almost identical. *Because the canines have a more massive development of the cingulum, clinical observation only gives an impression of greater curvature. This is an optical illusion which is dispelled when the outline of the canine is properly compared with other teeth on a graph.*

The maxillary premolar and molar show the same limited curvatures. The crest of curvature lingually on all posterior teeth is at or near the middle third of the crowns.

When curvatures are found that are greater in extent than 0.5 mm., rarely is the curvature as much as 1 mm., except lingually on mandibular posterior teeth and often lingually on maxillary posterior teeth. In these instances, the crest of contour will be found at the middle third of the crowns instead of at the cervical third (Fig. 5–23). These crests are always lingual.

The eye is easily confused at times when viewing certain aspects of the teeth because of the abrupt sweep of curvatures as they travel from the cervical line toward occlusal and incisal surfaces; *i.e.,* the buccal surfaces of mandibular posterior teeth, the lingual surfaces of posterior maxillary teeth, or the lingual surfaces of canines. When the actual photographs are placed on a background of squares, with the long

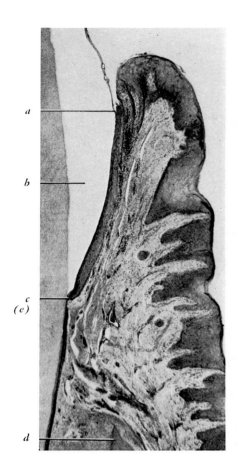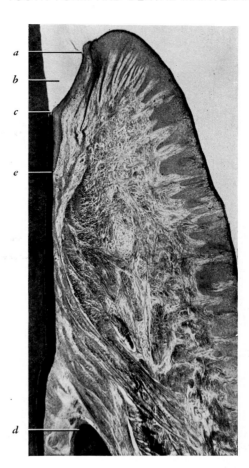

Figure 5–20. *A,* Epithelial attachment on the enamel (first stage in passive tooth exposure). Apical end of attachment is at cementoenamel junction. *B,* Epithelial attachment on enamel and cementum (second stage in passive tooth exposure). Apical end of attachment has proliferated along the cementum. *a,* Bottom of gingival sulcus; *b,* enamel; *c,* cementoenamel junction; *d,* alveolar crest; *e,* apical end of epithelial attachment. (From Orban, B.: *Periodontics,* 1958, The C. V. Mosby Company.)

axis of each tooth held vertically, one readily sees that the extent of curvature from the cervical line to the crest of curvature facially or lingually is slight. Quite often, in restorative procedures, it is *greatly overestimated and reproduced.*

Figure 5–24 shows a mandibular central incisor and canine from the mesial aspect. Here the curvature at the cervical third is less than that of the other teeth in the mouth, occasionally appearing so slight that it is hardly distinguishable. The canine often has very little more curvature immediately above the cervical line than the mandibular central or lateral incisor.

SUMMARY OF PROTECTIVE CONTOURS OF TOOTH CROWNS, FACIALLY AND LINGUALLY

All tooth crowns will exhibit some curvature above the cervical line. Again, this slight bulge at the cervical third is sometimes called the *cervical ridge.* Although the extent of curvature will vary in different individuals, apparently it is not normal for

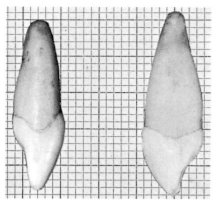

Figure 5–21. The maxillary central incisor exhibits a curvature of approximately 0.5 mm. labially and somewhat less lingually at the cervical third of the crown. Many specimens will show equal curvature on the two sides.

The maxillary canine exhibits approximately the same curvature. Note the limitation of the curvature at the cingulum area above the cervical line.

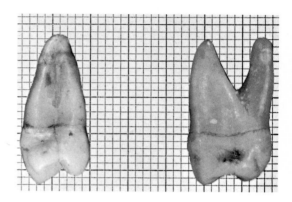

Figure 5–22. The maxillary first premolar has a curvature of approximately 0.5 mm. buccally and lingually. The crest of curvature buccally is located at the cervical third of the crown and lingually at the middle third.

The maxillary first molar has curvatures of the same degree at similar points on both sides.

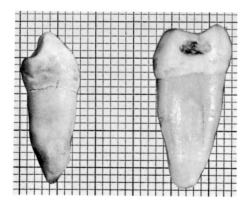

Figure 5–23. Mandibular first premolar and first molar. Both teeth have a curvature of approximately 0.5 mm. buccally at the cervical third of the crown and a curvature of approximately 1 mm. lingually, with the crest of curvature at the middle third.

Figure 5–24. Mandibular central incisor and canine. The central incisor curvature labially and lingually is less than 0.5 mm. in extent, and the crest of curvature is near the cervical line. The canine also exhibits less than 0.5 mm. curvatures, although the crest of curvature is higher up on the crown; however, it is still within the confines of the cervical third.

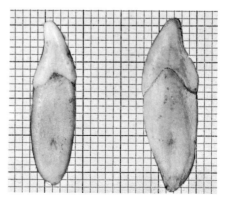

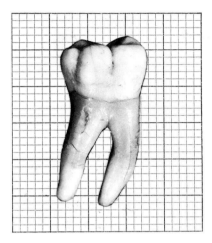
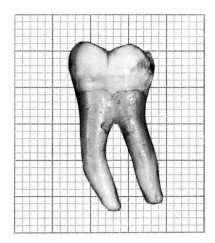
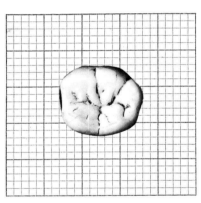
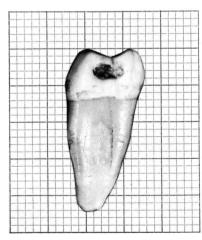
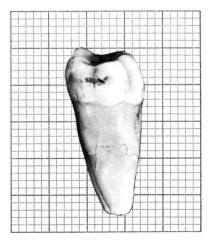

Figure 5–25.   Photographs of a natural specimen of a mandibular first molar, taken with a lens capable of two diameter registrations. Cut-outs of these photos were placed on graphs depicting squared millimeters. The result is an accurate graph in millimeters of tooth outlines from five aspects.

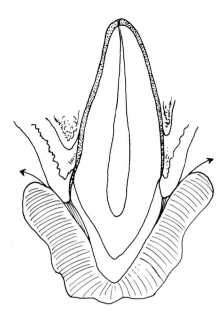

Figure 5–26. A schematic drawing which shows the effect periodontally when a tooth with normal curvature and attachment is forced through food material. If the elasticity of the food is consistent it will splay away from the cervical curvature even though it contacts the gum tissue. This contact normally seems to act as a stimulant rather than as a force for injury.

the curvatures on permanent teeth to extend out as much as 1 mm. beyond the cervical line; usually the curvature will be less.

The curvatures on the labial, buccal and lingual surfaces of all maxillary teeth and on the buccal surfaces of mandibular posterior teeth will be rather uniform; the average curvature as mentioned before is about 0.5 mm.

Mandibular posterior teeth will have a lingual curvature of approximately 1 mm., with the crest of curvature at the *middle third* of the crown instead of at the cervical third. Occasionally *maxillary posterior* teeth will have similar curvatures on the lingual aspect. (Compare the lingual curvatures in Figs. 5–22 and 5–23.)

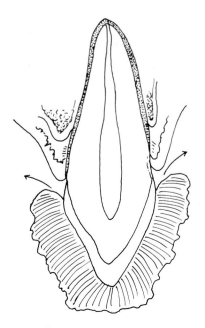

Figure 5–27. This figure, to be compared with Figure 5–26, shows what happens after physiological recession of gingival tissue on the tooth root beyond the cervical curvature on the crown facially and lingually. Here the curvature tends to protect the gingiva too much. More care must be taken to observe the rules of dental hygiene and gum stimulation when this relationship is present.

Mandibular anterior teeth will show less curvature on the crown above the cervical line than any of the other teeth. Usually it is less than 0.5 mm., and occasionally it is so slight that it is hardly distinguishable. The mandibular canines may show a little more curvature than central and lateral incisors.

Regardless of whether or not theories explaining the functional significance of these contours are correct, there is little doubt that they are important. If this were not so, there would be more variance in the presence or the extent of curvature. The curvatures as described seem to be as standard and as constant as any anatomical detail can be.

5. THE HEIGHT OF EPITHELIAL ATTACHMENT. CURVATURES OF THE CERVICAL LINES (CEMENTOENAMEL JUNCTION) MESIALLY AND DISTALLY

The *epithelial attachment* seals the soft tissue to the tooth hermetically. It is a remarkable system capable of adjustment to local physiological changes, but it is vulnerable to physical injury. Careless treatment can cause breaks in the attachment, making the tooth liable to further physical or pathologic injury. The teeth can be injured by careless probing during clinical examination; improper scaling during prophylactic treatment; tooth preparation techniques in operative procedures, and so forth (Figs. 5–29, 5–30).

Among treatment procedures, the possibilities for injury of periodontal attach-

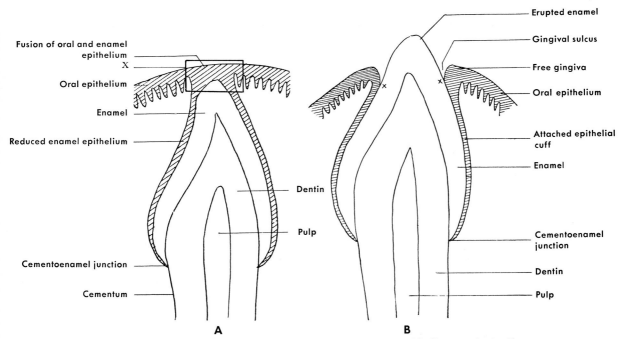

Figure 5–28. *A,* Diagrammatic illustration of the covering of enamel epithelium on the tooth crown fusing with the oral epithelium just prior to eruption. *B,* Diagrammatic illustration of the attached epithelial cuff and gingival sulcus at an early phase of tooth eruption. Bottom of sulcus at X. (From Orban, *Oral Histology and Embryology,* 7th Edition, C. V. Mosby Company, 1972.)

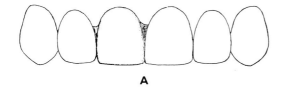

A

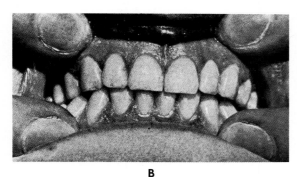

B

Figure 5–29. *A,* Unsightly appearance created after placement of anterior crown owing to the injury of the epithelial attachment during crown restoration.

B, Normal, healthy gums, showing the interdental tissue papillae reaching well up into the embrasures. (Courtesy of Dr. Russell W. Bunting. From Hill, *Textbook of Oral Pathology,* 2nd ed., Lea & Febiger, 1940.)

ment are greatest in full crown restoration procedure. The full crown preparation must be listed as radical because of complete encirclement, thereby removing the major portion of the functional form of the tooth crown. The attachment of epithelium near the free margin of gum all around the tooth is in constant danger during the process of tooth form removal. (Figs. 5–38, 5–39, 5–40, 5–41, and 5–42.)

Careless preparation is one way of injuring the tooth, but there is another way also. Careless reproduction of form in the final restoration will also act as a permanent injury. One way to avoid this is to leave margins exposed wherever possible; this facilitates smooth finish and proper form (Fig. 5–31, 5–32, 5–33, 5–34). Traditionally when margins of a restoration approached soft tissue, the margin was always supposed to disappear "beneath the gum." The location of all margins should be decided upon by a logical and scientific approach to diagnosis and prognosis. The functional form in teeth is difficult to replace when once removed.

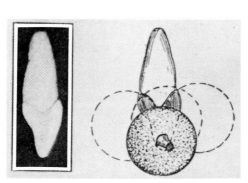

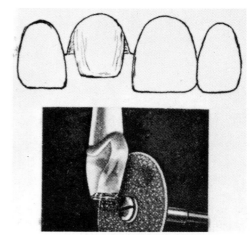

Figure 5–30. The possibility of injury of mesial and distal attachments is present during crown preparation.

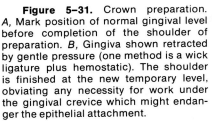

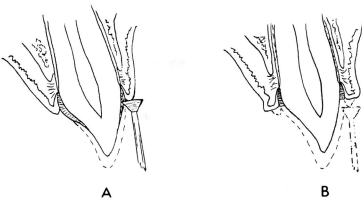

Figure 5–31. Crown preparation. *A,* Mark position of normal gingival level before completion of the shoulder of preparation. *B,* Gingiva shown retracted by gentle pressure (one method is a wick ligature plus hemostatic). The shoulder is finished at the new temporary level, obviating any necessity for work under the gingival crevice which might endanger the epithelial attachment.

A   B

Changes in the requirements for dental practice in recent years have been brought about by a greater knowledge of periodontal problems; changes derived in great part from a more enlightened attitude toward dental hygiene by the general public (even to the extent of requesting periodic examinations). Advances in periodontics and an enlightened attitude have made extensive removal of tooth tissue for restoration a *radical* rather than a *conservative* procedure. "Extension for Prevention," was once a good universal slogan in dentistry, but today it must be questioned before adopting it in many cases; the operator should keep a more favorable slogan in mind, and that is, at all times, "Conservation for Use."

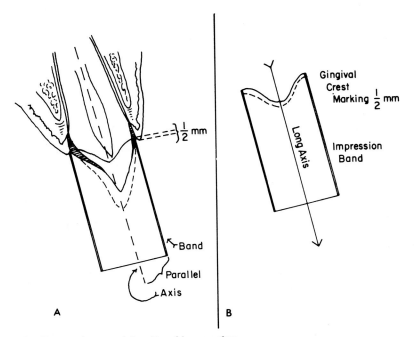

A   B

Figure 5–32. *The Proper Approach in a Band Impression.*

A, The carefully contoured and marked band carrying impression material is placed over the preparation in line with the long axis of the tooth and approximately ½ mm. into the gingival crevice evenly all around. If the band is forced unevenly and excessively root-wise, the epithelial attachment is likely to be broken, injuring the tooth. *B.* Illustration of the carefully contoured impression band, having been adapted to the cervical line required.

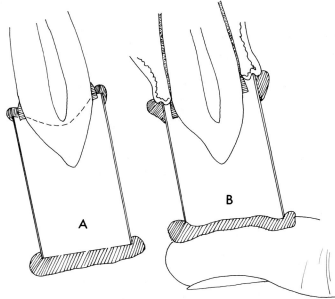

Figure 5–33. *An Improper Approach with a Band Impression.*

A. If the band used is too large, the band may cut the gingiva and be difficult to festoon properly. *B.* This shows what can happen when using an oversized impression band. When the band is filled with impression material, an accurate reproduction requires a closed end under finger pressure. The hydraulic pressure created in the oversized band can peel the gingiva away from the tooth by breaking the epithelial attachment.

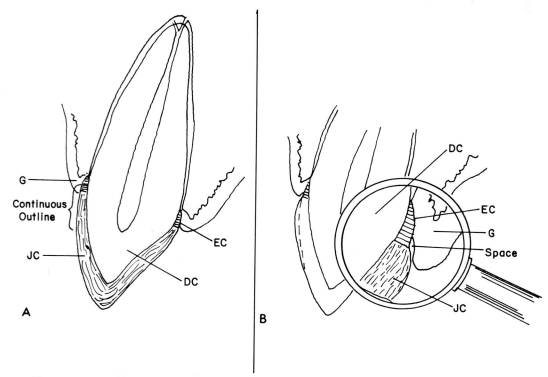

Figure 5–34. *A,* Properly contoured jacket crown. *JC,* Jacket crown; *DC,* dentin core; *EC,* enamel curvature with epithelial attachment; *G,* gingiva.

B, Crown over-contoured cervically, creating a double curvature in conjunction with the curvature left intact on the tooth. This arrangement would create an unnatural space subgingivally for the stasis of food and the harboring of bacteria.

The height of normal gingival tissue, mesially and distally on approximating teeth, is directly dependent upon the heights of the epithelial attachment on these teeth. Normal attachment follows the curvature of the cementoenamel junction if the teeth are in normal alignment and contact. This does not mean that the cementoenamel junction and the epithelial attachment are at the same level, but it does mean that they tend to follow the same curvature even though the epithelial attachment may be higher on the crown on its enamel surface (Fig. 5–38). A comparison of the curvatures of the cementoenamel junction mesially and distally on the teeth is therefore in order. Measurement and comparisons are shown in Figures 5–39 and 5–43. See also Measurement Table, page 20.

The extent of curvature seems to depend upon the height of the contact area above the crown cervix and also upon the diameter of the crown labiolingually or buccolingually. The crowns of anterior teeth, which are narrower and longer from these aspects, show the greatest curvature (Fig. 5–43). In using the words "height" and "above," the supposition is made that in either the maxillary or the mandibular arch the occlusal surfaces of the teeth are above the cervices. Any point approaching the incisal edge or occlusal surface of a crown is considered above the cervix, and the height is increased as it approaches occlusal levels.

Periodontal attachment which follows the curvature of the cementoenamel junction mesially and distally seems to be about as high on *mandibular* anterior teeth as on their counterparts that are larger in the maxillary arch. Although the crowns of the mandibular anterior teeth average 1 mm. less in labiolingual diameter (the lateral incisors excepted), the *contact areas* are higher accordingly, being near the incisal edges on centrals and laterals. Consequently, measurements will usually show less

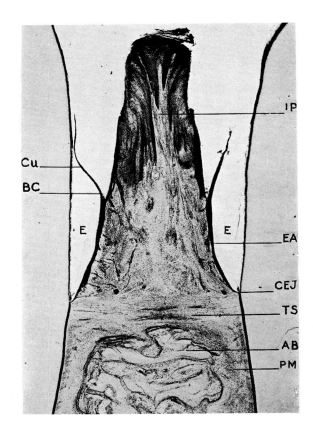

Figure 5–35. Interdental papilla and bone between two lower premolars of a child aged fourteen years. This photomicrograph shows the topographic relation between interdental papilla, epithelial attachment to the enamel of both bicuspids, transseptal fibers, interdental bone, and periodontal membrane. *IP*, interdental papilla; *EE*, space formerly occupied by the enamel; *EA*, epithelial attachment to the enamel; *Cu*, enamel cuticle, *BC*, bottom of gingival crevice; *CEJ*, cementoenamel junction; *TS*, transseptal fibers; *AB*, alveolar bone; *PM*, periodontal membrane. Magnification × 24. (Kronfeld, *Dental Histology and Comparative Dental Anatomy,* Lea & Febiger.)

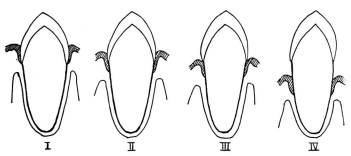

Figure 5–36. Four different stages of the relations existing between the tooth and the surrounding tissues, especially the epithelial attachment. I, Bottom of the gingival crevice on the enamel; deepest point of the epithelial attachment at the cementoenamel junction (see Fig. 5–20, A). II, Bottom of the crevice still on the enamel, but deepest point of attachment already on the cementum. III, Bottom of the crevice exactly at the cementoenamel junction and the epithelial attachment on the cementum. IV, Bottom of the crevice on the cementum with the deepest point of the epithelial attachment shifted farther apically but still attached. (Fig. 5–37). (Mueller and Orban, J. Am. Dent. A.)

than 1 mm. variation in mesial and distal curvatures between maxillary and mandibular anterior teeth.

Posterior teeth will show little variation in either arch. Figure 5–39 is a diagrammatic drawing of the outlines of the teeth on one side of the arch when viewed from the labial and buccal aspects. These outlines have been placed so that a direct comparison can be made with the graphs below them. The graphs demonstrate the relative height of individual attachments in the average normal case. They are based on cases having upper central incisors with crowns 10.5 to 11 mm. in length. Unless the teeth were very large or very small, the graphs would not vary from those illustrated by more than 0.5 mm.

The curvature of the cervical line of most teeth (cementoenamel junction) will be approximately 1 mm. less distally than mesially. The greater curvature will be found at the median line on central incisors, maxillary and mandibular. The height of attachment is dependent upon the height of the contact areas of the two teeth creating the interproximal space. If the mesial curvature of the central incisor is calibrated at 3.5 mm., then the distal curvature will be about 1 mm. less or 2.5 mm.

The six anterior teeth, both maxillary and mandibular, when compared with posteriors, exhibit the greatest curvature. Because the canine crowns function distally as posterior teeth their curvatures distally represented by the cementoenamel junction are slight, being about 1 mm. to 1.5 mm. on the average. Premolars and molars have rather uniform but slight curvatures. The contact levels are low in relation to total crown length, consequently these teeth do not have high periodontal attachments interproximally. The average premolar or molar has a curvature mesially of only 1 mm. or less, with no curvature, or even a "minus" curvature distally (Fig. 5–44).

From the operator's point of view, anterior teeth especially must be carefully approached (when attachment is normal) as, for example, in preparing them for restoration. Posterior teeth have curvatures that are less critical.

A summary of the height of periodontal attachment interproximally indicates the attachment to be highest at the median line on central incisors. In distal progression the height of attachment decreases along with the decrease in curvature of cementoenamel junctions until the mesial surface of the first premolar is reached. From this point distally through third molars curvatures are slight.

The possibility of injury to mesial and distal periodontal attachment during tooth

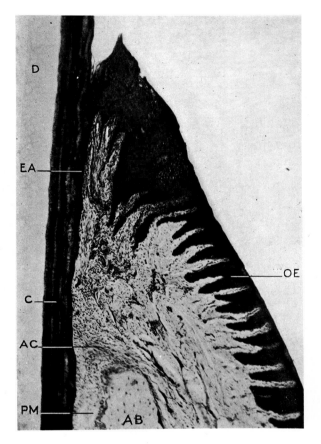

Figure 5–37. Epithelial attachment and gingival crevice of an adult human tooth. Lingual side of a lower bicuspid; age, fifty-two years. The bottom of the gingival crevice is located on the root surface. *D,* dentin; *C,* cementum; *EA,* epithelial attachment to the cementum; *OE,* oral epithelium; *AC,* alveolar crest fibers; *PM,* periodontal membrane; *AB,* alveolar bone. Magnification × 55. (Kronfeld, *Dental Histology and Comparative Dental Anatomy,* Lea & Febiger.)

preparation is indicated in Figures 5–29, 5–30, 5–31 and 5–32. The height of attachment must be ascertained by careful probing and by the continuous observation of landmarks during the operation. Careless manipulation of band impressions must be avoided also (Fig. 5–33).

In order to secure scientific data regarding comparative curvatures, it was necessary to examine many tooth specimens. It was found that, usually, a graph of the cementoenamel curvatures from the median line distally could be staggered as in

(*Text continued on page 133.*)

Figure 5–38. Curvatures of the cervical line (cementoenamel junction) mesially and distally on the maxillary central incisor, demonstrating the points of measurement in determining the relation between the curvatures of the cervical line mesially and distally. Other points of measurement of the crown and root, when one observes the mesial and distal aspects, are outlined and are considered average measurements for a mandibular central incisor. The shaded area in the form of a band on the enamel follows the cervical curvature and represents the epithelial attachment of gingival tissue to the enamel of the crown. Compare with Fig. 5–17.

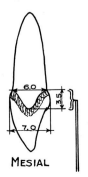

MESIAL

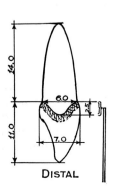

DISTAL

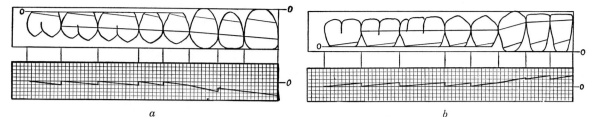

a   *b*

Figure 5–39.   Schematic drawings of the crowns of maxillary and mandibular teeth with associated graphs of the average extent of curvatures of the cervical line mesially and distally. *a,* Maxillary teeth. *b,* Mandibular teeth. Compare the graph of cervical curvatures with a line drawn through the center of contact areas. Note that the graph tends to run somewhat parallel to this line.

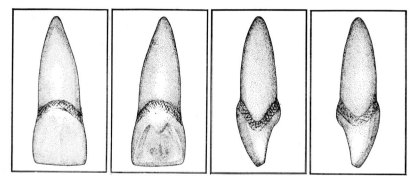

Figure 5–40.   Maxillary central incisor. The shaded area in the form of a band represents the epithelial attachment of gingival tissue to the enamel of the crown after the maturation of the process of eruption. This diagrammatic illustration is a further clarification of Fig. 5–38.

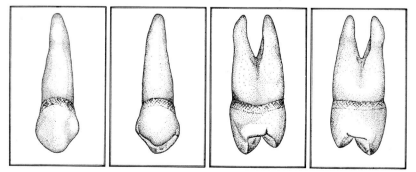

Figure 5–41.   Maxillary first premolar. Compare this illustration with Fig. 5–40. The band of attachment shows the greatest curvature buccally and lingually because of the greater curvature of the cemento-enamel junction in these areas.

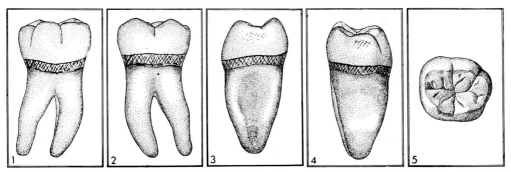

Figure 5–42. 1, 2, 3, 4, 5. Mandibular first molar. Because the cervical line encircles this tooth rather evenly, the epithelial band follows suit. Looking straight down on the occlusal surface in line with the long axis of the tooth, the band of attachment would not be in view because it would be root-wise beyond the crests of curvature.

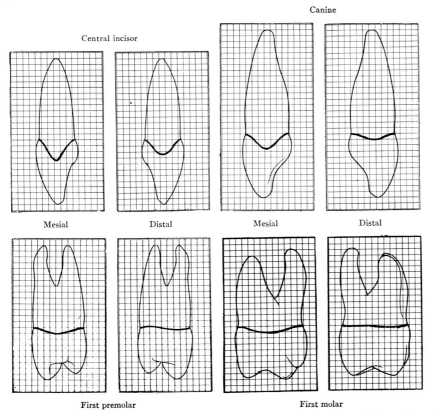

Figure 5–43. Graphs of typical forms of maxillary teeth accenting the outlines of cervical lines mesially and distally.

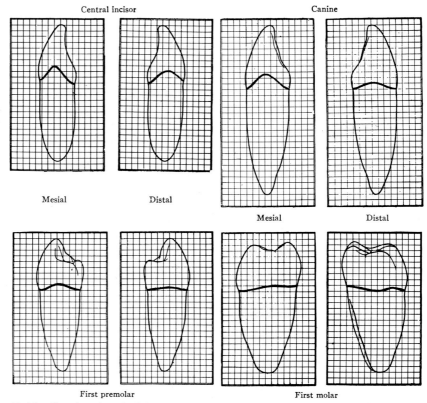

Central incisor

Canine

Mesial   Distal

Mesial   Distal

First premolar   First molar

Figure 5–44.   Graphs of typical forms of mandibular teeth accenting the outlines of cervical lines mesially and distally.

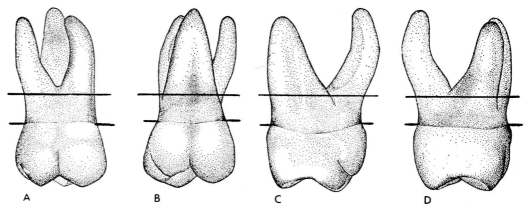

A   B   C   D

Figure 5–45.   Various aspects of the maxillary first molar serving as examples in order to show the complicated form of the root trunk of molars. *A*, Buccal. *B*, Lingual. *C*, Mesial. *D*, Distal. In restoration, no effort should be made to include the root trunk of a tooth with complicated form, especially if a full crown is planned. If the encroachment of caries or erosion demands care, the original form of the root trunk must be reproduced in order to maintain proper dental hygiene. (See also Figs. 5–46 and 5–47.)

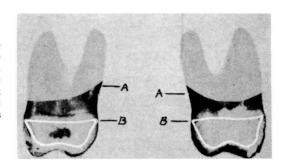

Figure 5–46. Outlines placed on actual photos of the mesial and distal aspects of a maxillary first molar. The white outline of the crown preparation shows the gingival margin (*B*) to be within the cervical third of the crown, preserving the difficult cervical contour. *A*, represents the root trunk exposed below the present gingival level and periodontal attachment. No attempt should be made to reproduce this complicated form in the restoration.

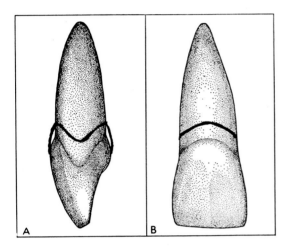

Figure 5–47. *A*, The mesial aspect of the maxillary central incisor. *B*, The labial aspect of the tooth. The crown form may be extended on the root trunk of single-rooted teeth.

Figure 5–39. It will be noticed that, in the posterior teeth, the variation in curvature is slight and the amount of curvature is minor, the variance ranging from 1 mm. mesially toward the occlusal surface to a slight curvature in the opposite direction. (Note the distal aspect of the mandibular first molar, Fig. 5–44.)

Figures 5–43 and 5–44 are graphs of maxillary and mandibular teeth demonstrating typical cervical curvatures mesially and distally.

The Permanent Teeth

*The anatomy of the permanent teeth
will be described in detail in Chapters 6 through 12.*

6

The Permanent
Maxillary Incisors

The maxillary incisors are *four* in number. The maxillary *central* or *first* incisors are centered in the maxilla, one on either side of the median line, with the mesial surface of each in contact with the mesial surface of the other. The maxillary and mandibular central incisors are the only neighboring teeth in the dental arches with mesial surfaces in contact. The right and left maxillary *lateral* or *second* incisors are distal to the central incisors.

The maxillary central incisor is larger than the lateral incisor. These teeth supplement each other in function, and they are similar anatomically. The incisors are shearing or cutting teeth. Their major function is to punch and cut food material during the process of mastication. These teeth have incisal *ridges* or *edges* rather than cusps such as are found on the canines and posterior teeth.

It might be well at this point to differentiate between the two terms, "incisal *ridge*" and "incisal *edge*." The incisal ridge is that portion of the crown which makes up the complete incisal portion. When an incisor is newly erupted, the incisal portion is rounded and merges with the mesio- and distoincisal angles and the labial and lingual surfaces. This ridge portion of the crown is called the *incisal ridge*. The term "edge" implies an angle formed by the merging of two flat surfaces. Therefore an incisal edge does not exist on an incisor until occlusal wear has created a flattened surface linguoincisally, which surface forms an angle with the labial surface. The *incisal edge* is formed by the junction of the linguoincisal surface, sometimes called the "incisal surface," and the labial surface. (Fig. 6–1.)

Preceding the description of each tooth in this and subsequent chapters, the chronology of *calcification* and *eruption* of the tooth will be given as in the table following. A table of measurements as suggested by the author for carving technique will follow. Average measurements of each tooth as found in the table should be memorized. Knowing the proportions of the individual tooth helps one learn the proportions of one tooth to another.

Outline drawings of the five aspects of the teeth, and following that tooth carving, are explained more fully in An Atlas of Tooth Form.*

---

*An Atlas of Tooth Form. W. B. Saunders Company.

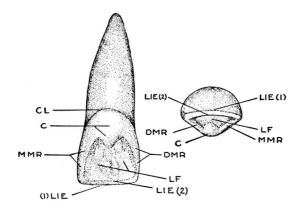

Figure 6–1. Maxillary right central incisor—lingual aspect and incisal aspect. *CL,* cervical line; *C,* cingulum; *MMR,* mesial marginal ridge; *LIE* (1), labioincisal edge, and *LIE* (2), linguoincisal edge (these (1) and (2), border the *incisal ridge*); *LF,* lingual fossa; *DMR,* distal marginal ridge.

The *Atlas of Tooth Form* will be of interest, not only to undergraduates in dentistry but also to dental ancillaries who are to be trained to work with graduate dental organizations.

The maxillary central incisor is the widest mesiodistally of any of the anterior teeth. The labial face is less convex than the maxillary lateral incisor or canine, which gives the central incisor a squared or rectangular appearance. From this aspect the crown nearly always looks symmetrical and regularly formed, having a nearly straight incisal edge, a cervical line with even curvature toward the root, a mesial side with straight outline, the distal side more curved. The mesial incisal angle is relatively sharp, the distal incisal angle rounded (Fig. 6–2).

Although the *labial* surface of the crown is usually convex, especially toward the cervical third, some central incisors will be flat at the middle and incisal portions. The enamel surface is relatively smooth. When the tooth is newly erupted, or if little wear is evident, mamelons will be seen on the incisal ridge. The middle one is the smallest. The developmental lines on the labial surface which divide the surface into three parts are most noticeable at the middle portion if they can be distinguished at all (Fig. 4–22).

MAXILLARY CENTRAL INCISOR

Maxillary Central Incisor

First evidence of calcification.....3 to 4 months
Enamel completed......................4 to 5 years
Eruption....................................7 to 8 years
Root completed............................10 years

Measurement Table

	Cervico-incisal Length of Crown	Length of Root	Mesio-distal Diameter of Crown	Mesio-distal Diameter of Crown at Cervix	Labio- or Bucco-lingual Diameter of Crown	Labio- or Bucco-lingual Diameter at Cervix	Curvature of Cervical Line—Mesial	Curvature of Cervical Line—Distal
Dimensions suggested for carving technic	10.5°	13.0	8.5	7.0	7.0	6.0	3.5	2.5

° Millimeters.

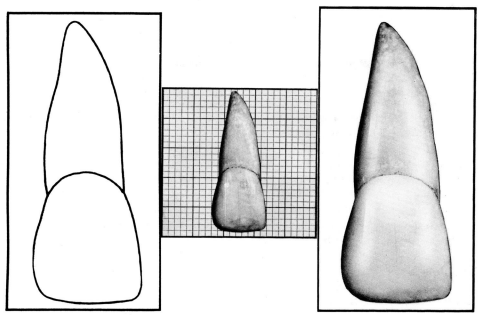

Figure 6–2. Maxillary right central incisor—labial aspect.

Lingually, the surface form of the maxillary central incisor is more irregular. The largest part of the middle and incisal portions of the lingual area is concave. The concavity is bordered by mesial and distal marginal ridges, the lingual portion of the incisal ridge, and the convexity rootwise of the cingulum. The lingual topography gives a scooplike form to the crown (Fig. 6–3).

The maxillary central incisor usually develops normally. One anomaly which sometimes occurs is a short root. Another variation is an unusually long crown. (Fig. 6–12, specimens 4 and 5.)

The maxillary central incisors are the most prominent teeth in the mouth. There are *two* basic forms: The first is relatively wide at the cervix when viewed from the labial aspect, in comparison with the mesiodistal width at the contact areas (Fig. 6–9, specimens 1 and 4); the second form is relatively narrow at the cervix, where the root joins the crown, in comparison with the mesiodistal width at the contact areas (Fig. 6–9, specimens 5, 7 and 9).

In the description of the central incisor an attempt will be made to strike an average between the extremes of the two forms.

DETAILED DESCRIPTION OF THE MAXILLARY CENTRAL INCISOR FROM ALL ASPECTS

Labial Aspect (Figs. 6–2 and 6–9)

The crown of the average central incisor will be 10 to 11 mm. long from the highest point on the cervical line to the lowest point on the incisal edge. The mesiodistal measurement will be 8 to 9 mm. wide at the contact areas. The mesiodistal measurement, where the root joins the crown, will be 1.5 to 2 mm. less. The crests of curvature mesially and distally on the crown represent the areas at which the central incisor contacts its neighbors. Any change in the position of this crest of contour affects the level of the contact area (Fig. 5–8, A).

The mesial outline of the crown is only slightly convex, with the crest of curvature (representing the contact area) approaching the mesioincisal angle. (See "Proximal Contact Areas," Chapter 5.)

The distal outline of the crown is more convex than the mesial outline, the crest of curvature being higher toward the cervical line. The distoincisal angle is not so sharp as the mesioincisal angle, the extent of curvature depending upon the typal form of the tooth.

The incisal outline is usually regular and straight in a mesiodistal direction after the tooth has been in function long enough to obliterate the mamelons. The incisal outline tends to curve downward toward the center of the crown outline, making the crown length greater at the center than at the two mesial angles.

The cervical outline of the crown follows a semicircular direction with the curvature rootwise, from the point at which the root outline joins the crown mesially to the point at which the root outline joins the crown distally.

The root of the central incisor from the labial aspect is cone-shaped, in most instances with a relatively blunt apex, the outline mesially and distally being regular. The root is usually 2 or 3 mm. longer than the crown, although it varies considerably. (See illustrations of typical central incisors and those of variations from the labial aspect (Figs. 6–9 and 6–12.).

A line drawn through the center of the root and crown of the maxillary central incisor tends to parallel the mesial outline of the crown and root.

Lingual Aspect (Fig. 6–3)

The lingual outline of the maxillary central incisor is the reverse of that found on the labial aspect. The lingual aspect of the crown is different, however, when one is

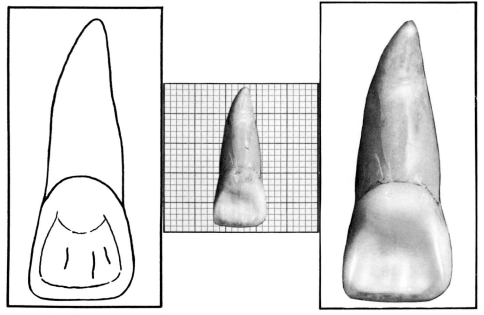

Figure 6–3. Maxillary right central incisor—lingual aspect.

comparing the surface of the lingual aspect with that of the labial aspect. From the labial aspect the surface of the crown is smooth generally. The lingual aspect has convexities and a concavity. The outline of the cervical line is similar, but immediately below the cervical line a smooth convexity is to be found; this is called the *cingulum* (Fig. 6–1).

Mesially and distally confluent with the cingulum are the *marginal ridges*. Between the marginal ridges, below the cingulum, a shallow concavity is present which is called the *lingual fossa.* Outlining the lingual fossa, the linguoincisal edge is raised somewhat, being on a level with the marginal ridges mesially and distally, completing the lingual portion of the incisal ridge of the central incisor.

From the foregoing description one notes that the lingual fossa is bordered mesially by the mesial marginal ridge, incisally by the lingual portion of the incisal ridge, distally by the distal marginal ridge and cervically by the cingulum. Usually there are developmental grooves extending from the cingulum into the lingual fossa.

The crown and root taper lingually, making the crown calibration at the two labial line angles greater than the calibration at the two lingual line angles, making the lingual portion of the root narrower than the labial portion. A cross section of the root at the cervix shows the root to be generally triangular with rounded angles: one side of the triangle is labial, with the mesial and distal sides pointing lingually. The mesial side of this triangle is a trifle longer than the distal side (Fig. 13–8, specimens C, 3, 4, 5, 6).

Mesial Aspect (Figs. 6–4 and 6–10)

The mesial aspect of this tooth has the fundamental form of an incisor: The crown is wedge-shaped, or triangular, with the base of the triangle at the cervix and the apex at the incisal ridge (Fig. 4–21).

Usually a line drawn through the crown and the root from the mesial aspect

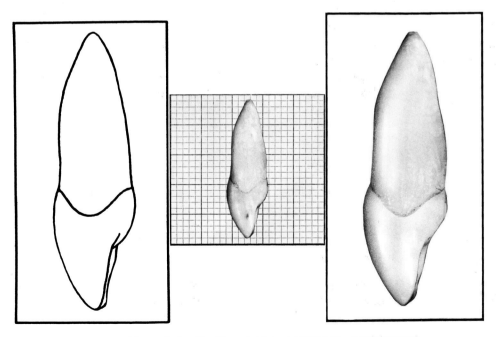

Figure 6–4. Maxillary right central incisor—mesial aspect.

through the center of the tooth will bisect the apex of the root and also the incisal ridge of the crown. The incisal ridge of the crown is therefore on a line with the center of the root. This alignment is characteristic of maxillary central and lateral incisors. A straight line drawn through the center of the crown and root from the mesial or distal aspects will rarely if ever pass lingual to the incisal edge. Maxillary incisors are occasionally seen with the incisal ridges *lingual* to the bisecting line (Fig. 6–12, specimen 1).

Labially and lingually, immediately coronal to the cervical line are the crests of curvature of these surfaces. These crests of contour give the crown its greatest labiolingual measurement.

Normally, the curvature labially and lingually is approximately 0.5 mm. in extent (Fig. 6–4) before continuing the outlines to the incisal ridge.

The labial outline of the crown from the crest of curvature to the incisal ridge is very slightly convex. The lingual outline is convex at the point where it joins the crest of curvature at the cingulum; it then becomes concave at the mesial marginal ridge, and it becomes slightly convex again at the linguoincisal ridge and the incisal edge.

The cervical line which outlines the cementoenamel junction mesially on the maxillary central incisor curves incisally to a noticeable degree. This cervical curvature is greater on the mesial surface of this tooth than on any surface of any other tooth in the mouth. The curvature varies in extent, depending upon the length of the crown and the measurement of the crown labiolingually. On an average central incisor of 10.5 to 11 mm. in crown length, the curvature will be 3 to 4 mm. (See "Curvatures of the Cervical Lines," Chapter 5.)

The root of this tooth from the mesial aspect is cone-shaped, and the apex of the root is usually bluntly rounded.

Distal Aspect (Fig. 6–5)

There is little difference between the distal and mesial outlines of this tooth. When looking at the central incisor from the distal aspect, one may note that the crown gives the impression of being somewhat thicker toward the incisal third. Because of the slope of the labial surface distolingually, more of that surface is seen from the distal aspect; this creates the illusion of greater thickness. Actually, most teeth are turned a little on their root bases, in order to adapt to the dental arch curvature. The maxillary central incisor is no exception.

The curvature of the cervical line outlining the cementoenamel junction is less in extent on the distal than on the mesial surfaces. Most teeth show this characteristic.

Incisal Aspect (Figs. 6–6 and 6–11)

The specimen of this tooth is posed in the illustrations so that the incisal edge is centered over the root. A view of the crown from this aspect superposes it over the root entirely, so that the latter is not visible.

The labial face of the crown, from this aspect, is relatively broad and flat in comparison with the lingual surface, especially toward the incisal third. Nevertheless, the cervical portion of the crown labially is convex, although the arc described is broad.

The incisal ridge may be seen clearly, and a differentiation between the incisal

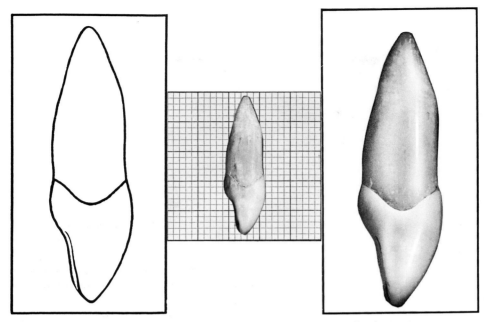

Figure 6–5.   Maxillary right central incisor—distal aspect.

edge and the remainder of the incisal ridge, with its slope toward the lingual, is easily distinguished.

The outline of the lingual portion tapers lingually toward the cingulum. The cingulum of the crown makes up the cervical portion of the lingual surface.

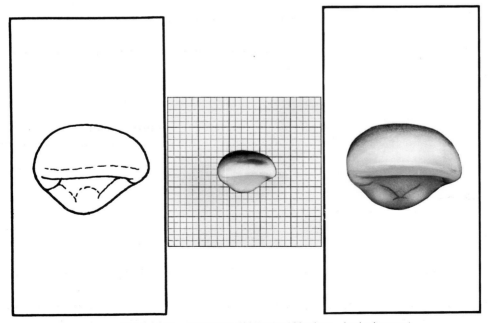

Figure 6–6.   Maxillary right central incisor—incisal aspect.

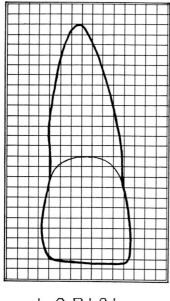

LABIAL

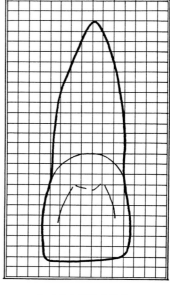

LINGUAL

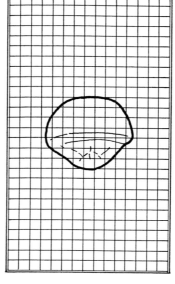

INCISAL

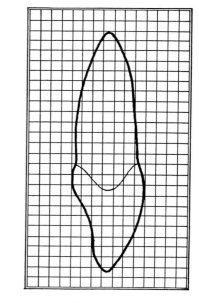

MESIAL

DISTAL

Figure 6–7. Maxillary right central incisor. Graph outlines of five aspects. In incisal view, labial aspect is at top of drawing.

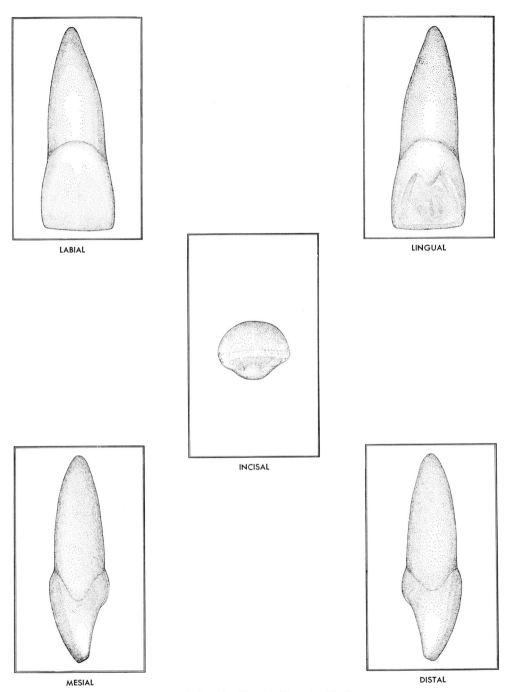

Figure 6–8.   Maxillary right central incisor.

The mesiolabial and distolabial line angles are prominent from the incisal aspect. The relative positions of these line angles should be compared with the mesiolingual and distolingual line angles—which are represented by the borders of the mesial and distal marginal ridges. The mesiodistal calibration of the crown at the labial line angles is greater than the same calibration at the lingual line angles.

The crown of this tooth shows more bulk from the incisal aspect than one would expect from viewing it from the mesial or distal aspect. There are relatively broad surfaces at the site of contact areas mesially and distally. Comparison should also be made between the dimensions of the crown labiolingually and mesiodistally. The labiolingual calibration of the crown is more than two thirds as great as the mesiodistal calibration. A cursory examination would not indicate this comparison.

Bilaterally, the outline of the incisal aspect is rather uniform. The lingual portion shows some variation, however, in that a line drawn from the mesioincisal angle to the center of the cingulum lingually will be a longer line than one drawn from the same point on the cingulum to the distoincisal angle. The crown conforms to a triangular outline reflected by the outline of the root cross section at the cervix mentioned formerly.

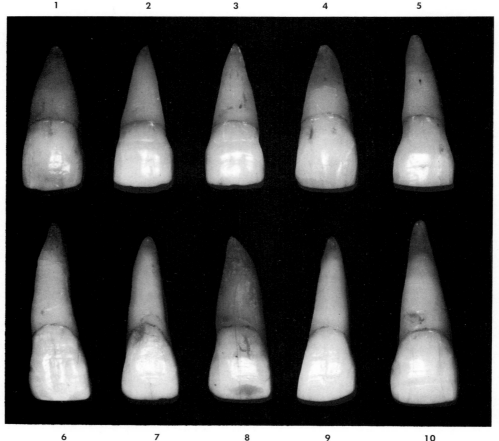

Figure 6–9.   Maxillary central incisor—ten typical specimens—labial aspect.

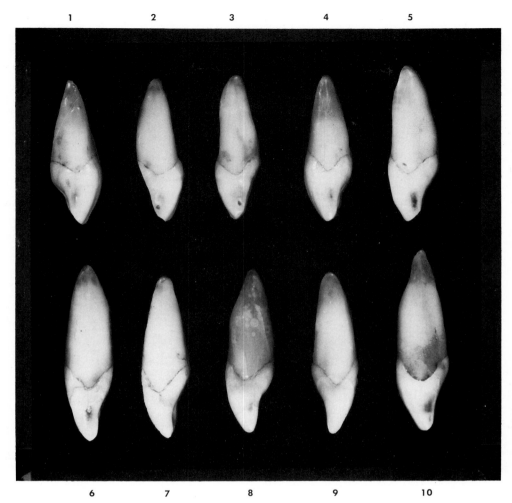

Figure 6–10.   Maxillary central incisor—ten typical specimens—mesial aspect.

MAXILLARY LATERAL INCISOR

The maxillary lateral incisor supplements the central incisor in function, so the crowns bear a close resemblance. The lateral incisor is smaller in all dimensions except root length. Since it resembles the maxillary central incisor in form, direct comparisons will be made with the central incisor in its description.

This tooth differs from the central incisor in this—its development may vary considerably. Maxillary lateral incisors vary in form more than any other tooth in the mouth except the third molar. If the variation is too great, it is considered a developmental anomaly. A not uncommon situation is to find maxillary lateral incisors with a nondescript, pointed form; such teeth are called "peg-shaped" laterals (Fig. 6–2l, specimens 7 and 8). In some individuals the lateral incisors are missing entirely; in these cases the maxillary central incisor may be in contact distally with the canine.

One type of malformed maxillary lateral incisor will have a large pointed tubercle

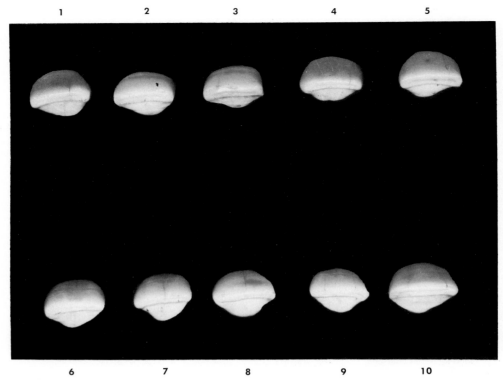

Figure 6–11. Maxillary central incisor—ten typical specimens—incisal aspect.

as part of the cingulum; some will have deep developmental grooves which extend down on the root lingually with a deep fold in the cingulum; some will show twisted roots, distorted crowns, and so forth (Fig. 6–21).

DETAILED DESCRIPTION OF THE MAXILLARY LATERAL INCISOR FROM ALL ASPECTS

Labial Aspect (Figs. 6–13 and 6–19)

Although the labial aspect of the maxillary lateral incisor may appear to favor that of the central incisor, usually it has more curvature, with a rounded incisal ridge and rounded incisal angles mesially and distally. Although the crown is smaller in all dimensions, its proportions usually correspond to those of the central incisor.

The mesial outline of the crown from the labial aspect resembles that of the central incisor, with a more rounded mesioincisal angle. The crest of contour mesially is usually at the point of junction of the middle and incisal thirds; occasionally, in the so-called square forms, the mesioincisal angle is almost as sharp as that found on most maxillary central incisors (Fig. 6–19, specimens 4 and 5). However, a more rounded mesioincisal angle is seen more frequently.

The distal outline of the crown from the labial aspect differs somewhat from that of the central incisor. The distal outline is always more rounded, and the crest of contour is more cervical, usually in the center of the middle third. Some forms describe a

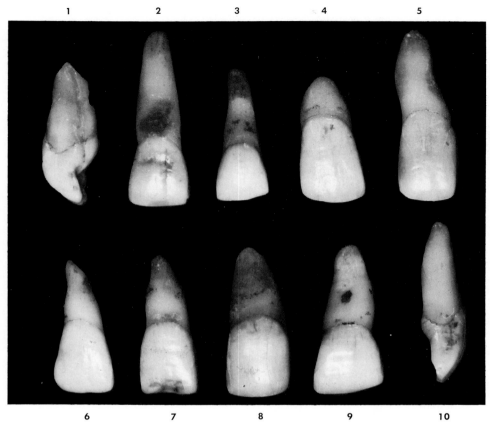

Figure 6–12. Maxillary central incisor—ten specimens showing uncommon variations. 1, Extreme lingual inclination of incisal portion of crown. Note developmental groove traversing root and part of crown. 2, Root extremely long. 3, Specimen small in all dimensions. 4, Crown extremely long—root very short. 5, Specimen malformed—crown unusually long—cervix very wide. 6, Root short and tapering. 7, Same as specimen 6. 8, Crown nearly as wide at the cervix as at contact areas—crown long—root short. 9, Root with unusual curvature. 10, Crown and root narrow labiolingually; root comparable to 2.

MAXILLARY LATERAL INCISOR

Maxillary Lateral Incisor

First evidence of calcification.....1 year
Enamel completed......................4 to 5 years
Eruption....................................8 to 9 years
Root completed...........................11 years

Measurement Table

	Cervico-incisal Length of Crown	Length of Root	Mesio-distal Diameter of Crown	Mesio-distal Diameter of Crown at Cervix	Labio- or Bucco-lingual Diameter of Crown	Labio- or Bucco-lingual Diameter at Cervix	Curvature of Cervical Line— Mesial	Curvature of Cervical Line— Distal
Dimensions suggested for carving technic	9.0°	13.0	6.5	5.0	6.0	5.0	3.0	2.0

°Millimeters.

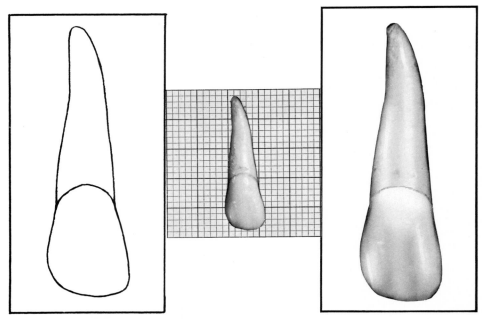

Figure 6–13. Maxillary right lateral incisor—labial aspect.

semicircular outline distally from the cervix to the center of the incisal ridge (Fig. 6–19, specimens 3 and 7).

The labial surface of the crown is more convex than that of the central incisor except in some square and flat-faced forms.

This tooth is relatively narrow mesiodistally, usually about 2 mm. narrower than the central incisor. The crown on the average will measure from 2 to 3 mm. shorter cervicoincisally than that of the central incisor, although the root is usually as long if not somewhat longer than that of the central incisor.

As a rule its root length is greater in proportion to its crown length than that of the central incisor. The root is often about one and one-half times the length of the crown.

The root tapers evenly from the cervical line to a point approximately two-thirds of its length apically. In most cases it curves sharply from this location in a distal direction and ends in a pointed apex. Although the curvature distally is typical, some roots are straight (Fig. 6–19, specimens 4, 7, and 9), and some may be found curving mesially. As mentioned previously, this tooth may show considerable variance in its crown form; the root form may be more characteristic.

Lingual Aspect (Fig. 6–14)

Mesial and distal marginal ridges are marked, and the cingulum is usually prominent, with a tendency toward deep developmental grooves within the lingual fossa, where it joins the cingulum. The linguoincisal ridge is well developed, and the lingual fossa is more concave and circumscribed than that found on the central incisor.

The tooth tapers toward the lingual, resembling a central incisor in this respect. It is not uncommon to find a deep developmental groove at the side of the cingulum, usually on the distal side, which may extend up on the root for part or all of its length.

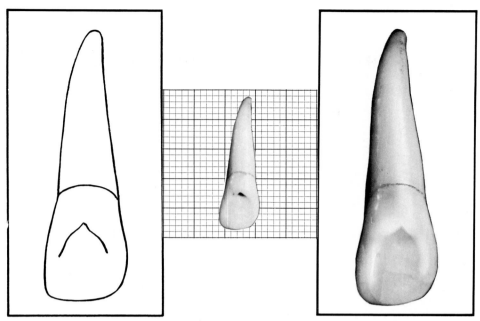

Figure 6–14. Maxillary right lateral incisor—lingual aspect.

Faults in the enamel of the crown are often found in the deep portions of these developmental grooves (Fig. 6–21, specimens 3 and 4).

Mesial Aspect (Figs. 6–15 and 6–20)

The mesial aspect of the maxillary lateral incisor is similar to that of a small central incisor except that the root appears longer. The crown is shorter; the root is relatively longer, and the labiolingual measurement of the crown and root is a millimeter or so less than the maxillary central incisor of the same mouth.

The curvature of the cervical line is marked in the direction of the incisal ridge, although because of the small size of the crown the actual extent of curvature is less than that found on the central incisor. The heavy development of the incisal ridge accordingly makes the incisal portion appear somewhat thicker than that of the central incisor.

The root appears as a tapered cone from this aspect, with a bluntly rounded, apical end. This varies in individuals, sometimes being quite blunt, while at other times it is pointed. In a good many cases the labial outline of the root from this aspect is straight. As in the central incisor, a line drawn through the center of the root tends to bisect the incisal ridge of the crown.

Distal Aspect (Fig. 6–16)

Because of the placement of the crown on the root, the width of the crown distally appears thicker than it does on the mesial aspect from marginal ridge to labial face. The curvature of the cervical line is usually a millimeter or so less in depth than on the mesial side. It is not uncommon to find a developmental groove distally on this crown extending on the root for part or all of its length.

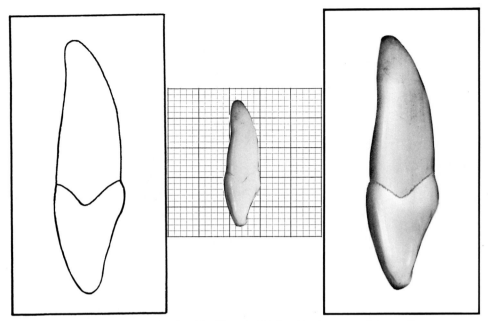

Figure 6–15.   Maxillary right lateral incisor — mesial aspect.

Incisal Aspect (Figs. 6–17 and 6–18)

The incisal aspect of this tooth sometimes resembles that of the central incisor, or it may resemble that of a small canine. If the tooth conforms in development to its central incisor neighbor in other respects, it will, from the incisal aspect, resemble a

(Text continued on page 154.)

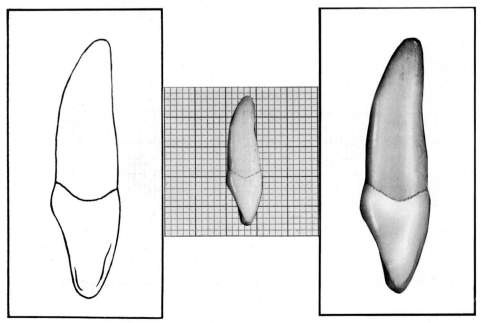

Figure 6–16.   Maxillary right lateral incisor — distal aspect.

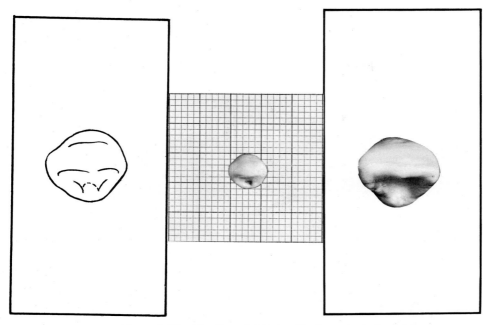

Figure 6–17.   Maxillary right lateral incisor—incisal aspect.

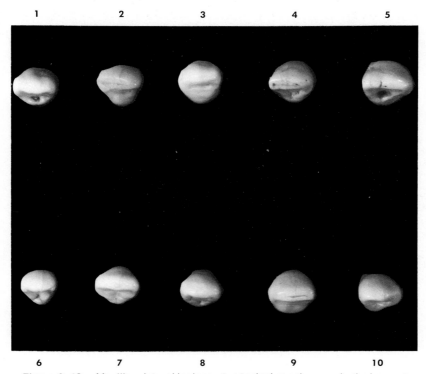

Figure 6–18.   Maxillary lateral incisor—ten typical specimens—incisal aspect.

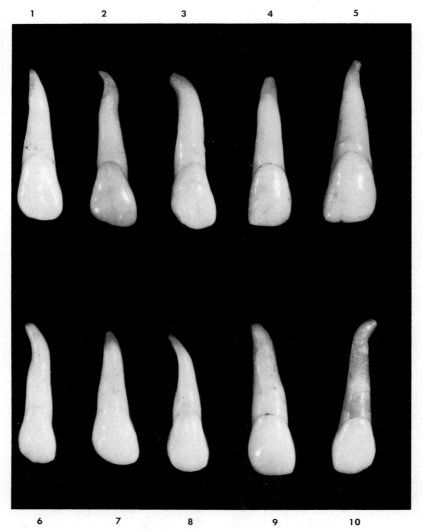

Figure 6–19.   Maxillary lateral incisor — ten typical specimens — labial aspect.

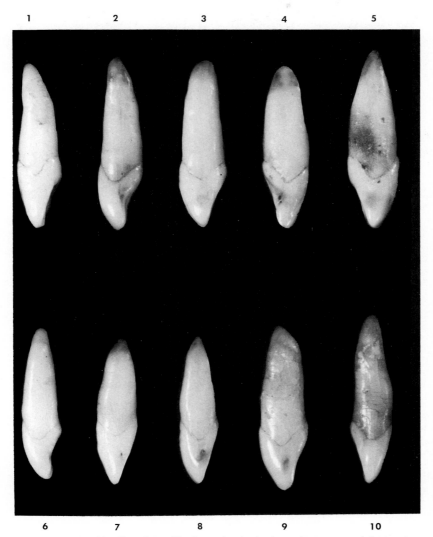

Figure 6–20.   Maxillary lateral incisor—ten typical specimens—mesial aspect.

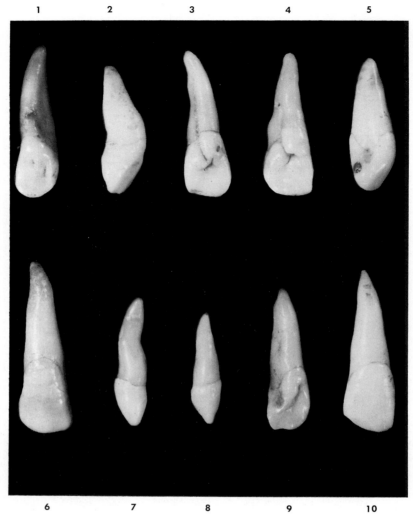

Figure 6–21.   Maxillary lateral incisor—ten specimens showing uncommon variations. 1, Odd twist to crown and root. 2, Malformed generally. 3, Deep developmental groove distally; note pit in lingual fossa. 4, Same as specimen 3 with pit and groove connected. 5, Deep concavity above contact area of the crown. 6, Abnormally large but well formed. 7, Single-cusp development and malformed root—so-called "peg lateral incisor." 8, Same as specimen 7 except root is straight. 9, Same as specimen 5, with deep lingual pit in addition. 10, Resemblance to a small maxillary central incisor more marked than the average.

central incisor except in size (Fig. 6–18, specimens 5 and 9). The cingulum, however, may be large; the incisal ridge also; the labiolingual dimension may be greater than usual in comparison with the mesiodistal dimension. If these variations are present, the tooth has a marked resemblance to a small canine (Fig. 6–18, specimens 3 and 10).

All maxillary lateral incisors exhibit more convexity labially and lingually from the incisal aspect than maxillary central incisors.

7

The Permanent
Mandibular Incisors

The mandibular incisors are *four* in number. The mandibular *central* or *first* incisors are centered in the mandible, one on either side of the median line, with the mesial surface of each one in contact with the mesial surface of the other. The right and left mandibular *lateral* or *second* incisors are distal to the central incisors. They are in contact with the central incisors mesially and with the canines distally.

The mandibular incisors have smaller mesiodistal dimensions than any of the other teeth. The central incisor is somewhat smaller than the lateral incisor, which is the reverse of the situation in the maxilla.

These teeth are similar in form and have smooth crown surfaces which show few traces of developmental lines. Mamelons on the incisal ridges are worn off soon after eruption, if the occlusion is normal, leaving the incisal ridges smooth and straight (compare specimens 7 and 8, Fig. 7–9). The contact areas are near the incisal ridges mesially and distally, and lines drawn through the contact areas are near the same level on both central and lateral incisors; here also the situation is unlike the maxillary incisors. The mandibular incisors show uniform development, with few instances of malformations or anomalies.

The anatomic form of these teeth differs entirely from that of the maxillary incisors. The inclination of the crowns differs from the mesial and distal aspects; the labial faces are inclined lingually so that the incisal ridges are lingual to a line bisecting the root. After normal wear has taken place, obliterating the mamelons, the incisal surfaces thus created show a *labial inclination* when the occlusion has been normal. It will be remembered that the incisal surfaces of maxillary incisors have a *lingual* inclination. With this arrangement the incisal planes of the mandibular and maxillary incisors are parallel with each other, fitting together during incising action.

MANDIBULAR CENTRAL INCISOR

Normally, the mandibular central incisor is the smallest tooth in the dental arches. The crown has little more than half the mesiodistal diameter of the maxillary central incisor; however, the labiolingual diameter is only about 1 mm. less. The lines of greatest masticatory stress are brought to bear on the mandibular incisors in a labiolingual direction, making this reinforcement necessary.

Mandibular Central Incisor

First evidence of calcification.....3 to 4 months
Enamel completed ....4 to 5 years
Eruption.....................................6 to 7 years
Root completed..........................9 years

Measurement Table

	Cervico-incisal Length of Crown	Length of Root	Mesio-distal Diameter of Crown	Mesio-distal Diameter of Crown at Cervix	Labio- or Bucco-lingual Diameter of Crown	Labio- or Bucco-lingual Diameter of Crown at Cervix	Curva-ture of Cervical Line — Mesial	Curva-ture of Cervical Line — Distal
Dimensions suggested for carving technic	9.0°	12.5	5.0	3.5	6.0	5.3	3.0	2.0

° Millimeters.

The single root is very narrow mesiodistally and corresponds to the narrowness of the crown, although the root and crown are wide labiolingually. The length of the root is as great, if not greater, than that of the maxillary central incisor.

DETAILED DESCRIPTION OF THE MANDIBULAR CENTRAL INCISOR FROM ALL ASPECTS

Labial Aspect (Figs. 7–2, 7–7, 7–8, and 7–9)

The labial aspect of the mandibular central incisor is regular, tapering evenly from the relatively sharp mesial and distal incisal angles to the apical portion of the root. The incisal ridge of the crown is straight and is at approximately a right angle to the long axis of the tooth. Usually the mesial and distal outlines of the crown make a straight drop downward from the incisal angles to the contact areas, which are incisal to the junction of incisal and middle thirds of the crown. The mesial and distal sides of the crown taper evenly from the contact areas to the narrow cervix.

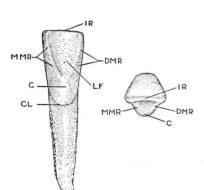

Figure 7–1. Mandibular right central incisor—lingual aspect and incisal aspect. *IR*, incisal ridge; *DMR*, distal marginal ridge; *LF*, lingual fossa; *CL*, cervical line; *C*, cingulum; *MMR*, mesial marginal ridge.

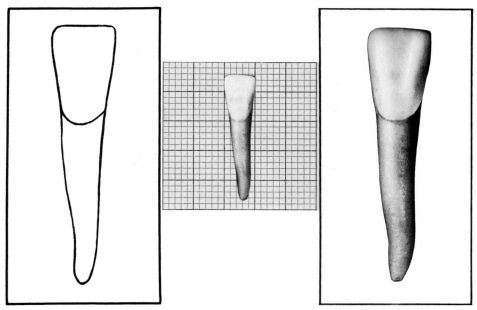

Figure 7–2.   Mandibular right central incisor — labial aspect.

The mesial and distal root outlines are straight with the mesial and distal outlines of the crown down to the apical portion. The apical third of the root terminates in a small pointed taper, in most cases curving distally. Sometimes the roots are straight (Fig. 7–9, specimens 2 and 10).

The labial face of the mandibular central incisor crown is ordinarily smooth, with a flattened surface at the incisal third; the middle third is more convex, narrowing down to the convexity of the root at the cervical portion.

Except in newly erupted teeth, central incisors show few traces of developmental lines.

The labial surface of the root of the mandibular central incisor is regular and convex.

Lingual Aspect (Figs. 7–1, 7–3, 7–7, and 7–8)

The *lingual* surface of the crown is smooth, with very slight concavity at the incisal third between the inconspicuous marginal ridges. In some instances the marginal ridges are more prominent near the incisal edges (Fig. 7–11, specimens 2 and 8). In these cases the concavity between the marginal ridges is more distinct.

The lingual surface becomes flat and then convex as progression is made from the incisal third to the cervical third.

No developmental lines mark the cingulum development on this tooth at the cervical third. No other tooth in the mouth, except the mandibular lateral incisor, shows so few developmental lines and grooves. The outlines and surfaces of the mandibular incisors are regular and symmetrical.

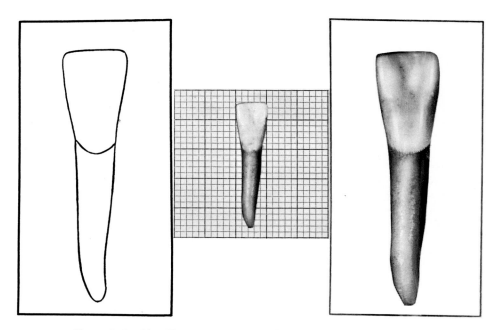

Figure 7–3. Mandibular right central incisor—lingual aspect.

Mesial Aspect (Figs. 7–4, 7–7, 7–8 and 7–10)

The curvature labially and lingually above the cervical line is less than that found on maxillary incisors.

The outline of the labial face of the crown is straight above the cervical curvature, sloping rapidly from the crest of curvature to the incisal ridge. The lingual outline of the crown is a straight line inclined labially for a short distance above the smooth convexity of the cingulum; the straight outline joins a concave line at the middle third of the crown, which extends upward to join the rounded outline of a narrow incisal ridge. The incisal ridge is rounded or worn flat, and its center is usually lingual to the center of the root.

The curvature of the cervical line representing the cementoenamel junction on the mesial surface is marked, curving incisally approximately one-third the length of the crown.

The root outlines from the mesial aspect are straight with the crown outline from the cervical line, keeping the root diameter uniform through the cervical third and part of the middle third; the outline of the root begins to taper in the middle third area, tapering rapidly in the apical third to either a bluntly rounded or a pointed root end.

The mesial surface of the crown is convex and smooth at the incisal third and becomes broader and flatter at the middle third cervical to the contact area; it then becomes quite flat, with a tendency toward concavity immediately below the middle third of the crown and above the cervical line (Fig. 7–10, specimens 5, 8 and 10).

The mesial surface of the root is flat just below the cervical line. Most of these roots have a broad developmental depression for most of the root length. The depressions usually are deeper at the junction of the middle and apical thirds (Fig. 7–10, specimens 3 and 9).

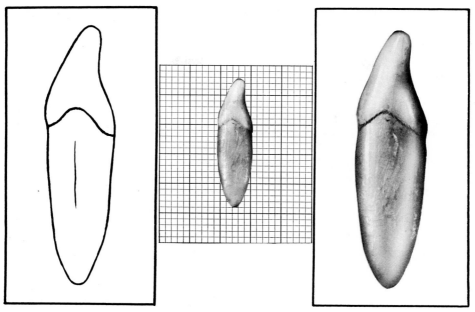

Figure 7–4. Mandibular right central incisor—mesial aspect.

Distal Aspect (Figs. 7–5, 7–7, and 7–8)

The cervical line representing the cementoenamel junction curves incisally about 1 mm. less than on the mesial.

The distal surface of the crown and root of the mandibular central incisor is simi-

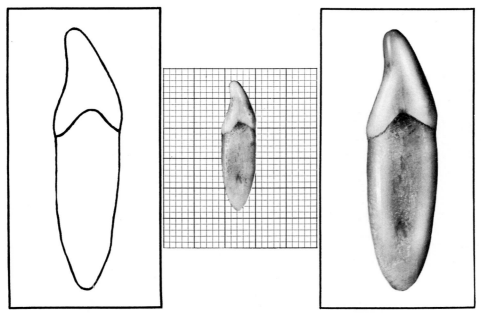

Figure 7–5. Mandibular right central incisor—distal aspect.

lar to that of the mesial surface. The developmental depression on the distal surface of the root may be more marked, with a deeper and more well-defined developmental groove at its center.

Incisal Aspect (Figs. 7–1, 7–6, 7–7, 7–8, and 7–11)

This aspect illustrates the bilateral symmetry of the mandibular central incisor. The mesial half of the crown is almost identical with the distal half.

The incisal edge is almost at right angles to a line bisecting the crown labiolingually. This feature is characteristic of the tooth and serves as a mark of identification in differentiation between mandibular central and lateral incisors (see "Mandibular Lateral Incisor"). Note the comparison between the diameter of these crowns labiolingually and their diameters mesiodistally. The labiolingual diameter is always *greater*.

The labial surface of the crown is wider mesiodistally than the lingual surface. The crown is usually wider labially than lingually at the cervical third, which latter area is represented by a smooth cingulum.

The labial surface of the crown at the incisal third, although rather broad and flat in comparison with the cervical third, has a tendency toward *convexity*, whereas the lingual surface of the crown at the incisal third has an inclination toward *concavity*.

When this tooth is posed from the incisal aspect so that the line of vision is on a line with the long axis of the tooth, more of the labial surface may be seen than of the lingual surface.

(Text continued on page 165.)

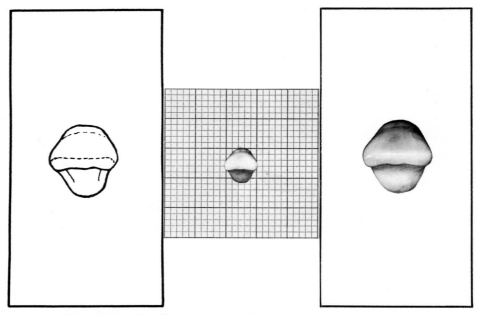

Figure 7–6.   Mandibular right central incisor—incisal aspect.

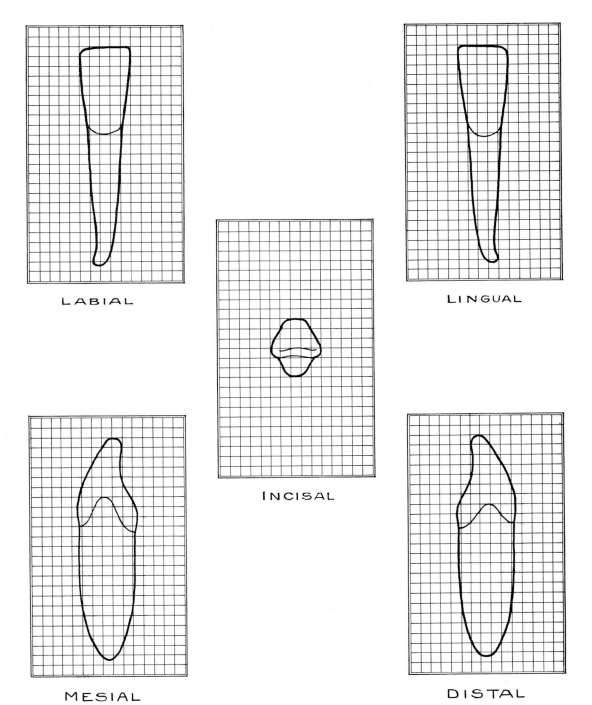

LABIAL

LINGUAL

INCISAL

MESIAL

DISTAL

Figure 7–7.   Mandibular right central incisor. Graph outlines of five aspects.

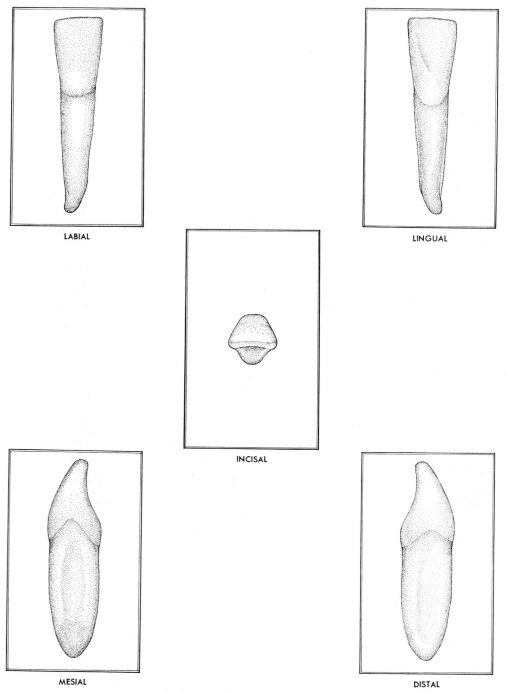

LABIAL

LINGUAL

INCISAL

MESIAL

DISTAL

Figure 7–8. Mandibular right central incisor.

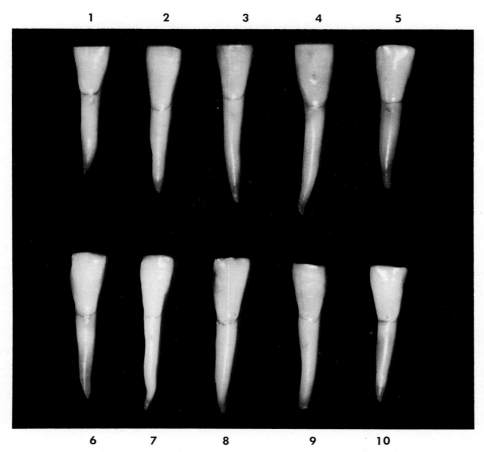

Figure 7–9.   Mandibular central incisor — ten typical specimens — labial aspect.

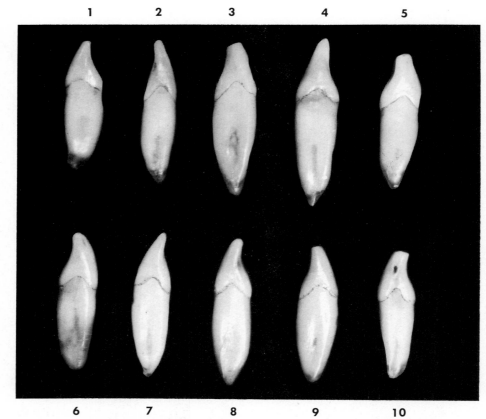

Figure 7–10. Mandibular central incisor—ten typical specimens—mesial aspect.

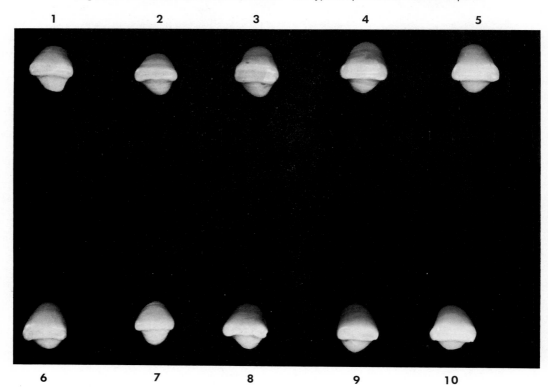

Figure 7–11. Mandibular central incisor—ten typical specimens—incisal aspect.

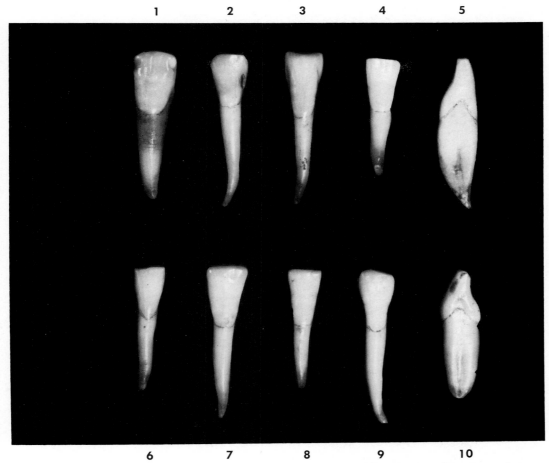

Figure 7–12.   Mandibular central incisor—ten specimens showing uncommon variations. 1, Crown and root very broad mesiodistally, malformed enamel at incisal third of crown. 2, Crown wide at incisal third, with short crown. Root length extreme. 3, Unusual contours at middle third of crown, cervix narrow. 4, Well-formed crown, short root. 5, No curvature labially at cervical third, extreme labial curvature at root end. 6, Specimen well formed but undersized. 7, Contact areas pointed at incisal edge. Crown and root very long. 8, Crown long and narrow, root short. 9, Crown measurement at cervical third same as root; crown and root of extreme length. 10, Crown and root very wide labiolingually, greater curvature than average above cervical line at the cervical third of the crown.

MANDIBULAR LATERAL INCISOR

The mandibular lateral incisor is the second mandibular tooth from the median line, right or left (Figs. 7–13 to 7–21). It resembles the mandibular central incisor so closely that a detailed description of each aspect of the lateral incisor is unnecessary. Direct comparison will be made with the mandibular central incisor, and the variations will be mentioned. The two incisors operate in the dental arch as a team, therefore their functional form is related.

The mandibular lateral incisor is somewhat larger than the mandibular central incisor (compare measurements) but, generally speaking, its form closely resembles the central.

The labial and lingual aspects show the added fraction of approximately 1 mm. of crown diameter mesiodistally added to the distal half. This, however, is not always true (see Fig. 7–19, specimens 3 and 6).

Mandibular Lateral Incisor

First evidence of calcification.....3 to 4 months
Enamel completed ....4 to 5 years
Eruption ....7 to 8 years
Root completed..........................10 years

Measurement Table

	Cervico-incisal Length of Crown	Length of Root	Mesio-distal Diameter of Crown	Mesio-distal Diameter of Crown at Cervix	Labio- or Bucco-lingual Diameter of Crown	Labio- or Bucco-lingual Diameter of Crown at Cervix	Curva-ture of Cervical Line— Mesial	Curva-ture of Cervical Line— Distal
Dimensions suggested for carving technic	9.5°	14.0	5.5	4.0	6.5	5.8	3.0	2.0

°Millimeters.

The mesial side of the crown is often longer than the distal side, causing the incisal ridge, which is straight, to slope downward in a distal direction (Fig. 7–19, specimen 1). The distal contact area is more toward the cervical than the mesial contact area to contact properly the mesial contact area of the mandibular canine.

Except for size, there is no marked difference between the mesial and distal surfaces of central and lateral incisors. Even the curvatures of the cervical line mesially and distally are similar in extent. There is a tendency toward a deeper concavity im-

(Text continued on page 170.)

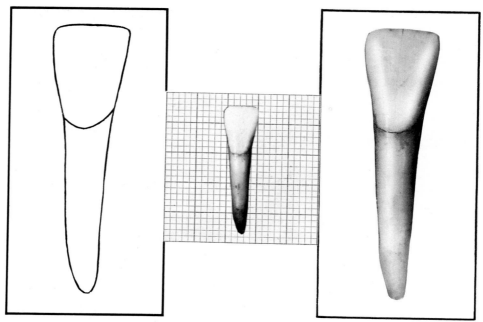

Figure 7–13. Mandibular right lateral incisor—labial aspect.

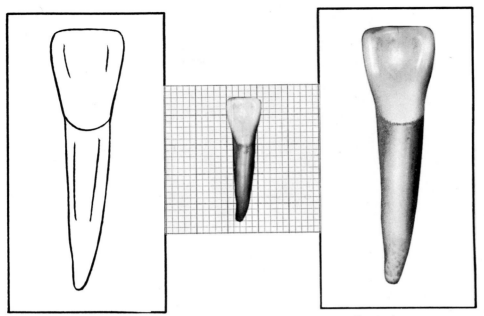

Figure 7–14.   Mandibular right lateral incisor—lingual aspect.

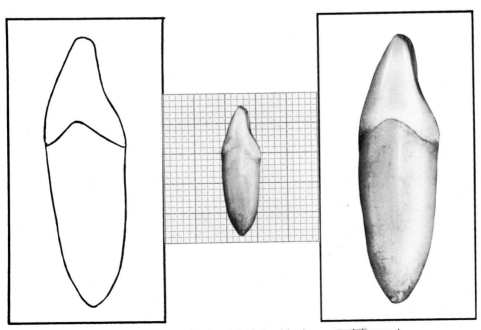

Figure 7–15.   Mandibular right lateral incisor—mesial aspect.

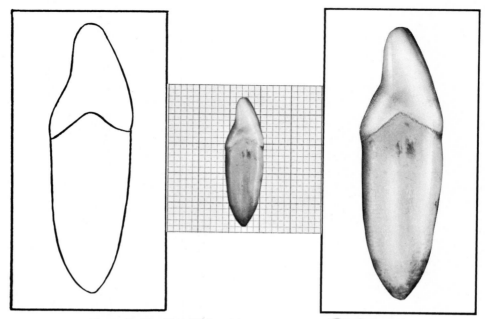

Figure 7–16. Mandibular right lateral incisor—distal aspect.

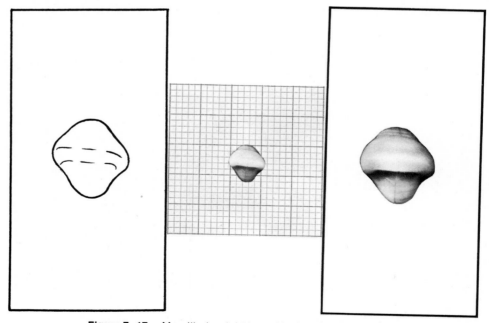

Figure 7–17. Mandibular right lateral incisor—incisal aspect.

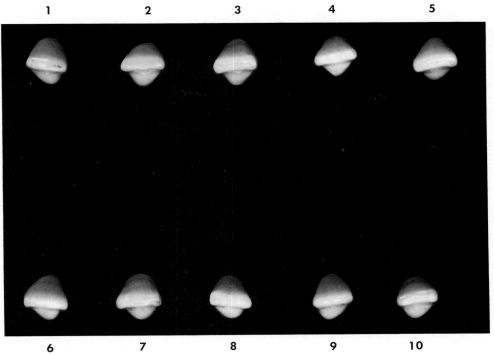

Figure 7–18. Mandibular lateral incisor—ten typical specimens—incisal aspect.

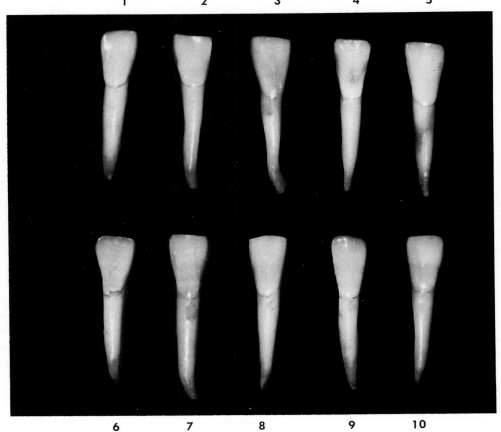

Figure 7–19. Mandibular lateral incisor—ten typical specimens—labial aspect.

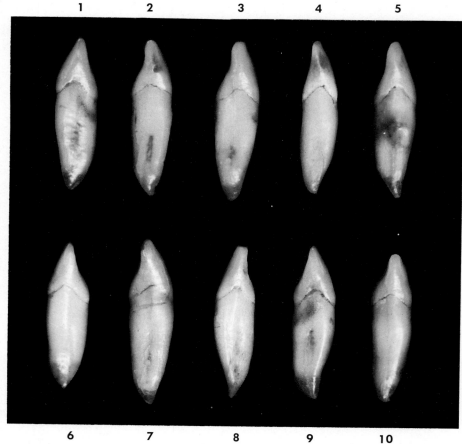

Figure 7–20.   Mandibular lateral incisor—ten typical specimens—mesial aspect.

mediately above the cervical line on the distal surface of the mandibular lateral incisor.

Although the crown of the mandibular lateral incisor is somewhat longer than that of the central incisor (usually a fraction of a millimeter), the root may be considerably longer. The tooth is, therefore, in most instances, a little larger in all dimensions. The root form is similar to that of the central incisor, including the developmental depressions mesially and distally.

The *incisal aspect* of the mandibular lateral incisor provides a feature which can usually serve to identify this tooth. The incisal edge is not at approximate right angles to a line bisecting the crown and root labiolingually, as was found when observing the central incisor: The edge follows the curvature of the mandibular dental arch, giving the crown of the mandibular lateral incisor the appearance of being twisted slightly on its root base. It is interesting to note that the labiolingual root axes of mandibular central and lateral incisors remain almost parallel in the alveolar process, even though the incisal ridges are not directly in line (see mandibular alveoli, Chapter 14, Fig. 14–25).

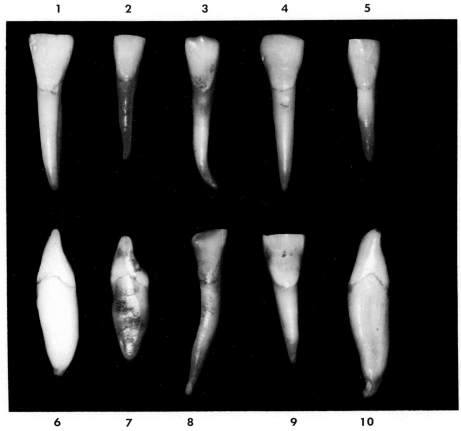

Figure 7–21.   Mandibular lateral incisor—ten specimens showing uncommon variations. 1, Tooth very large, cervix constricted in comparison with crown width. 2, Specimen well formed, smaller than average. 3, Root extra long, extreme curvature at apical third, mesial and middle mamelons intact on incisal ridge. 4, Extreme mesiodistal measurement for crown length, contact areas very broad cervico-incisally. 5, Specimen undersized. 6, Incisal ridge thin, little or no curvature at cervical third of crown. 7, Incisal edge labial to center of root, root rounded, cingulum with more curvature above root than average. 8, Malformed crown and root, root with extreme length. 9, Crown very wide, root short. 10, Very slight curvature at cervical third of crown, entire tooth oversize, malformation at root end.

8

The Permanent Canines, Maxillary and Mandibular

The maxillary and mandibular canines bear a close resemblance to each other, and their functions are closely related. The four canines are placed at the "corners" of the mouth, each one the third tooth from the median line, right and left, in the maxilla and mandible. They are the longest teeth in the mouth; the crowns are usually as long as those of the maxillary central incisors, and the single roots are longer than those of any of the other teeth. The middle labial lobes have been highly developed incisally into strong well-formed cusps. Crowns and roots are markedly convex on most surfaces.

The shape of the crowns, with their single pointed cusps, their locations in the mouth, and the extra anchorage furnished by the long, strongly developed roots, makes these canines resemble those of the Carnivora. This resemblance to the prehensile teeth of Carnivora gives rise to the term *canine.*

Because of the labiolingual thickness of crown and root and the anchorage in the alveolar process of the jaws, these teeth are perhaps the most stable in the mouth. The crown portions of the canines are shaped in a manner which promotes cleanliness. This self-cleansing quality, along with the efficient anchorage in the jaws, tends to preserve these teeth throughout life. When teeth are lost, the canines are usually the last ones to go. They are very valuable teeth, either when considered as units of the natural dental arches, or as possible assistants in stabilizing replacements of lost teeth in prosthetic procedures.

Both maxillary and mandibular canines have another quality which must not be overlooked: The positions and forms of these teeth and their anchorage in the bone, along with the bone ridge over the labial portions of the roots, called the *canine eminence,* have a cosmetic value. They help to form a foundation that insures normal facial expression at the "corners" of the mouth. Loss of all of these teeth makes it extremely difficult, if not impossible, to make replacements that will restore the natural appearance of the face for any length of time. It would therefore be difficult to place a value on the canines, their importance being made manifest by their efficiency in function, their stability, and their help in maintaining natural facial expression.

In *function*, the canines support the incisors and the premolars, since they are located between those groups. The canine crowns have some characteristics of functional form which will bear a resemblance to incisor form, and some which resemble the premolar form.

MAXILLARY CANINE

The outline of the labial or lingual aspect of the maxillary canine is a series of curves or arcs except for the angle made by the tip of the cusp. This cusp has a mesial incisal ridge and a distoincisal ridge.

The mesial half of the crown makes contact with the lateral incisor, and the distal half contacts the first premolar. Therefore the contact areas of the maxillary canine are at different levels cervicoincisally.

From a labial view, the mesial half of the crown resembles a portion of an incisor, whereas the distal half resembles a portion of a premolar. This tooth seems to be a compromise in the change from anterior to posterior teeth in the dental arch.

It is apparent that the construction of this tooth has reinforcement, labiolingually, to offset directional lines of the force brought against it when in use. The incisal portion is thicker labiolingually than that of either the maxillary central or the lateral incisor.

The labiolingual measurement of the crown is about 1 mm. greater than that of the maxillary central incisor. The mesiodistal measurement is approximately 1 mm. less.

The cingulum shows greater development than that of the central incisor.

The root of the maxillary canine is usually the longest of any root with the possible exception of that of the mandibular canine, which may be as long at times. The root is thick labiolingually, with developmental depressions mesially and distally which help to furnish the secure anchorage this tooth has in the maxilla.

Maxillary Canine

First evidence of calcification .... 4 to 5 months
Enamel completed .... 6 to 7 years
Eruption................................... 11 to 12 years
Root completed .... 13 to 15 years

Measurement Table

	Cervico-incisal Length of Crown	Length of Root	Mesio-distal Diameter of Crown	Mesio-distal Diameter of Crown at Cervix	Labio- or Bucco-lingual Diameter of Crown	Labio- or Bucco-lingual Diameter at Cervix	Curvature of Cervical Line— Mesial	Curvature of Cervical Line— Distal
Dimensions suggested for carving technic	10.0°	17.0	7.5	5.5	8.0	7.0	2.5	1.5

°Millimeters.

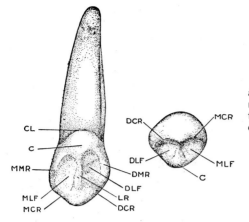

Figure 8–1. Maxillary right canine—lingual aspect—incisal aspect. *CL,* cervical line; *C,* cingulum; *MMR,* mesial marginal ridge; *MLF,* mesiolingual fossa; *MCR,* mesial cusp ridge; *DCR,* distal cusp ridge; *LR,* lingual ridge; *DLF,* distolingual fossa; *DMR,* distal marginal ridge.

DETAILED DESCRIPTION OF THE MAXILLARY CANINE FROM ALL ASPECTS

Labial Aspect (Figs. 8–2, 8–7, 8–8, and 8–9)

The crown and root are narrower mesiodistally than those of the maxillary central incisor. The difference is about 1 mm. in most mouths. The cervical line labially is convex, with the convexity toward the root portion.

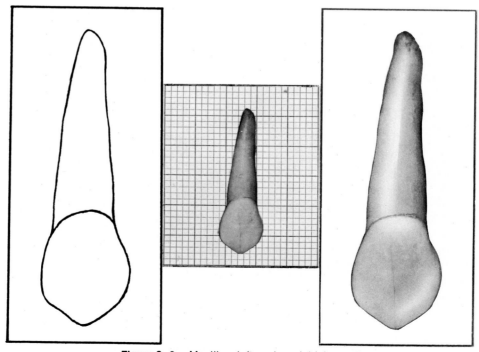

Figure 8–2. Maxillary left canine—labial aspect.

Mesially, the outline of the crown may be convex from the cervix to the center of the mesial contact area; or the crown may exhibit a slight concavity above the contact area from the labial aspect. The center of the contact area mesially is approximately at the junction of middle and incisal thirds of the crown.

Distally, the outline of the crown is usually concave between the cervical line and the distal contact area. The distal contact area is usually at the center of the middle third of the crown. The two levels of contact areas mesially and distally should be noted (Fig. 5–8, B and C).

Unless the crown has been worn unevenly, the cusp tip is on a line with the center of the root. The cusp has a mesial slope and a distal slope, the mesial slope being the shorter of the two. Both slopes show a tendency toward concavity before wear has taken place (Fig. 8–9, specimens 5 and 6). These depressions are developmental in character.

The labial surface of the crown is smooth, with no developmental lines of note except shallow depressions mesially and distally, dividing the three labial lobes. The middle labial lobe shows much greater development than the other lobes. This produces a ridge on the labial surface of the crown. A line drawn over the crest of this ridge, from the cervical line to the tip of the cusp, is a curved one inclined mesially at its center. All areas mesial to the crest of this ridge exhibit convexity except for insignificant developmental lines in the enamel. Distally to the labial ridge (see incisal aspect), there is a tendency toward concavity at the cervical third of the crown, although convexity is noted elsewhere in all areas approaching the labial ridge (Fig. 8–11, specimens 7, 8 and 9).

The root of the maxillary canine appears slender from the labial aspect when compared with the bulk of the crown; it is conical in form with a bluntly pointed apex. It is not uncommon for this root to have a sharp curve in the vicinity of the apical third. This curvature may be in a mesial or distal direction—in most instances the latter (Fig. 8–9, compare specimens 1 and 6). The labial surface of the root is smooth and convex at all points.

Lingual Aspect (Figs. 8–3, 8–7, and 8–8)

The crown and root are narrower lingually than labially.

The cervical line from this aspect differs somewhat from the curvature found labially. The cervical line shows a more even curvature. The line may be straight for a short interval at this point.

The cingulum is large, and in some instances is pointed like a small cusp (see Fig. 8–10, No. 7). In the latter types, definite ridges are found on the lingual surface of the crown below the cingulum and between strongly developed marginal ridges. Although depressions are to be found between these ridge forms, there are seldom any deep developmental grooves.

Very often a well-developed lingual ridge is seen which is confluent with the cusp tip; this extends to a point near the cingulum. There may be shallow concavities between this ridge and the marginal ridges. When these concavities are present, they are called mesial and distal lingual fossae (Figs. 8–1 and 8–8).

Sometimes the lingual surface of the canine crown is so smooth that fossae or minor ridges are difficult to distinguish. There is a tendency toward concavities, however, where the fossae are usually found, and heavy marginal ridges with a well formed cingulum are to be expected. The smooth cingulum, marginal ridges and the lingual portion of the incisal ridges are confluent usually, with little evidence of developmental grooves.

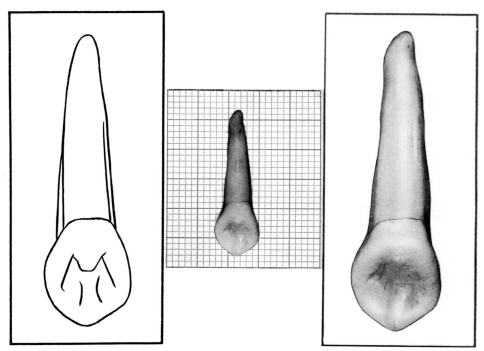

Figure 8–3. Maxillary left canine—lingual aspect.

The lingual portion of the root of the maxillary canine is narrower than the labial portion. Because of this formation, much of the mesial and distal surfaces of the root is visible from the lingual aspect. Developmental depressions mesially and distally may be seen on most of these roots, extending most of the root length. The lingual ridge of the root is rather narrow, but it is smooth and convex at all points from the cervical line to the apical end (Fig. 8–3).

Mesial Aspect (Figs. 8–4, 8–7, 8–8, and 8–10)

The mesial aspect of the maxillary canine presents the outline of the functional form of an anterior tooth. It shows greater bulk generally, however, and greater labiolingual measurement than any of the other anterior teeth.

The outline of the crown is wedge-shaped, the greatest measurement being at the cervical third and the wedge point being represented by the tip of the cusp.

The curvature of the crown below the cervical line labially and lingually corresponds in extent to the curvature of maxillary central and lateral incisors. Nevertheless, the crest of that curvature is found at a level more incisal, since the middle labial and the lingual lobes are more highly developed (Fig. 8–10, specimens 5 and 10). Many canines show a flattened area labially at the cervical third of the crown, which appears as a straight outline from the mesial aspect. It is questionable just how much wear has to do with this effect (Fig. 8–10, specimens 1 and 2).

Below the cervical third of the crown, the labial face may be represented by a line only slightly convex from the crest of curvature at the cervical third to the tip of the cusp. The line usually becomes straighter as it approaches the cusp.

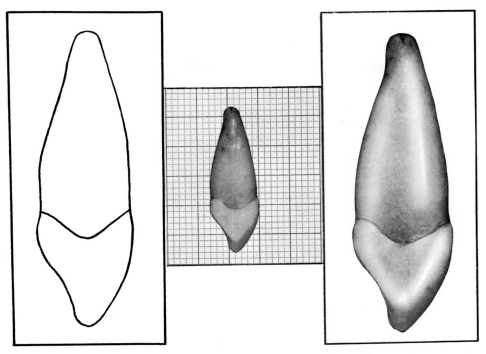

Figure 8–4.   Maxillary left canine — mesial aspect.

The entire labial outline from the mesial aspect exhibits more convexity from the cervical line to the cusp tip than the maxillary central incisor does from cervix to incisal edge.

The lingual outline of the crown from the mesial aspect may be represented by a convex line describing the cingulum, which convexity straightens out as the middle third is reached, becoming convex again in the incisal third (Fig. 8–10, specimen 10).

The cervical line which outlines the base of the crown from this aspect curves toward the cusp, on the average, approximately 2.5 mm. (cementoenamel junction).

The outline of the root from this aspect is conical, with a tapered or bluntly pointed apex. The root may curve labially toward the apical third. The labial outline of the root may be almost perpendicular, with most of the taper appearing on the lingual side (Fig. 8–10, specimens 4 and 9).

The position of the tip of the cusp in relation to the long axis of the root is different from that of maxillary central and lateral incisors. Although the specimen illustrations in Figures 8–4 and 8–5 do not show this difference, most specimens shown in Figure 8–10 show it conclusively. A line bisecting the cusp is labial to a line bisecting the root. Lines bisecting the roots of central and lateral incisors also bisect the incisal ridges.

The mesial surface of the canine crown presents convexities at all points except for a small circumscribed area above the contact area, where the surface is concave or flat between that area and the cervical line.

The mesial surface of the root appears broad, with a shallow developmental depression for part of the root length. Developmental depressions on the heavy roots help to anchor the teeth in the alveoli and help to prevent rotation and displacement.

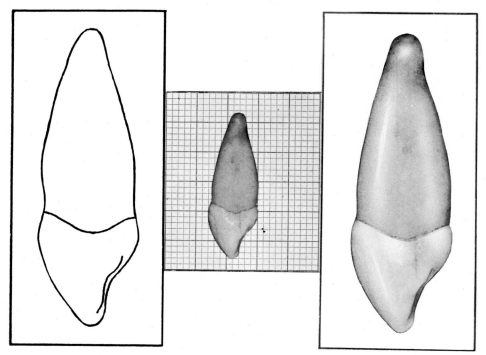

Figure 8–5.   Maxillary left canine – distal aspect.

Distal Aspect (Figs. 8–5, 8–7, and 8–8)

The distal aspect of the maxillary canine shows somewhat the same form as the mesial aspect, with the following variations: The cervical line exhibits less curvature toward the cusp ridge; the distal marginal ridge is heavier and more irregular in outline; the surface displays more concavity, usually, above the contact area, and the developmental depression on the distal side of the root is more pronounced.

Incisal Aspect (Figs. 8–6, 8–7, 8–8, and 8–11)

The incisal aspect of the maxillary canine emphasizes the proportions of this tooth mesiodistally and labiolingually. In general, the labiolingual dimension is greater than the mesiodistal. Occasionally the two measurements are about equal (Fig. 8–11, specimen 8). Other instances appear with the crown larger than usual in a *labiolingual* direction (Fig. 8–11, specimen 10).

From the incisal aspect, if the tooth is correctly posed so that the long axis of the root is directly in the line of vision, the tip of the cusp is *labial* to the *center* of the *crown labiolingually* and *mesial* to the *center mesiodistally*.

If the tooth were to be sectioned labiolingually, beginning at the center of the cusp of the crown, the two sections would show the root rather evenly bisected, with the mesial portion carrying a narrower portion of the crown mesiodistally than that carried by the distal section of the tooth. (Note the proportions demonstrated by the fracture line in the enamel of specimen 9, Fig. 8–11.) Nevertheless, the mesial section

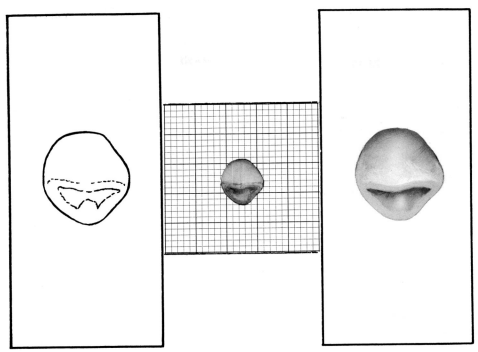

Figure 8–6.   Maxillary left canine—incisal aspect.

shows a crown portion with greater labiolingual bulk. The crown of this tooth gives the impression of having all of the *distal portion stretched* to make *contact* with the first premolar.

The ridge of the middle labial lobe is very noticeable labially from the incisal aspect. It attains its greatest convexity at the cervical third of the crown, becoming broader and flatter at the middle and incisal thirds.

The cingulum development makes up the cervical third of the crown lingually. The outline of the cingulum may be described by a shorter arc than the one labially from this aspect. This comparison coincides with the relative mesiodistal dimensions of the root lingually and labially.

A line bisecting the cusp and cusp ridges drawn in a mesiodistal direction is almost straight and bisects the short arcs representative of the mesial and distal contact areas. This fact emphasizes the close relation between maxillary canines and some lateral incisors, since they resemble each other in this characteristic (compare specimen 7, Fig. 8–11, with specimen 1, Fig. 6–18, Chapter 6). As was mentioned in Chapter 6, there are two types of maxillary lateral incisors: Some resemble canines from the incisal aspect and some resemble central incisors. The latter are supposed to be in the majority. Naturally the lateral incisors that resemble canines are those which are relatively wide labiolingually, and those that resemble central incisors are those which are narrow in that direction.

The incisal aspect of most canines, maxillary or mandibular, may be outlined in many cases by a series of arcs. Specimen 6, Figure 8–11, for example, could be drawn almost perfectly with the aid of a "French curve," a drawing instrument used by draftsmen to draw arcs of varying degrees.

(Text continued on page 184.)

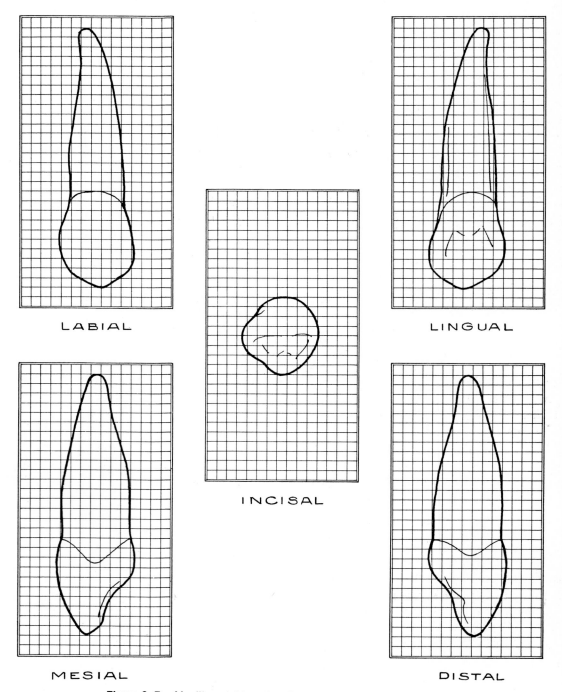

LABIAL

LINGUAL

INCISAL

MESIAL

DISTAL

Figure 8–7.   Maxillary right canine. Graph outlines of five aspects.

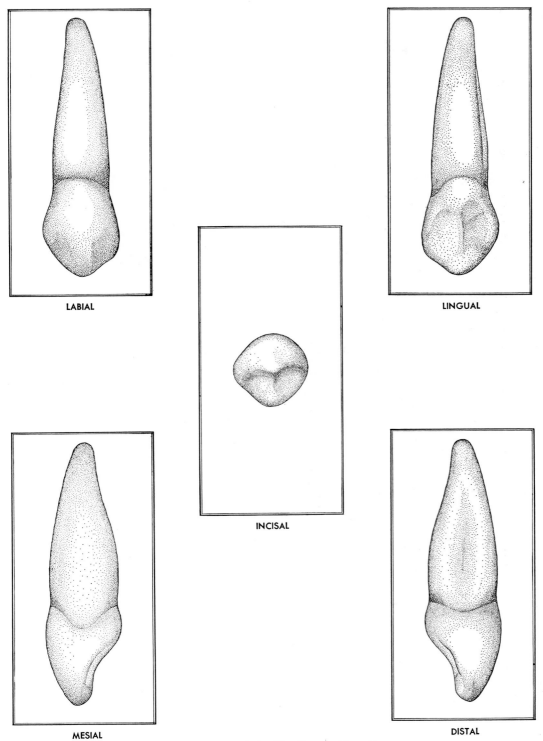

LABIAL

LINGUAL

INCISAL

MESIAL

DISTAL

Figure 8–8. Maxillary right canine.

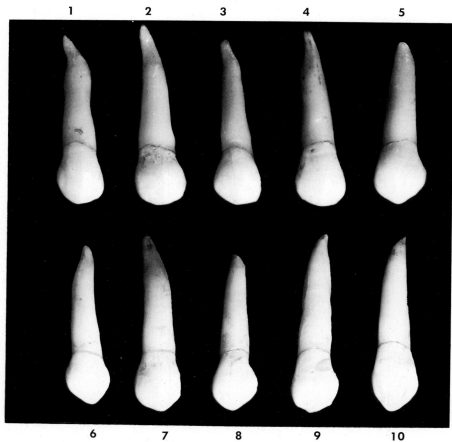

Figure 8–9. Maxillary canine—ten typical specimens—labial aspect.

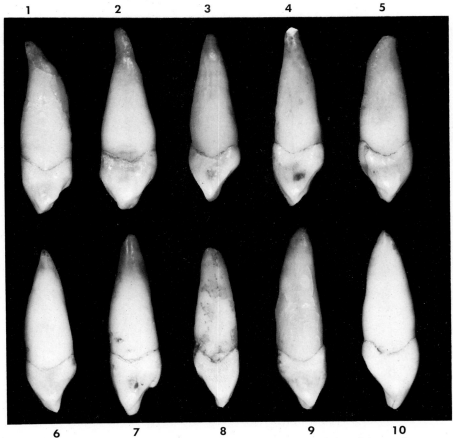

Figure 8–10.   Maxillary canine—ten typical specimens—mesial aspect.

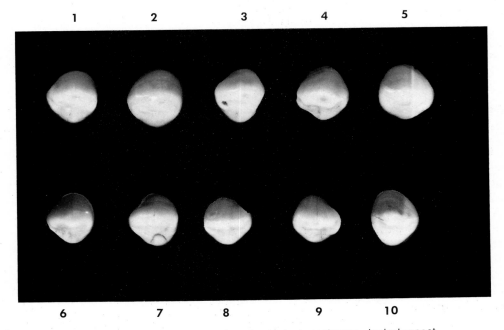

Figure 8–11.   Maxillary canine—ten typical specimens—incisal aspect.

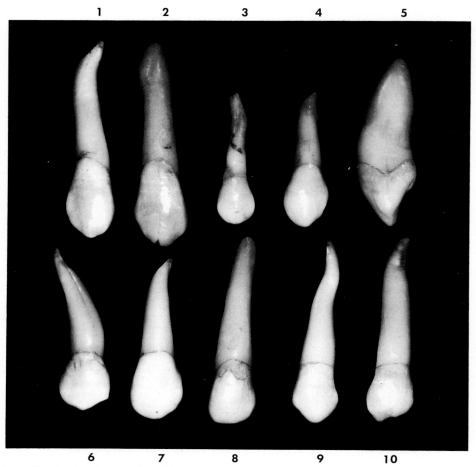

Figure 8–12.   Specimens of maxillary canine—variations. 1, Crown very long, with extreme curvature at apical third of the root. 2, Entire tooth unusually long. Note hypercementosis at root end. 3, Very short crown, root small and malformed. 4, Mesiodistal dimension of crown at contact area extreme, calibration at cervix narrow in comparison; root short for crown of this size. 5, Extreme labiolingual calibration, root with unusual curvature. 6, Tooth malformed generally. 7, Large crown, short root. 8, Root overdeveloped and very blunt at apex. 9, Odd curvature to root, extra length. 10, Crown poorly formed, root extra long.

MANDIBULAR CANINE

Because maxillary and mandibular canines bear a close resemblance to each other, direct comparisons will be made with the maxillary canine in describing the mandibular canine.

The mandibular canine crown is narrower mesiodistally than that of the maxillary canine, although it is just as long in most instances and in many instances is longer by 0.5 to 1 mm. The root may be as long as the maxillary canine, but usually it is somewhat shorter. The labiolingual diameter of crown and root is usually a fraction of a millimeter less, adapting this measurement to the other anteriors.

The lingual surface of the crown is smoother, with less cingulum development and less bulk to the marginal ridges. The lingual portion of this crown resembles the form of the lingual surfaces of mandibular lateral incisors.

Mandibular Canine

First evidence of calcification.... 4 to 5 years
Enamel completed..................... 6 to 7 years
Eruption .... 9 to 10 years
Root completed........................12 to 14 years

Measurement Table

	Cervico-incisal Length of Crown	Length of Root	Mesio-distal Diameter of Crown	Mesio-distal Diameter of Crown at Cervix	Labio- or Bucco-lingual Diameter of Crown	Labio- or Bucco-lingual Diameter at Cervix	Curvature of Cervical Line — Mesial	Curvature of Cervical Line — Distal
Dimensions suggested for carving technic	11.0°	16.0	7.0	5.5	7.5	7.0	2.5	1.0

°Millimeters.

The cusp of the mandibular canine is not so well developed as that of the maxillary canine, and the cusp ridges are thinner labiolingually. Usually the cusp tip is on a line with the center of the root, from the mesial or distal aspect, but sometimes it lies lingual to the line, comparable to mandibular incisors.

A variation in the form of the mandibular canine is *bifurcated* roots. This variation is not rare (Fig. 8–24, specimens 1, 2, 5 and 6).

DETAILED DESCRIPTION OF MANDIBULAR CANINE FROM ALL ASPECTS

Labial Aspect (Figs. 8–14, 8–19, 8–20, and 8–21)

The mesiodistal dimensions of the mandibular canine are less than those of the maxillary canine. The difference is usually about 1 mm. The mandibular canine is

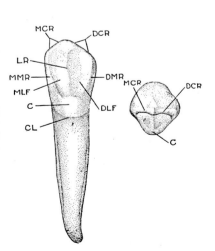

Figure 8–13. Mandibular right canine—lingual aspect—incisal aspect. *DCR*, Distal cusp ridge; *DMR*, distal marginal ridge; *DLF*, distolingual fossa; *CL*, cervical line; *C*, cingulum; *MLF*, mesiolingual fossa; *MMR*, mesial marginal ridge; *LR*, lingual ridge; *MCR*, mesial cusp ridge.

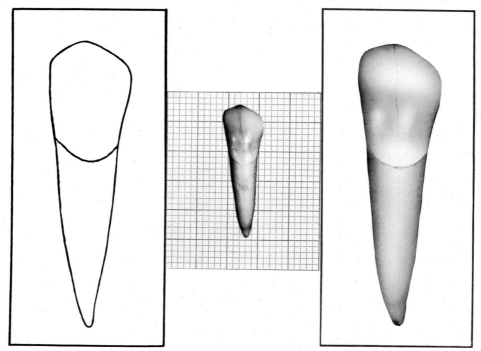

Figure 8–14. Mandibular left canine—labial aspect.

broader mesiodistally than either of the mandibular incisors; for example, about 1 mm. wider than the mandibular lateral incisor.

The essential differences between mandibular and maxillary canines viewed from the labial aspect may be described as follows:

The crowns of the mandibular canines *appear* longer. Sometimes they are longer, but the effect of greater length is emphasized by the narrowness of the crown mesiodistally and the height of the contact areas above the cervix.

The mesial outline of the crown of the mandibular canine is nearly straight with the mesial outline of the root, the mesial contact area being near the mesioincisal angle.

When the cusp ridges have not been affected by wear, the cusp angle is on a line with the center of the root, as on the maxillary canine. The mesial cusp ridge is the shorter.

The distal contact area of the mandibular canine is more toward the incisal than that of the maxillary canine, but not up to the level of the mesial area.

The cervical line labially has a semicircular curvature apically.

Many mandibular canines give the impression from this aspect of being bent distally on the root base. The maxillary canine crowns are more likely to be in line with the root.

The mandibular canine root is shorter by 1 or 2 mm. on the average than that of the maxillary canine, and its apical end is more sharply pointed. When curvature of root ends is present, it is often in a mesial direction. (Fig. 8–21, specimens 1, 2, 3, 4.)

Lingual Aspect (Figs. 8–15, 8–19, and 8–20)

In comparing the lingual aspect of the mandibular canine with the maxillary canine the following differences are noted:

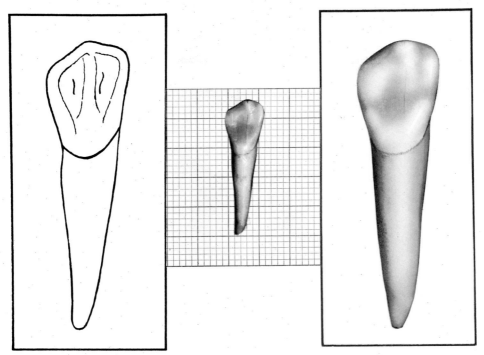

Figure 8–15.   Mandibular left canine—lingual aspect.

The lingual surface of the crown of the mandibular canine is flatter, simulating the lingual surfaces of mandibular incisors. The cingulum is smooth and poorly developed. The marginal ridges are less distinct. This is true also of the lingual ridge except toward the cusp tip, where it is raised. Generally speaking, the lingual surface of the crown is smooth and regular.

The lingual portion of the root is narrower relatively than that of the maxillary canine. It narrows down to little more than half the width of the labial portion.

Mesial Aspect (Figs. 8–16, 8–19, 8–20, and 8–22)

The characteristic differences between the two teeth in question from the mesial aspect are as follows:

The mandibular canine has less curvature labially on the crown, with very little curvature directly above the cervical line. The curvature at the cervical portion is, as a rule, less than 0.5 mm.

The lingual outline of the crown is curved in the same manner as that of the maxillary canine, but it differs in degree. The cingulum is not so pronounced, and the incisal portion of the crown is thiner labiolingually, which allows the cusp to appear more pointed and the cusp ridge more slender. The tip of the cusp is more nearly centered over the root, with a lingual placement in some cases comparable to the placement of incisal ridges on mandibular incisors.

The cervical line curves more toward the incisal portion than does the cervical line on the maxillary canine.

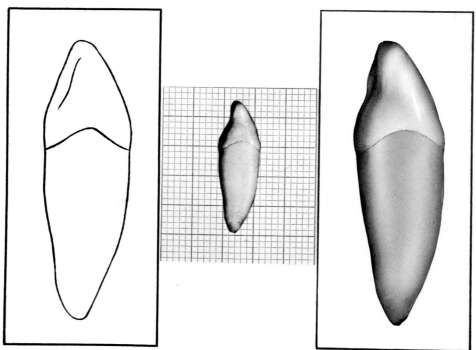

Figure 8–16.   Mandibular left canine—mesial aspect.

The roots of the two teeth are quite similar from the mesial aspect, with the possible exception of a more pointed root tip. The developmental depression mesially on the root of the mandibular canine is more pronounced and sometimes quite deep.

Distal Aspect (Figs. 8–17, 8–19, and 8–20)

There is little difference from the distal aspect between mandibular and maxillary canines except those features mentioned under *mesial aspect*, which are common to both.

Incisal Aspect (Figs. 8–18, 8–19, 8–20, and 8–23)

The outlines of the crowns of mandibular and maxillary canines from the incisal aspect are often similar. The main differences to be noted are these:

The mesiodistal dimension of the mandibular canine is less than the labiolingual dimension. In this, there is a similarity, but the outlines of the mesial surface are less curved. The cusp tip and mesial cusp ridge are more likely to be inclined in a lingual direction, in the mandibular canine with the distal cusp ridge and the contact area extension distinctly so. It will be remembered that the cusp ridges of the maxillary canine with the contact area extensions were more nearly in a straight line mesiodistally from the incisal aspect.

(See following pages for Figures 8–17 through 8–24.)

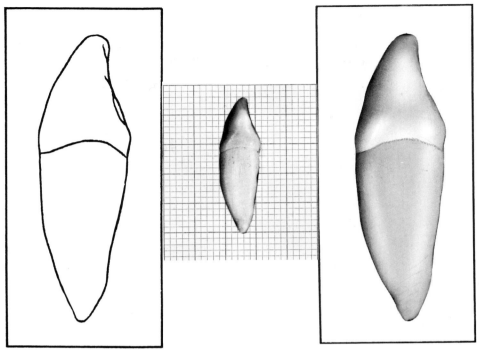

Figure 8–17. Mandibular left canine—distal aspect.

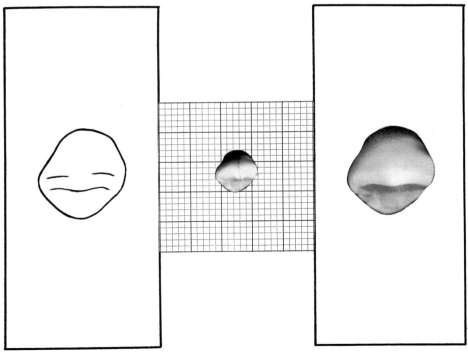

Figure 8–18. Mandibular left canine—incisal aspect.

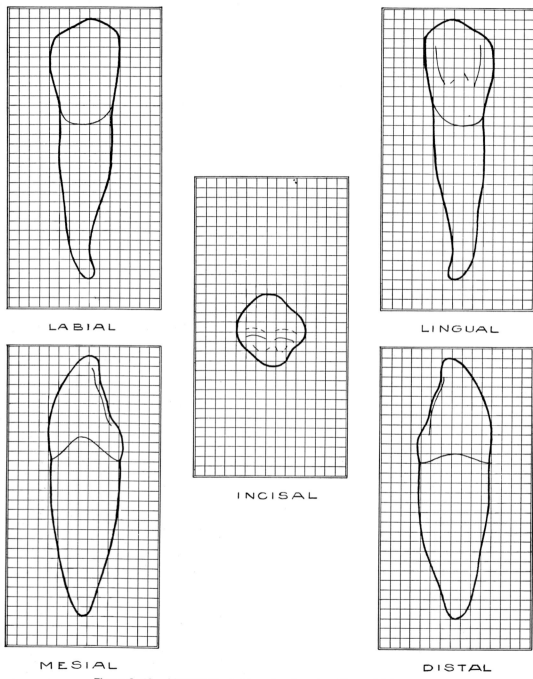

Figure 8–19.   Mandibular right canine. Graph outlines of five aspects.

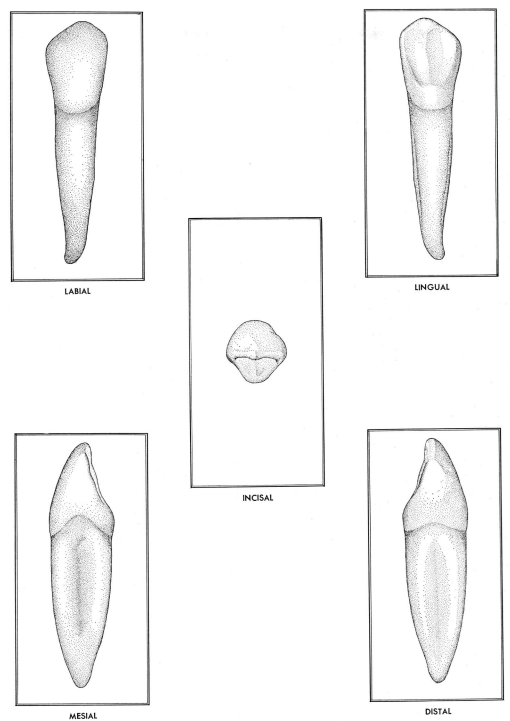

LABIAL

LINGUAL

INCISAL

MESIAL

DISTAL

Figure 8–20. Mandibular right canine.

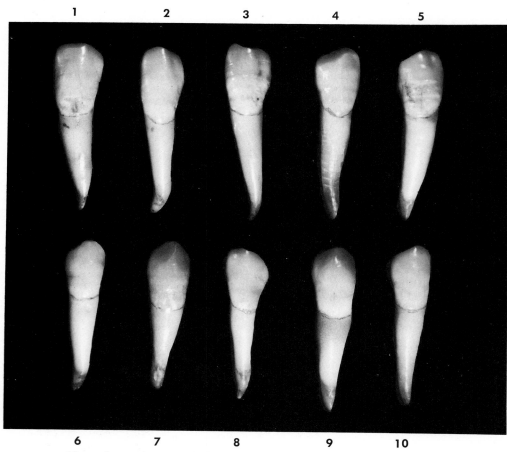

Figure 8–21.   Mandibular canine—ten typical specimens—labial aspect.

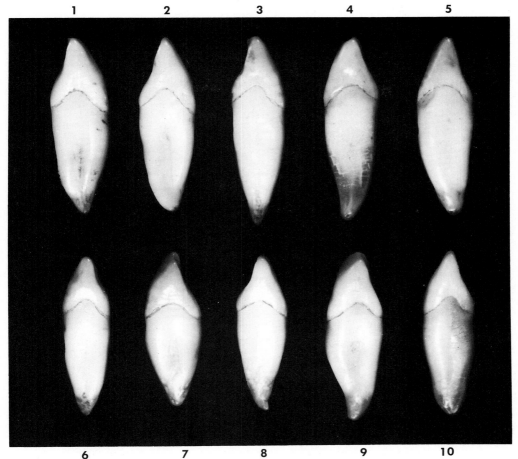

Figure 8–22. Mandibular canine—ten typical specimens—mesial aspect.

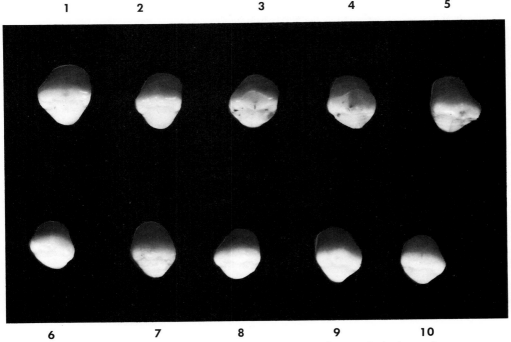

Figure 8–23. Mandibular canine—ten typical specimens—incisal aspect.

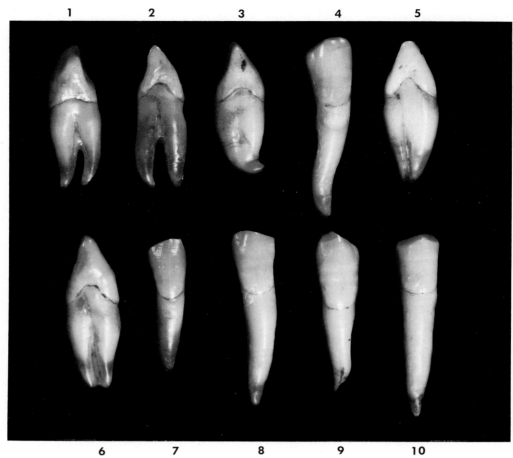

Figure 8–24.   Specimens of mandibular canine—variations. 1, Well-formed crown; two roots, one lingual and one labial. 2, Same as specimen 1, with longer roots. 3, Well-formed crown portion, poorly formed root. 4, Root longer than average, with extreme curvature. 5, Deep developmental groove dividing the root. 6, Same as specimen 5. 7, Crown resembling mandibular lateral incisor, root short. 8, Root extra long, with odd mesial curvature starting at cervical third. 9, Crown extra long and irregular in outline. Root short and poorly formed at apex. 10, Crown with straight mesial and distal sides, wide at cervix, with a root of extreme length.

9

The Permanent
Maxillary Premolars

The maxillary premolars are four in number: two in the right maxilla and two in the left maxilla. They are posterior to the canines and immediately anterior to the molars.

The premolars are so named because they are anterior to the molars in the permanent dentition. In zoology, the premolars are those teeth which succeed the deciduous molars regardless of the number to be succeeded. The term *bicuspid*, which is widely used when one describes human teeth, presupposes two cusps, a supposition which makes the term misleading, since mandibular premolars in the human subject may show a variation in the number of cusps from one to three. Among Carnivora, in the study of comparative dental anatomy, premolar forms differ so greatly that a more descriptive single term than premolar is out of the question. Since the term *premolar* is the one most widely used by all sciences interested in dental anatomy, human and comparative, it is the one which will be given preference here.

The maxillary premolars are developed from the same number of lobes as anterior teeth, which is four. The primary difference in development is the well-formed lingual cusp, developed from the lingual lobe, which is represented by the cingulum development on incisors and canines. The middle buccal lobe on the premolars, corresponding to the middle labial lobe of the canines, remains highly developed, the maxillary premolars resembling the canines when viewed from the buccal aspect. The buccal cusp of the maxillary first premolar, especially, is long and sharp, assisting the canine as a prehensile or tearing tooth. The mandibular first premolar assists the mandibular canine in the same manner.

The *second* premolars, both maxillary and mandibular, have cusps less sharp than the others, and their cusps intercusp with opposing teeth when the jaws are brought together; this makes them more efficient as grinding teeth and they function much like the molars, to a lesser degree.

The maxillary premolar crowns are shorter than those of the maxillary canines, and the roots are shorter also. The root lengths equal those of the molars. The crowns are a little longer than those of the molars.

Because of the cusp development buccally and lingually, the marginal ridges are in a more horizontal plane and are considered part of the occlusal surface of the crown rather than of the lingual surface, as in the case of incisors and canines.

When premolars have two roots, one is placed buccally and one lingually.

MAXILLARY FIRST PREMOLAR

Maxillary First Premolar

First evidence of calcification.....$1\frac{1}{2}$ to $1\frac{3}{4}$ years
Enamel completed......................5 to 6 years
Eruption ....10 to 11 years
Root completed.........................12 to 13 years

Measurement Table

	Cervico-occlusal Length of Crown	Length of Root	Mesio-distal Diam-eter of Crown	Mesio-distal Diam-eter of Crown at Cervix	Labio- or Bucco-lingual Diameter of Crown	Labio- or Bucco-lingual Diameter at Cervix	Curvature of Cervical Line — Mesial	Curvature of Cervical Line — Distal
Dimensions suggested for carving technic	8.5°	14.0	7.0	5.0	9.0	8.0	1.0	0.0

°Millimeters.

The maxillary first premolar has two cusps, a buccal and a lingual, each being sharply defined. The buccal cusp is usually about 1 mm. longer than the lingual cusp. The crown is angular and the buccal line angles prominent.

The crown is shorter than the canine by 1.5 to 2 mm. on the average. Although this tooth resembles the canine from the buccal aspect, it differs in that the contact areas mesially and distally are at about the same level. The root is shorter. If the buccal cusp form has not been changed by wear, the mesial slope of the cusp is longer than the distal slope. The opposite arrangement is true of the maxillary canine. Generally the first premolar is not so wide in a mesiodistal direction as the canine.

Most maxillary first premolars have two roots (Fig. 9–10) and two pulp canals. When only one root is present, two pulp canals are usually found anyway.

The maxillary first premolar has some characteristics common to all posterior teeth. Briefly, these characteristics as differentiated from those of anterior teeth are as follows:

1. Greater relative faciolingual measurement as compared with the mesiodistal measurement.
2. Broader contact areas.
3. Contact areas more nearly at the same level.
4. Less curvature of the cervical line mesially and distally.
5. Shorter crown, cervico-occlusally when compared with anterior teeth.

DETAILED DESCRIPTION OF THE MAXILLARY FIRST PREMOLAR FROM ALL ASPECTS

Buccal Aspect (Figs. 9–2, 9–7, 9–8 and 9–9)

From this aspect the crown is roughly trapezoidal (Chapter 4, Fig. 4–26, C). The crown exhibits little curvature at the cervical line. The crest of curvature of the cervical line buccally is near the center of the root buccally.

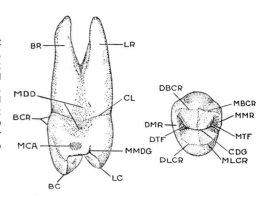

Figure 9–1. Maxillary right first premolar—mesial aspect and occlusal aspect. *LR,* lingual root; *CL,* cervical line; *MMDG,* mesial marginal developmental groove; *LC,* lingual cusp; *BC,* buccal cusp; *MCA,* mesial contact area; *BCR,* buccal cervical ridge; *MDD,* mesial developmental depression; *BR,* buccal root; *MBCR,* mesiobuccal cusp ridge; *MMR,* mesial marginal ridge; *MTF,* mesial triangular fossa (shaded area); *CDG,* central developmental groove; *MLCR,* mesiolingual cusp ridge; *DLCR,* distolingual cusp ridge; *DTF,* distal triangular fossa; *DMR,* distal marginal ridge; *DBCR,* distobuccal cusp ridge.

The mesial outline of the crown is slightly concave from the cervical line to the mesial contact area. The contact area is represented by a relatively broad curvature, the crest of which lies immediately occlusal to the halfway point from the cervical line to the tip of the buccal cusp.

The mesial slope of the buccal cusp is rather straight and longer than the distal slope, which is shorter and more curved. This arrangement places the tip of the buccal cusp distal to a line bisecting the buccal surface of the crown. The mesial slope of the buccal cusp is sometimes notched; in other instances a concave outline is noted at this point (Fig. 9–9, specimens 7, 9 and 10).

The distal outline of the crown below the cervical line is straighter than that of the mesial, although it may be somewhat concave also. The distal contact area is represented by a broader curvature than is found mesially, and the crest of curvature of the contact area tends to be a little more occlusal when the tooth is posed with its long axis vertical. Even so, the contact areas are more nearly level with each other than those found on anterior teeth.

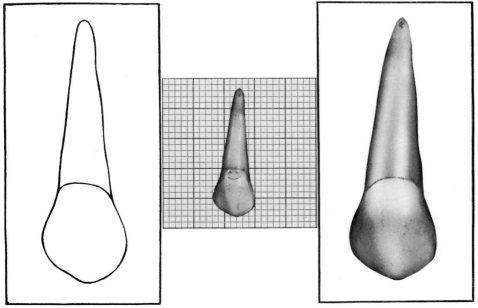

Figure 9–2. Maxillary left first premolar—buccal aspect.

The width of the crown of the maxillary first premolar mesiodistally is about 2 mm. less at the cervix than at its width at the points of its greatest mesiodistal measurement.

The buccal cusp is long, coming to a pointed tip and resembling the canine in this respect, although contact areas in this tooth are near the same level.

The buccal surface of the crown is convex, showing strong development of the middle buccal lobe. The continuous ridge from cusp tip to cervical margin on the buccal surface of the crown is called the *buccal ridge*.

Mesial and distal to the buccal ridge, at or occlusal to the middle third, developmental depressions are usually seen which serve as demarcations between the middle buccal lobe and the mesio- and distobuccal lobes. Although the latter lobes show less development, they are nevertheless prominent and serve to emphasize strong mesiobuccal and distobuccal line angles on the crown (Chapter 4, Fig. 4–22, E).

The roots are 3 or 4 mm. shorter than those of the maxillary canine, although the outline of the buccal portion of the root form bears a close resemblance.

Lingual Aspect (Fig. 9–3, 9–7 and 9–8)

From the lingual aspect, the gross outline of the maxillary first premolar is the reverse of the gross outline of the buccal aspect.

The crown tapers toward the lingual, since the lingual cusp is narrower mesiodistally than the buccal cusp. The lingual cusp is smooth and spheroidal from the cervical portion to the area near the cusp tip. The cusp tip is pointed, with mesial and distal slopes meeting at an angle of about 90 degrees.

Naturally the spheroidal form of the lingual portion of the crown is convex at all points. Sometimes the crest of the smooth lingual portion which terminates at the point of the lingual cusp is called the *lingual ridge*.

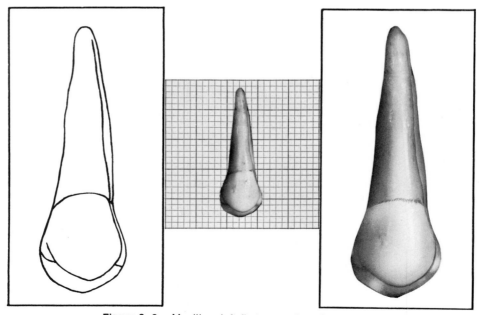

Figure 9–3.   Maxillary left first premolar—lingual aspect.

The mesial and distal outlines of the lingual portion of the crown are convex, these outlines being continuous with the mesial and distal slopes of the lingual cusp, straightening out as they join the mesial and distal sides of the lingual root at the cervical line.

The cervical line lingually is regular, with slight curvature toward the root and the crest of curvature centered on the root. Since the lingual portion of the crown is narrower than the buccal portion, it is possible to see part of the mesial and distal surfaces of crown and root from the lingual aspect, depending upon the posing of the tooth and the line of vision.

Since the lingual cusp is not so long as the buccal cusp, the tips of both cusps, with their mesial and distal slopes, may be seen from the lingual aspect.

The lingual portion of the root, or the lingual portion of the lingual root if two roots are present, is smooth and convex at all points. The apex of the lingual root of a two-root specimen tends to be more blunt than the buccal root apex.

Mesial Aspect (Figs. 9–4, 9–7, 9–8 and 9–10)

The mesial aspect of the crown of the maxillary first premolar is also roughly trapezoidal. However, the longest of the uneven sides is toward the cervical portion and the shortest toward the occlusal portion (Chapter 4, Fig. 4–26, E).

Another characteristic which is representative of all posterior maxillary teeth is that the tips of the cusps are well within the confines of the root trunk (for a definition of root trunk, see Figures 11–3, and 11–8). That is, the measurement from the tip of the buccal cusp to the tip of the lingual cusp is less than the buccolingual measurement of the root at its cervical portion.

Most maxillary first premolars have two roots, one buccal and one lingual; these are clearly outlined from the mesial aspect.

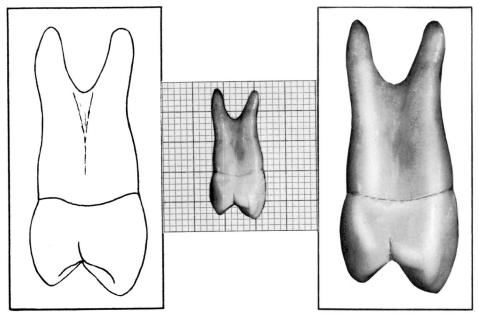

Figure 9–4. Maxillary left first premolar—mesial aspect.

The cervical line may be regular in outline (Fig. 9–10, specimen 1) or irregular (Fig. 9–10, specimen 4). In either case the curvature occlusally is less (about 1 mm. on the average) than the cervical curvature on the mesial of any of the anterior teeth. The extent of the curvature of the cervical line mesially on these teeth is constant within a fraction of a millimeter and is similar to the average curvature to the mesial of all posterior teeth.

The buccal outline of the crown from the mesial aspect curves outward below the cervical line; the crest of curvature is often located approximately at the junction of cervical and middle thirds. Or the crest of curvature may be located within the cervical third (Fig. 9–10, specimens 1 and 10). From the crest of curvature the buccal outline continues as a line of less convexity to the tip of the buccal cusp, which is directly below the center of the buccal root (when two roots are present).

The lingual outline of the crown may be described as a smoothly curved line starting at the cervical line and ending at the tip of the lingual cusp. The crest of this curvature is most often near the center of the middle third. Some specimens show a more abrupt curvature at the cervical third (Fig. 9–10, specimens 2 and 9).

The tip of the lingual cusp is on a line, in most cases, with the lingual border of the lingual root. The lingual cusp is always shorter than the buccal cusp, the average difference being about 1 mm. This difference, however, may be greater (Fig. 9–10, specimens 1, 4, and 10). From this aspect it is noted that the cusps of the maxillary first premolar are long and sharp, with the mesial marginal ridge at about the level of the junction of the middle and occlusal thirds

A distinguishing feature of this tooth is found on the mesial surface of the crown. Immediately cervical to the mesial contact area, centered on the mesial surface, is a marked depression, which continues up to and includes the cervical line (Fig. 9–1). This *mesial developmental depression* is bordered buccally and lingually by the mesiobuccal and mesiolingual line angles. The concavity continues upward beyond the cervical line, joining a deep developmental depression between the roots which ends at the root bifurcation. On single-root specimens, the concavity on the crown and root is plainly seen also, although it may not be so deeply marked. Maxillary second premolars do not have this feature.

Another distinguishing feature of the maxillary first premolar is a well-defined developmental groove in the enamel of the mesial marginal ridge. This groove is in alignment with the developmental depression on the mesial surface of the root but is not usually connected with it. This marginal groove is continuous with the central groove of the occlusal surface of the crown, crossing the marginal ridge immediately lingual to the mesial contact area and terminating a short distance cervical to the mesial marginal ridge on the mesial surface (Fig. 9–10, specimen 10).

The buccal outline of the buccal root, above the cervical line, is straight, with a tendency toward a lingual inclination. On those buccal roots which have a buccal inclination above the root bifurcation, the outline may be relatively straight up to the apical portion of the buccal root, or it may curve buccally at the middle third. Buccal roots may take a buccal or lingual inclination, apical to middle thirds.

The lingual outline of the lingual root is rather straight above the cervical line. It may not exhibit much curvature between the cervix and the apex. Many cases, however, show considerable curvature to lingual roots apical to the middle thirds. It may take a buccal or lingual inclination (Fig. 9–10, specimens 1, 2 and 9).

The root trunk is long on this tooth, making up about half of the root length. The bifurcation on those teeth with two roots begins at a more occlusal point mesially than distally. Generally speaking, when bifurcated, the root is bifurcated for half its total length.

Except for the deep developmental groove and depression at or below the bifurcation, the mesial surface of the root portion of this tooth is smoothly convex buccally and lingually. Even when one root only is present, the developmental depression is very noticeable for most of the root length. The latter instances show roots with buccal and lingual outlines ending in a blunt apex above the center of the crown (Fig. 9–10, specimens 4 and 5).

Distal Aspect (Figs. 9–5, 9–7, and 9–8)

From the distal aspect the anatomy of crown and root of the maxillary first premolar differs from that of the mesial aspect as follows.

The crown surface is convex at all points except for a small flattened area just cervical to the contact area and buccal to the center of the distal surface.

The curvature of the cervical line is less on the distal than on the mesial surface, often showing a line straight across from buccal to lingual.

There is no evidence of a deep developmental groove crossing the distal marginal ridge of the crown. If a developmental groove should be noticeable, it is shallow and insignificant.

The root trunk is flattened on the distal surface above the cervical line with no outstanding developmental signs.

The bifurcation of the roots is abrupt near the apical third, with no developmental groove leading to it such as one finds mesially.

Occlusal Aspect (Figs. 9–6, 9–7, 9–8, 9–11, 9–13, 9–14, and 9–15)

The occlusal aspect of the maxillary first premolar resembles roughly a six-sided or hexagonal figure (Fig. 9–13). The six sides are made up of the mesiobuccal (which

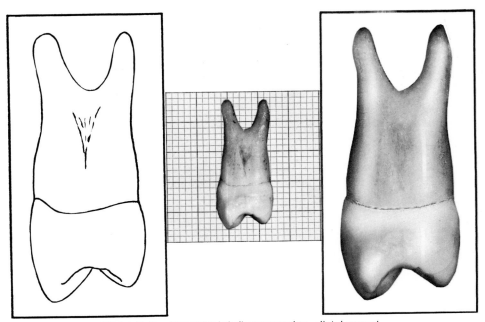

Figure 9–5. Maxillary left first premolar—distal aspect.

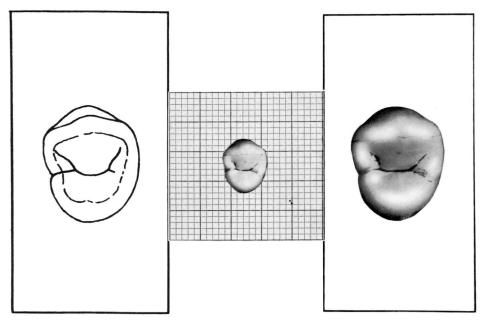

Figure 9–6. Maxillary left first premolar—occlusal aspect.

is mesial to the buccal ridge), mesial, mesiolingual (which is mesial to the lingual ridge), distolingual, distal and distobuccal. This hexagonal figure is not, however, equilateral. The two buccal sides are nearly equal, the mesial side is shorter than the distal side and the mesiolingual side is shorter than the distolingual side (Fig. 9–13).

The relation and position of various anatomic points are to be considered from the occlusal aspect. A drawing of the outline of this occlusal aspect, when placed within a rectangle the dimensions of which represent the mesiodistal and buccolingual width of the crown, demonstrates the relative positions of the mesial and distal contact areas and also those of the buccal and lingual ridges (Fig. 9–14). (See also Fig. 9–6.)

The crest of the distal contact area is somewhat buccal to that of the mesial contact area, and the crest of the buccal ridge is somewhat distal to that of the lingual ridge. The crests of curvature represent the highest points on the buccal and lingual ridges and the mesial and distal contact areas.

Close observation of the crown from this aspect reveals the following characteristics (Fig. 9–14).

1. The distance from the buccal crest (*A*) to the mesial crest (*C*) is slightly longer than the distance from the buccal crest to the distal crest (*D*).

2. The distance from the mesial crest to the lingual crest is much shorter than the distance from the distal crest to the lingual crest.

3. The crown is wider on the buccal than on the lingual.

4. The buccolingual dimension of the crown is much greater than the mesiodistal dimension.

The occlusal surface of the maxillary first premolar is circumscribed by the cusp ridges and marginal ridges. The mesiobuccal and distobuccal cusp ridges are in line with each other, and their alignment is in a distobuccal direction. In other words, even though they are in the same alignment, the distobuccal cusp ridge is buccal to the mesiobuccal cusp ridge (Fig. 9–15).

INDIVIDUAL TOOTH FORM

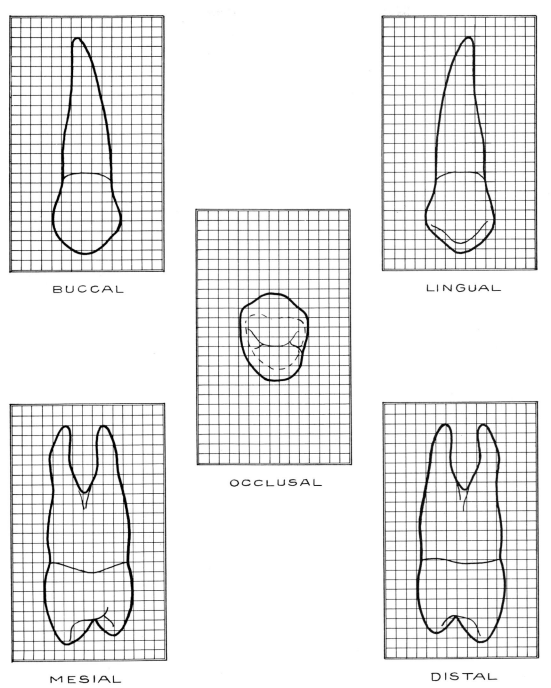

BUCCAL

LINGUAL

OCCLUSAL

MESIAL

DISTAL

Figure 9–7.   Maxillary right first premolar. Graph outlines of five aspects.

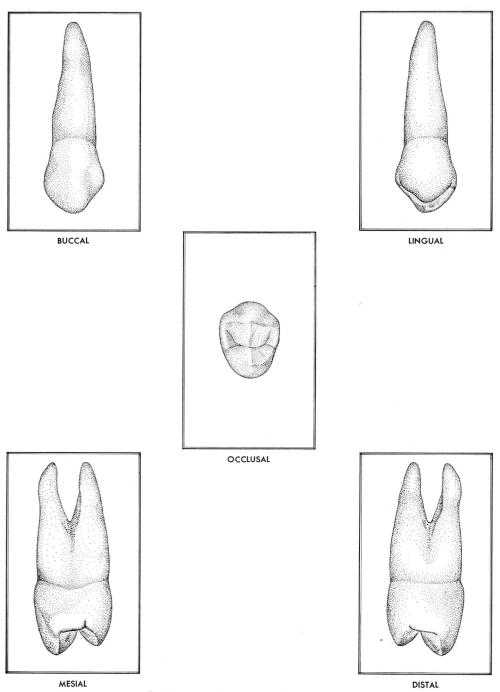

BUCCAL

LINGUAL

OCCLUSAL

MESIAL

DISTAL

Figure 9–8.   Maxillary right first premolar.

1   2   3   4   5

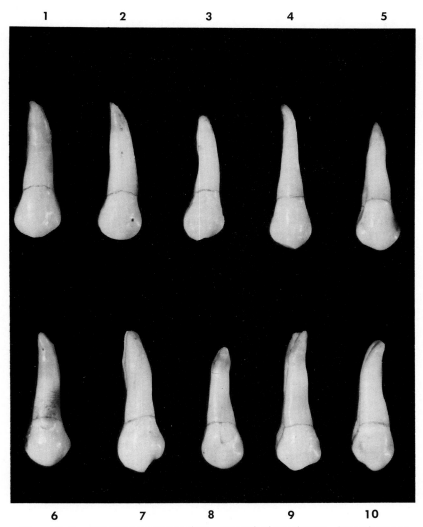

6   7   8   9   10

Figure 9–9.   Maxillary first premolars—ten typical specimens—buccal aspect.

The angle formed by the convergence of the mesiobuccal cusp ridge and the mesial marginal ridge approaches a right angle. The angle formed by the convergence of the distobuccal cusp ridge and the distal marginal ridge is acute. The mesiolingual and distolingual cusp ridges are confluent with the mesial and distal marginal ridges; these cusp ridges are curved, following a semicircular outline from the marginal ridges to their convergence at the tip of the lingual cusp.

When looking at the occlusal aspect of the maxillary first premolar, posing the tooth so that the line of vision is in line with the long axis, one sees more of the buccal surface of the crown than of the lingual surface. It should be remembered that when one looks at the tooth from the mesial aspect, the tip of the buccal cusp is nearer the center of the root trunk than is the lingual cusp.

The occlusal surface of this tooth has no supplemental grooves in most cases, a fact which makes the surface relatively smooth. A well-defined central developmental groove divides the surface evenly buccolingually. This groove is called the *central*

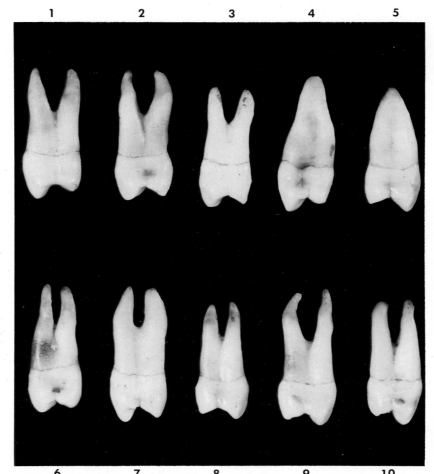

Figure 9–10. Maxillary first premolars — ten typical specimens — mesial aspect.

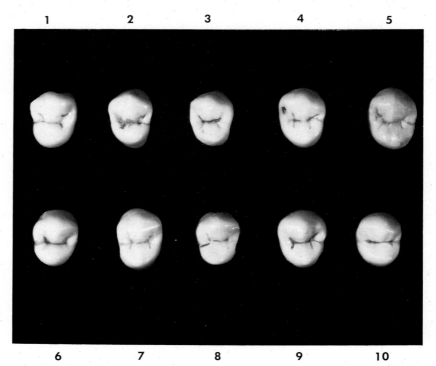

Figure 9–11. Maxillary first premolars — ten typical specimens — occlusal aspect.

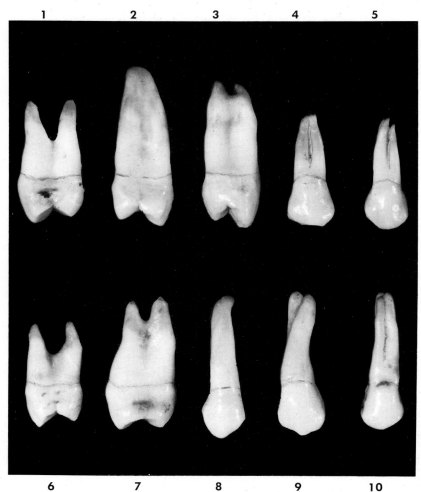

Figure 9–12. Maxillary first premolars—ten specimens showing uncommon variations. 1, Constricted occlusal surface, short roots. 2, Single root of extreme length. 3, Constricted occlusal surface, mesial developmental groove indistinct on mesial surface of root. 4, Short root form, with two buccal roots fused. 5, Short root form, with two buccal roots showing bifurcation. 6, Short roots, with considerable separation. 7, Buccolingual calibration greater than usual. 8, Root extremely long, distal contact area high. 9, Twisted buccal root. 10, Three roots fused; uncommonly long also.

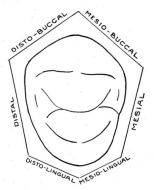

Figure 9–13. Maxillary first premolar—hexagonal figure—occlusal aspect.

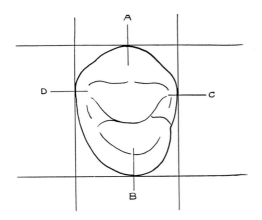

Figure 9–14. Maxillary first premolar—occlusal aspect. *A*, crest of buccal ridge. *B*, crest of lingual ridge. *C*, crest of mesial contact area. *D*, crest of distal contact area.

developmental groove. It is located at the bottom of the central sulcus of the occlusal surface, extending from a point just mesial to the distal marginal ridge to the mesial marginal ridge, where it joins the *mesial marginal developmental groove;* this latter crosses the mesial marginal ridge and ends on the mesial surface of the crown (Figs. 9–1 and 9–4).

Two collateral developmental grooves join the central groove just inside the mesial and distal marginal ridges. These grooves are called the *mesiobuccal developmental groove* and the *distobuccal developmental groove.* The junctions of the grooves are deeply pointed and are named the *mesial* and *distal developmental pits.*

Just distal to the mesial marginal ridge, the triangular depression which harbors the mesiobuccal developmental groove is called the *mesial triangular fossa.* The depression in the occlusal surface, just mesial to the distal marginal ridge, is called the *distal triangular fossa.*

Although no supplemental grooves are present in most instances, smooth developmental depressions may be visible radiating from the central groove and giving the occlusal surface an uneven appearance.

The *buccal triangular ridge* of the buccal cusp is prominent, arising near the center of the central groove and converging with the tip of the buccal cusp. The *lingual triangular ridge* is less prominent; it also arises near the center of the central groove and converges with the tip of the lingual cusp.

The lingual cusp is pointed more sharply than the buccal cusp.

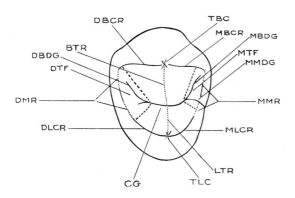

Figure 9–15. Maxillary first premolar—occlusal aspect. *TBC*, tip of buccal cusp; *MBCR*, mesiobuccal cusp ridge; *MBDG*, mesiobuccal developmental groove; *MTF*, mesial triangular fossa; *MMDG*, mesial marginal developmental groove; *MMR*, mesial marginal ridge; *MLCR*, mesiolingual cusp ridge; *LTR*, lingual triangular ridge; *TLC*, tip of lingual cusp; *CG*, central groove; *DLCR*, distolingual cusp ridge; *DMR*, distal marginal ridge; *DTF*, distal triangular fossa; *DBDG*, distobuccal developmental groove; *BTR*, buccal triangular ridge; *DBCR*, distobuccal cusp ridge. (Compare with Fig. 9–1.)

MAXILLARY SECOND PREMOLAR

Maxillary Second Premolar

First evidence of calcification.....2 to 2¼ years
Enamel completed......................6 to 7   years
Eruption..................................10 to 12   years
Root completed........................12 to 14   years

Measurement Table

	Cervico-occlusal Length of Crown	Length of Root	Mesio-distal Diam-eter of Crown	Mesio-distal Diam-eter of Crown at Cervix	Labio- or Bucco-lingual Diameter of Crown	Labio- or Bucco-lingual Diameter at Cervix	Curvature of Cervical Line — Mesial	Curvature of Cervical Line — Distal
Dimensions suggested for carving technic	8.5°	14.0	7.0	5.0	9.0	8.0	1.0	0.0

°Millimeters.

The maxillary second premolar supplements the maxillary first premolar in function (Figs. 9–16 to 9–24). The two teeth resemble each other so closely that detailed description of each aspect of the second premolar will be unnecessary. Direct comparison will be made between it and the first premolar, variations being mentioned.

Compare, therefore, the accompanying illustrations of the two teeth and observe following variations:

The maxillary second premolar is less angular, giving a more rounded effect to the crown from all aspects. It has a single root.

Considerable variations in the relative sizes of the two teeth may be seen, since the second premolar does not appear true to form as often as does the first premolar. The maxillary second premolar may have a crown which is noticeably smaller cervico-occlusally and also mesiodistally. On the other hand, it may be larger in those dimensions. Usually the root length of the second premolar is as great, if not a millimeter or so greater, than that of the first premolar. The two teeth have about the same dimensions *on the average,* except for the tendency toward greater length to the second premolar root.

From the buccal aspect it may be noticed that the buccal cusp of the second premolar is not so long as that of the first premolar, and it appears less pointed. Also, the mesial slope of the buccal cusp ridge is usually shorter than the distal slope. The opposite is true of the first premolar.

In a good many instances the crown and root of the second premolar are thicker at their cervical portions. This is not, however, the rule (Fig. 9–21, specimens 5, 6, 7 and 9). The buccal ridge of the crown may not be so prominent when compared with the first premolar.

From the lingual aspect little variation may be seen except that the lingual cusp is longer, making the crown longer on the lingual side.

(Text continued on page 214.)

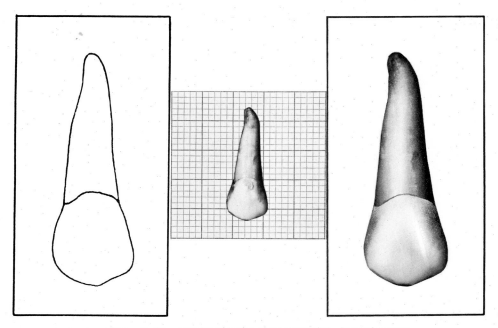

Figure 9–16.   Maxillary left second premolar — buccal aspect.

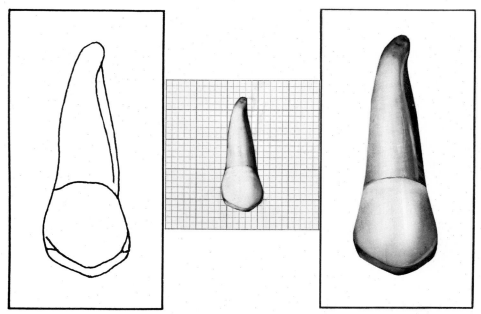

Figure 9–17.   Maxillary left second premolar — lingual aspect.

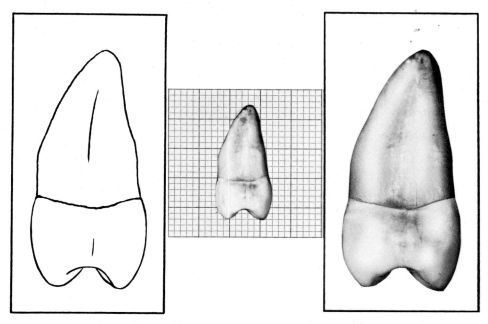

Figure 9–18.   Maxillary left second premolar—mesial aspect.

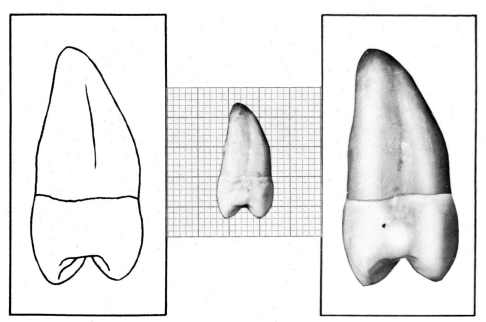

Figure 9–19.   Maxillary left second premolar—distal aspect.

212

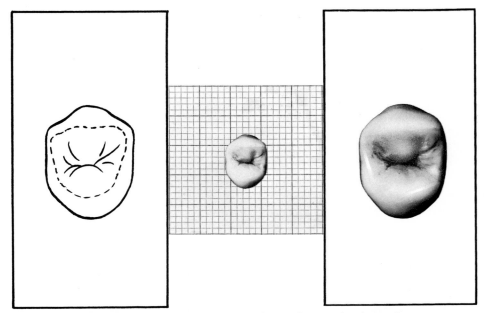

Figure 9–20. Maxillary left second premolar — occlusal aspect.

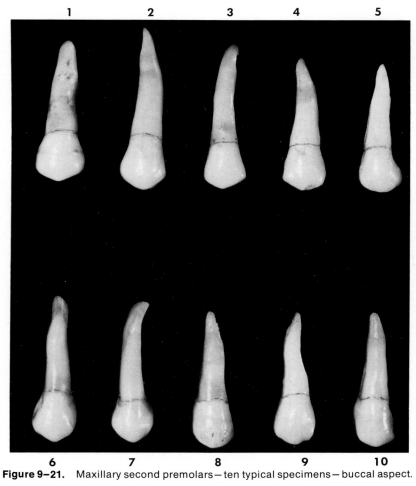

Figure 9–21. Maxillary second premolars — ten typical specimens — buccal aspect.

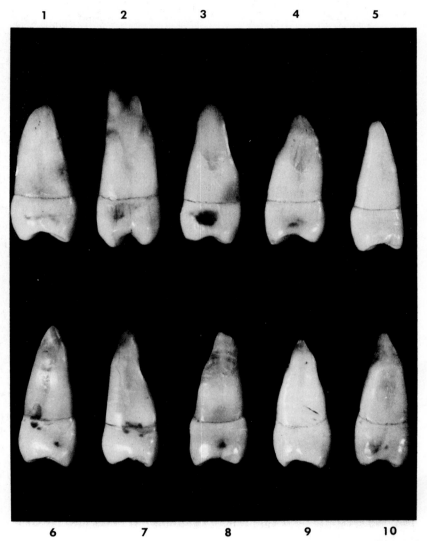

Figure 9–22.   Maxillary second premolar — ten typical specimens — mesial aspect.

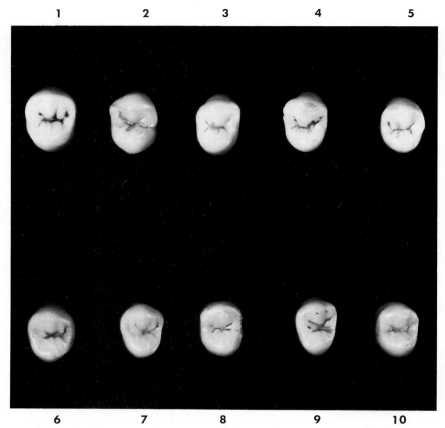

Figure 9–23. Maxillary second premolars — ten typical specimens — occlusal aspect.

The mesial aspect shows the difference in cusp length between the two teeth. The cusps of the second premolar are shorter, with the buccal and lingual cusps more nearly the same length. There may be greater distance between cusp tips — a condition which widens the occlusal surface buccolingually.

There is no deep developmental depression on the mesial surface of the crown as on the first premolar; the crown surface is convex instead. A shallow developmental groove appears on the single tapered root.

There is no deep developmental groove crossing the mesial marginal ridge, and except for the variation in root form there is no outstanding variation to be noted when one views the distal aspect.

From the *occlusal* aspect, some differences are to be noted between the two premolars: the outline of the crown is more rounded or oval, rather than angular. There are, of course, exceptions. The central developmental groove is shorter and more irregular, and there is a tendency toward multiple supplementary grooves radiating from the central groove. These supplementary grooves terminate in shallow depressions in the enamel which may extend out to the cusp ridges.

This arrangement makes for an irregular occlusal surface and gives the surface a very wrinkled appearance.

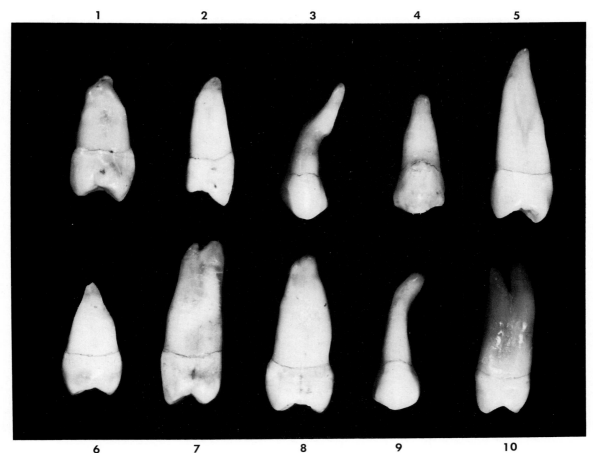

Figure 9–24. Maxillary second premolars—ten specimens showing uncommon variations. 1, Root dwarfed and malformed. 2, Broad occlusal surface, lingual outline of crown straight. 3, Malformed root. 4, Crown very broad mesiodistally, root dwarfed. 5, Root extremely long. 6, Root dwarfed and very pointed at apex. 7, Root extremely long, bifurcation at root end. 8, Crown wider than usual buccolingually, curvature at cervical third extreme. 9, Root malformed, thick at apical third. 10, Root unusually long, bifurcated at apical third.

10

The Permanent
Mandibular Premolars

The mandibular premolars are four in number: Two are situated in the right side of the mandible and two in the left side. They are immediately posterior to the mandibular canines and anterior to the molars.

The mandibular first premolars are developed from four *lobes* as were the maxillary premolars. The mandibular second premolars are, in most instances, developed from five lobes, three buccal and two lingual lobes.

The first premolar has a large buccal *cusp,* which is long and well formed, with a small nonfunctioning lingual cusp that in some specimens is no larger than the cingulum found on some maxillary canines (Fig. 10–10, specimens 3 and 8; Fig. 10–12, specimens 4 and 7). The second premolar has three well-formed cusps in most cases, one large buccal cusp and two smaller lingual cusps. The form of both mandibular premolars fails to conform to the implications of the term "bicuspid," which term implies two functioning cusps.

The mandibular first premolar has many of the characteristics of a small canine, since its sharp buccal cusp is the only part of it occluding with maxillary teeth. It functions along with the mandibular canine. The mandibular second premolar has more of the characteristics of a small molar, because its lingual cusps are well developed, a fact which places both marginal ridges high and which produces a more efficient occlusion with antagonists in the opposite jaw. It functions by being supplementary to the mandibular first molar.

The first premolar is always the smaller of the two *mandibular* premolars, whereas the opposite is true, in many cases, of the *maxillary* premolars.

MANDIBULAR FIRST PREMOLAR

The mandibular first premolar is the fourth tooth from the median line and the first posterior tooth in the mandible. This tooth is situated between the canine and second premolar and has some characteristics common to each of them.

The characteristics which resemble those of the *mandibular canine* are as follows:

1. The buccal cusp is long and sharp and is the only occluding cusp.

216

Mandibular First Premolar

First evidence of calcification... 1¾ to 2 years
Enamel completed................... 5   to 6 years
Eruption.............................10   to 12 years
Root completed.......................12   to 13 years

Measurement Table

	Cervico-occlusal Length of Crown	Length of Root	Mesio-distal Diam-eter of Crown	Mesio-distal Diam-eter of Crown at Cervix	Labio- or Bucco-lingual Diameter of Crown	Labio- or Bucco-lingual Diameter of Crown at Cervix	Curvature of Cervical Line – Mesial	Curvature of Cervical Line – Distal
Dimensions suggested for carving technic	8.5°	14.0	7.0	5.0	7.5	6.5	1.0	0.0

°Millimeters.

2. The buccolingual measurement is similar to that of the canine.

3. The occlusal surface slopes sharply lingually in a cervical direction.

4. The mesiobuccal cusp ridge is shorter than the distobuccal cusp ridge.

5. The outline form of the occlusal aspect resembles the outline form of the incisal aspect of the canine. (Compare Figs. 10–6 and 8–18.)

The characteristics which resemble those of the *second mandibular premolar* are as follows:

1. Except for the longer cusp, the outline of crown and root from the buccal aspect resembles the second premolar.

2. The contact areas, mesially and distally, are near the same level.

3. The curvatures of the cervical line mesially and distally are similar.

4. It has more than one cusp.

Although the root of the mandibular first premolar is shorter as a rule than that of the mandibular second premolar, it is closer to the length of the second premolar root than it is to that of the mandibular canine.

DETAILED DESCRIPTION OF THE MANDIBULAR FIRST PREMOLAR FROM ALL ASPECTS

Buccal Aspect (Figs. 10–2, 10–7, 10–8 and 10–9)

From the buccal aspect, the form of the mandibular first premolar crown is nearly symmetrical bilaterally. The middle buccal lobe is well developed, resulting in a large, pointed buccal cusp. The mesial cusp ridge is shorter than the distal cusp ridge. The contact areas are broad from this aspect; they are almost at the same level mesially and distally, this level being a little more than half the distance from cervical line to cusp tip. The measurement mesiodistally at the cervical line is small when it is compared with the measurement at the contact areas.

From the buccal aspect, the crown is roughly trapezoidal (Chapter 4, Fig. 4–26, C). The cervical margin is represented by the shortest of the uneven sides.

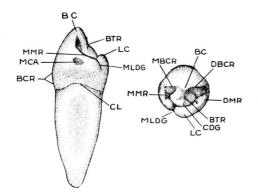

Figure 10–1.   Mandibular right first premolar—mesial aspect and occlusal aspect. *BC*, buccal cusp; *BTR*, buccal triangular ridge; *LC*, lingual cusp; *MLDG*, mesiolingual developmental groove; *CL*, cervical line; *BCR*, buccal cervical ridge; *MCA*, mesial contact area; *MMR*, mesial marginal ridge; *MBCR*, mesiobuccal cusp ridge.

The crown exhibits little curvature at the cervical line buccally, caused by the slight curvature of the cervical line on the mesial and distal surfaces of the tooth. The crest of curvature of the cervical line buccally approaches the center of the root buccally.

The mesial outline of the crown is straight or slightly concave above the cervical line to a point where it joins the curvature of the mesial contact area. The center of the contact area mesially is occlusal to the cervical line, a distance equal to a little more than half the crown length. The outline of the mesial slope of the buccal cusp usually shows some concavity unless wear has obliterated the original form.

The tip of the buccal cusp is pointed and is, in most cases, located a little mesial

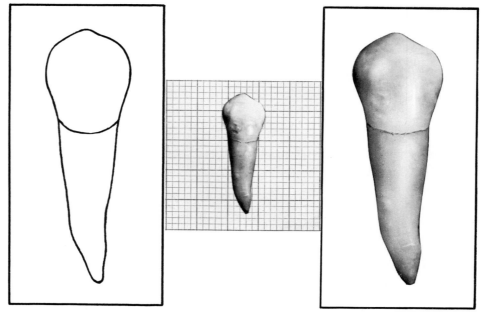

Figure 10–2.   Mandibular right first premolar—buccal aspect.*

---

*The specimen in this photograph shows a mesial inclination of the root. Mandibular premolars and canines have this tendency although most of the roots of these teeth will curve, if at all, in a distal direction.

to the center of the crown buccally (Fig. 9–9, specimens 3, 7, 8 and 9). The mandibular canine has the same characteristic to a greater degree.

The distal outline of the crown is slightly concave above the cervical line to a point where it is confluent with the curvature describing the distal contact area. This curvature is broader than that describing the curvature of the mesial contact area. The distal slope of the buccal cusp usually exhibits some concavity.

The cervix of the mandibular first premolar crown is narrow mesiodistally when compared with the crown width at the contact areas.

The root of this tooth is 3 or 4 mm. shorter than that of the mandibular canine, although the outline of the buccal portion of the root bears a close resemblance to the canine.

The buccal surface of the crown is more convex than in the maxillary premolars, especially at the cervical and middle thirds.

The development of the middle buccal lobe is outstanding, ending in a pointed buccal cusp. Developmental depressions are often seen between the three lobes (Fig. 9–9, specimens 2, 3, 8, and 10).

The continuous ridge from the cervical margin to the cusp tip is called the *buccal ridge.*

In general, the enamel of the buccal surface of the crown is smooth and shows no developmental grooves and few developmental lines. If the latter are present, they are seen as very fine horizontal cross lines at the cervical portion.

Lingual Aspect (Figs. 10–3, 10–7, and 10–8)

The crown of the mandibular first premolar tapers toward the lingual, since the lingual measurement mesiodistally is less than that buccally. The lingual cusp is

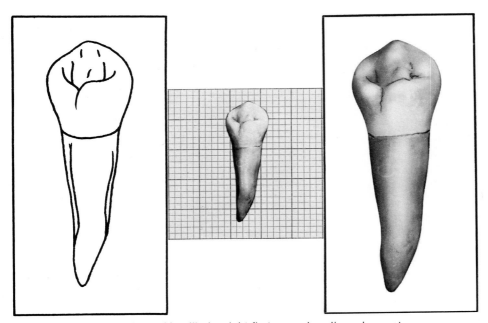

Figure 10–3.   Mandibular right first premolar—lingual aspect.

always small. The major portion of the crown is made up of the middle buccal lobe (Fig. 10–11). This makes it resemble the canine.

The crown and the root taper markedly toward the lingual, so that most of the mesial and distal surfaces of both may be seen from the lingual aspect.

The occlusal surface slopes greatly toward the lingual in a cervical direction down to the short lingual cusp. Most of the occlusal surface of this tooth can therefore be seen from this aspect.

The cervical portion of the crown lingually is narrow and convex, with concavities in evidence between the cervical line and the contact areas on the lingual portion of mesial and distal surfaces. The contact areas and marginal ridges are pronounced and extend out above the narrow cervical portion of the crown.

Although the lingual cusp is short and poorly developed (resembling a strongly developed cingulum at times), it usually shows a pointed tip. This cusp tip is in alignment with the buccal triangular ridge of the occlusal surface, which is in plain view. The mesial and distal occlusal fossae are on each side of the triangular ridge (See Fig. 10–1.)

A characteristic of the lingual surface of the mandibular first premolar is the *mesiolingual developmental groove*. This groove acts as a line of demarcation between the mesiobuccal lobe and the lingual lobe and extends into the mesial fossa of the occlusal surface.

The root of this tooth is much narrower on the lingual side, and there is a narrow ridge, smooth and convex, the full length of the root. This formation allows most of the mesial and distal surfaces of the root to be seen. Often developmental depressions in the root may be seen with developmental grooves mesially. The root of this tooth tapers evenly from the cervix to a pointed apex.

Mesial Aspect (Figs. 10–4, 10–7, 10–8 and 10–10)

From the mesial aspect, the mandibular first premolar shows an outline which is fundamental and characteristic of all mandibular posterior teeth when viewed from the mesial or distal aspect. The crown outline is roughly rhomboidal (Chapter 4, Fig. 4–26, *E*), and the tip of the buccal cusp is nearly centered over the root. The convexity of the outline of the lingual lobe is lingual to the outline of the root. The surface of the crown presents an overhang above the root trunk in a lingual direction. The tip of the cusp will be on a line approximately with the lingual border of the root. This differs from the condition found in maxillary posterior teeth, where both buccal and lingual cusp tips are well within the confines of the root trunks.

The mandibular first premolar, when viewed from the mesial aspect, often shows the buccal cusp centered over the root (Fig. 10–4). In other instances the buccal cusp tip is a little buccal to the center, corresponding to the typical placement of buccal cusps on all mandibular posterior teeth.

The buccal outline of the crown from this aspect is prominently curved from the cervical line to the tip of the buccal cusp; the crest of curvature is near the middle third of the crown. This accented convexity and the location of the crest of contour are characteristic of all mandibular posterior teeth on the buccal surfaces.

The lingual outline of the crown, representative of the lingual outline of the lingual cusp, is a curved outline of less convexity than that of the buccal surface. The crest of curvature lingually approaches the middle third of the crown, the curvature

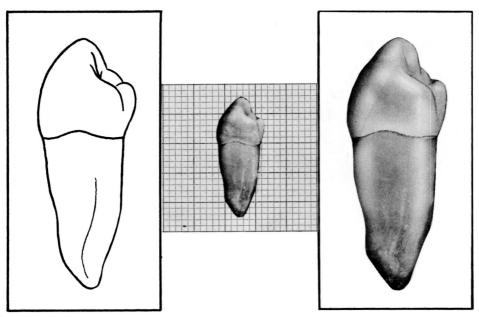

Figure 10–4. Mandibular right first premolar — mesial aspect.

ending at the tip of the lingual cusp which is in line with the lingual border of the root.

The distance from the cervical line lingually to the tip of the lingual cusp is about two-thirds of that from the cervical line buccally to the tip of the buccal cusp.

The mesiobuccal lobe development is prominent from this aspect; it creates by its form the mesial contact area and the mesial marginal ridge, which in turn has a sharp inclination lingually in a cervical direction. The lingual border of the mesial marginal ridge merges with the developmental depression mesiolingually; this harbors the mesiolingual developmental groove.

Some of the occlusal surface of the crown mesially may be seen with the mesial portion of the buccal triangular ridge. The slope of this ridge parallels the mesial marginal ridge, although the crest of the triangular ridge is above it. The sulcus formed by the convergence of buccal and lingual triangular ridges is directly above the mesiolingual groove from this aspect.

The cervical line on the mesial surface is rather regular, curving occlusally. The crest of the curvature is centered buccolingually, the average curvature being about 1 mm. in extent. It may, however, be a fraction of a millimeter, or the line may be straight across buccolingually.

The surface of the crown mesially is smooth except for the mesiolingual groove. The surface is plainly convex at the mesial contact area, which is centered on a line with the tip of the buccal cusp. Immediately below the convexity of the contact area the surface is sharply concave between that area and the cervical line. The distance between the contact area and the cervical line is very short.

The root outline from the mesial aspect is a tapered form from the cervix, ending in a relatively pointed apex in line with the tip of the buccal cusp. The lingual outline may be straight, the buccal outline more curved.

The mesial surface of the root is smooth and flat from the buccal margin to the center. From this point, it too converges sharply toward the root center lingually, often displaying a deep developmental groove in this area. Shallow grooves are nearly always in evidence, and occasionally a deep developmental groove will end in a bifurcation at the apical third (Fig. 10–12, specimens 5 and 7).

Distal Aspect (Figs. 10–5, 10–7 and 10–8)

The distal aspect of the mandibular first premolar differs from the mesial aspect in some respects. The distal marginal ridge is higher above the cervix, and it does not have the extreme lingual slope of the mesial marginal ridge, being more nearly at right angles to the axis of crown and root. The marginal ridge is confluent with the lingual cusp ridge; it has no developmental groove on the distal marginal ridge. The major portion of the distal surface of the crown is smoothly convex, the spheroidal form having an unbroken curved surface. Below this curvature and just above the cervical line, a concavity is to be noted which is linear in form and which extends buccolingually. The distal contact area is broader than the mesial, although it is centered in the same relation to the crown outlines. The center of the distal contact area is at a point midway between buccal and lingual crests of curvature and midway between the cervical line and the tip of the buccal cusp.

The curvature of the cervical line distally may be the same as that found mesially, although less curvature distally is the general rule when one is describing all posterior teeth.

The surface of the root distally exhibits more convexity than was found mesially. A shallow developmental depression is centered on the root, but rarely does it contain a deep developmental groove.

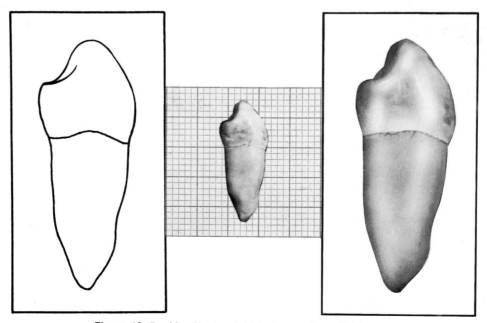

Figure 10–5. Mandibular right first premolar—distal aspect.

The distal surface slopes from the buccal margin toward the center of the root lingually, but the slope is more gradual than that found mesially.

Occlusal Aspect (Figs. 10–6, 10–7, 10–8 and 10–11)

The occlusal aspects of many specimens show considerable variation in the gross outlines of this tooth. Both mandibular premolars exhibit more variations in form occlusally than the maxillary premolars.

The usual outline form of the mandibular first premolar from the occlusal aspect is roughly diamond-shaped and similar to the incisal aspect of mandibular canines (Fig. 10–11, specimens 1, 3, 4, 7, 8, 9 and 10). Some of these teeth have a circular form similar to that of some mandibular second premolars (specimen 2); others conform to the gross outlines of the more common second premolars (specimens 5 and 6).

The characteristics common to all mandibular first premolars, regardless of type, when viewed from the occlusal aspect are these:

1. The middle buccal lobe makes up the major bulk of the tooth crown.

2. The buccal ridge is prominent.

3. The mesiobuccal and distobuccal line angles are prominent even though rounded.

4. The curvatures representing the contact areas, immediately lingual to the buccal line angles, are relatively broad, the distal area being the broader of the two.

5. The crown converges sharply to the center of the lingual surface, starting from points approximating the mesial and distal contact areas. This formation makes that part of the crown represented by buccal cusp ridges, marginal ridges and lingual lobe triangular in form, with the base of the triangle at the buccal cusp ridges and the point of the triangle at the lingual cusp.

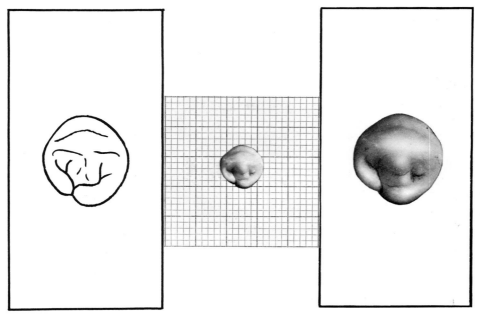

Figure 10–6.   Mandibular right first premolar — occlusal aspect.

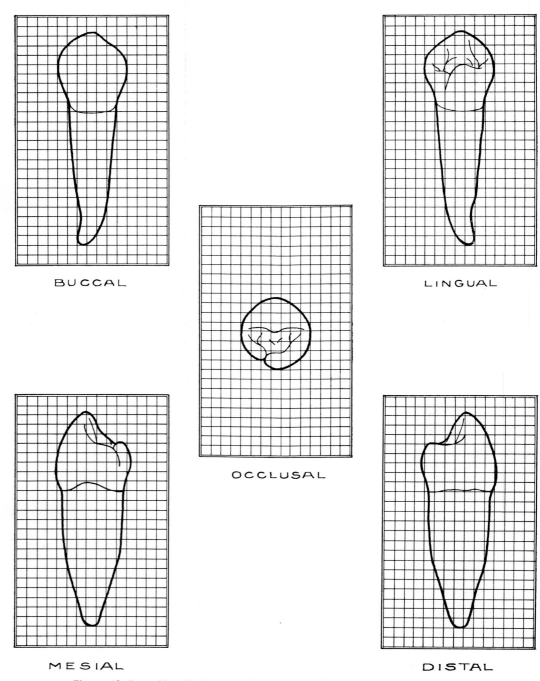

BUCCAL

LINGUAL

OCCLUSAL

MESIAL

DISTAL

Figure 10–7. Mandibular right first premolar. Graph outlines of five aspects.

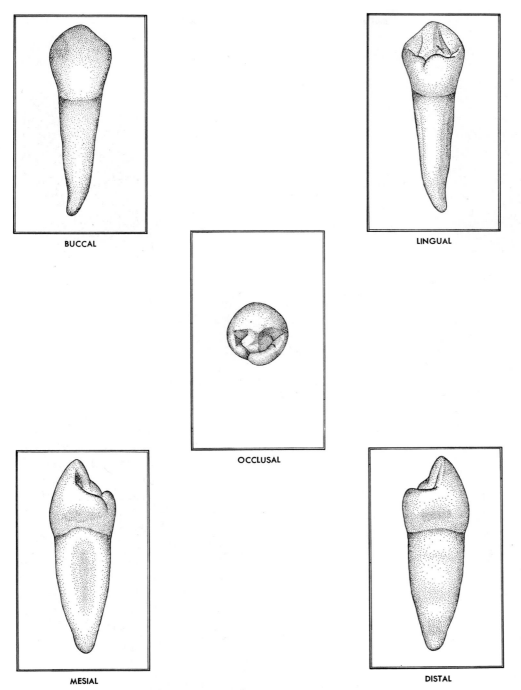

BUCCAL

LINGUAL

OCCLUSAL

MESIAL

DISTAL

Figure 10–8.   Mandibular right first premolar.

1   2   3   4   5

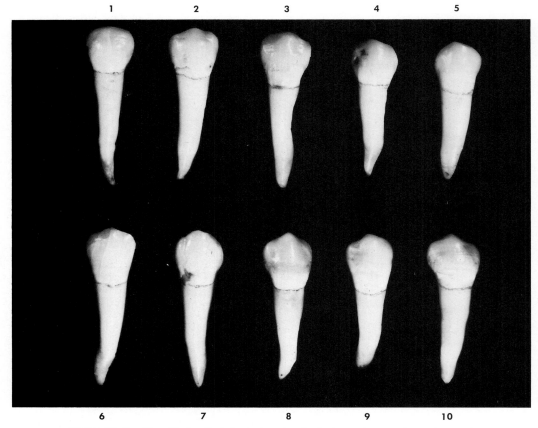

6   7   8   9   10

Figure 10–9.   Mandibular first premolar—ten typical specimens—buccal aspect.

6. The marginal ridges are well developed.

7. The lingual cusp is small.

8. The occlusal surface shows a heavy buccal triangular ridge and a small lingual triangular ridge.

9. The occlusal surface harbors two depressions which are called the *mesial* and *distal fossae* because of their irregularity of form, although they correspond in location to the mesial and distal triangular fossae of other posterior teeth.

The most common type of mandibular first premolars shows a mesiolingual developmental depression and groove. These constrict the mesial surface of the crown and create a smaller mesial contact area which is in contact with the mandibular canine. The distal portion of the crown is described by a larger arc which creates a broader contact area in contact with the second mandibular premolar, which has a broader proximal surface than the canine. (See Fig. 5–2.)

The mesial fossa is more linear in form, being more sulcate and containing the *mesial developmental groove,* which extends buccolingually. This groove is confluent with its extension, which becomes the *mesiolingual developmental groove* as it passes over to the mesiolingual surface. The distal fossa is more circular in most cases and is circumscribed by the distobuccal cusp ridge, the distal marginal ridge, the buccal triangular ridge and the distolingual cusp ridge.

The distal fossa may contain a distal developmental groove which is crescent-

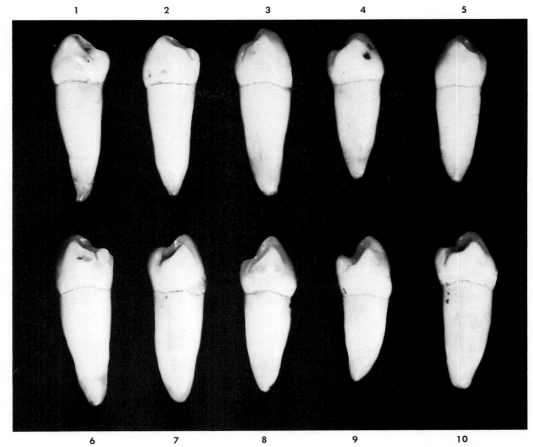

Figure 10–10. Mandibular first premolar—ten typical specimens—mesial aspect.

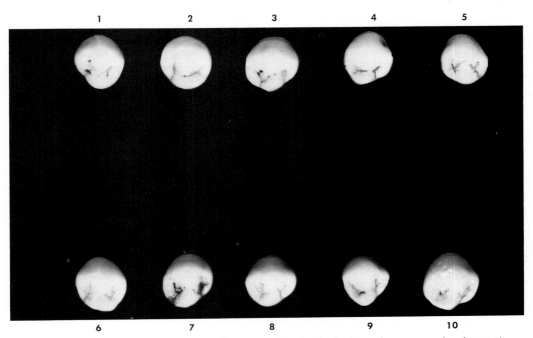

Figure 10–11. Mandibular first premolar—ten typical specimens— occlusal aspect.

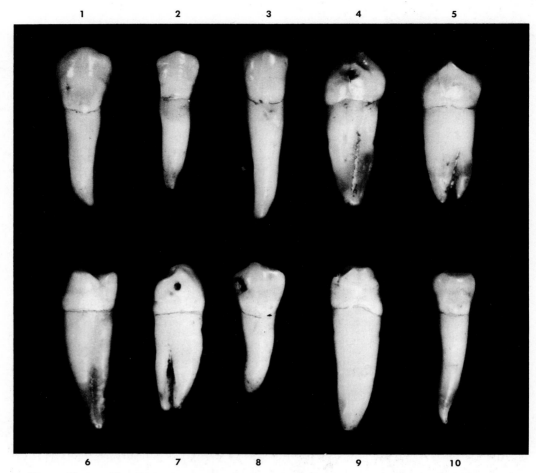

Figure 10–12. Mandibular first premolar—ten specimens showing uncommon variations. 1, Crown oversize. 2, Crown and root diminutive. 3, Mesial and distal sides of crown straight, cervix wide mesiodistally, root extra long. 4, Unusual formation of lingual portion of crown, root with deep developmental groove mesially. 5, Bifurcated root. 6, Lingual cusp long, little lingual curvature, root of extra length. 7, No lingual cusp, root bifurcated. 8, Dwarfed root. 9, Crown poorly formed, root unusually long. 10, Very long curved root for crown so small.

shaped (Fig. 10–11, specimen 2). It may harbor a distal developmental pit with accessory supplemental grooves radiating from it (specimen 10), or it may contain a linear groove running mesiodistally with an arrangement resembling the typical triangular fossa (specimens 4, 5 and 6).

Because of the position of this crown over the root, most of the buccal surface may be seen from the occlusal aspect, whereas very little of the lingual surface is in view.

MANDIBULAR SECOND PREMOLAR

The mandibular second premolar resembles the mandibular first premolar from the buccal aspect only. Although the buccal cusp is not so pronounced, the mesiodistal measurement of the crown and its general outline are similar. The tooth is larger

Mandibular Second Premolar

First evidence of calcification... 2¼ to 2½ years
Enamel completed .... 6 to 7 years
Eruption ....11 to 12 years
Root completed ....13 to 14 years

Measurement Table

	Cervico-occlusal Length of Crown	Length of Root	Mesio-distal Diameter of Crown	Mesio-distal Diameter of Crown at Cervix	Labio- or Bucco-lingual Diameter of Crown	Labio- or Bucco-lingual Diameter at Cervix	Curvature of Cervical Line – Mesial	Curvature of Cervical Line – Distal
Dimensions suggested for carving technic	8.0°	14.5	7.0	5.0	8.0	7.0	1.0	0.0

° Millimeters.

and has better development in other respects. There are two common forms which this tooth assumes: The first form, which probably occurs most often, is the *three-cusp* type, which appears more angular from the occlusal aspect (Fig. 10–17). The second form is the *two-cusp* type, which appears more rounded from the occlusal aspect. (Fig. 10–20, specimens 1, 2, 7 and 10.)

The two types differ mainly in the occlusal design. The outlines and general appearance from all other aspects are similar.

The single root of the second premolar is larger and longer than that of the first premolar. The root is seldom if ever bifurcated, although some specimens show a deep developmental groove buccally (Fig. 10–18, specimens 3 and 6). Often a flattened area appears in this location.

DETAILED DESCRIPTION OF THE MANDIBULAR SECOND PREMOLAR FROM ALL ASPECTS

In describing the separate aspects of this tooth, direct comparisons are made with the mandibular first premolar except for the occlusal aspect.

Buccal Aspect (Figs. 10–13 and 10–18)

From the buccal aspect the mandibular second premolar presents a shorter buccal cusp than the first premolar, with mesiobuccal and distobuccal cusp ridges presenting angulation of less degree. The contact areas, both mesial and distal, are broad. The contact areas appear to be higher because of the short buccal cusp.

The root is broader mesiodistally than that of the first premolar, the extra breadth appearing for most of its length, and the root ends in an apex which is more blunt. In other respects the two teeth are quite similar from this aspect.

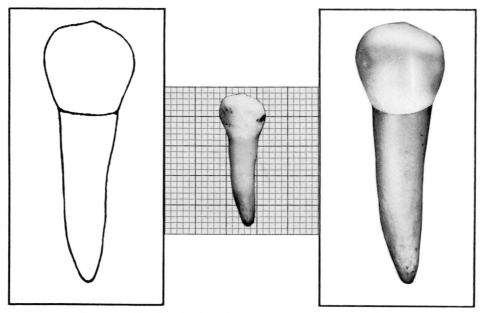

Figure 10–13. Mandibular left second premolar—buccal aspect.

Lingual Aspect (Fig. 10–14)

From the lingual aspect, the second premolar crown shows considerable variation from the crown portion of the first premolar. The variations are as follows:

1. The lingual lobes are developed to a greater degree, making the cusp or cusps (depending on the type) longer.

2. Less of the occlusal surface may be seen from this aspect. Nevertheless, since the lingual cusps are not as long as the buccal cusp, part of the buccal portion of the occlusal surface may be seen.

3. In the three-cusp type, the lingual development brings about the greatest variation between the two teeth. There are a mesiolingual and a distolingual cusp, the former being the larger and the longer one in most cases. There is a groove between them extending a very short distance on the lingual surface and usually centered over the root (Fig. 10–20, specimen 8).

In the two-cusp type, the single lingual cusp development attains equal height with the three-cusp type. The two-cusp type has no groove, but it shows a developmental depression distolingually where the lingual cusp ridge joins the distal marginal ridge (Fig. 10–20, specimens 2 and 3).

The lingual surface of the crown of all mandibular second premolars is smooth and spheroidal, having a bulbous form above the constricted cervical portion.

The root is wide lingually, although not quite so wide as the buccal portion. There is less difference in dimension than was found on the first premolar, a fact which creates much less convergence toward the lingual.

Since in most instances the lingual portion of the crown converges little from the buccal portion, less of the mesial and distal sides of this tooth may be seen from this aspect than are seen from the lingual aspect of the first premolar.

The lingual portion of the root is smoothly convex for most of its length.

Considered overall, the second premolar is the larger of the two mandibular premolars.

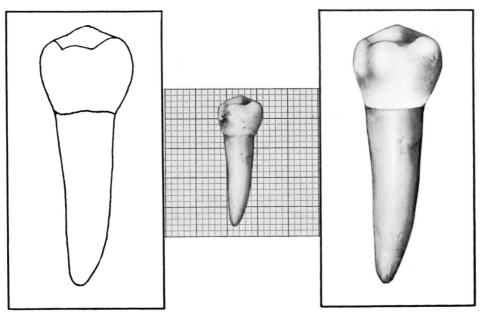

Figure 10–14.   Mandibular left second premolar—lingual aspect.

Mesial Aspect (Figs. 10–15 and 10–19)

The second premolar differs from the first premolar from the mesial aspect as follows:

1. The crown and root are wider buccolingually than in the first premolar.
2. The buccal cusp is not so nearly centered over the root trunk, and it is shorter.

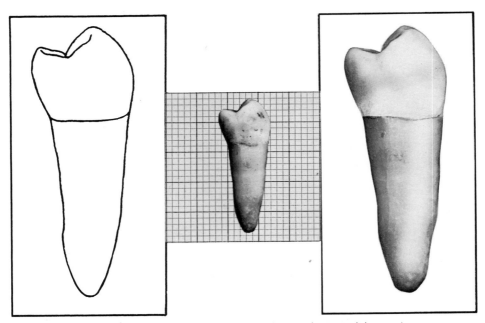

Figure 10–15.   Mandibular left second premolar—mesial aspect.

3. The lingual lobe development is greater.
4. The marginal ridge is at right angles to the long axis of the tooth.
5. Less of the occlusal surface may be seen.
6. There is no mesiolingual developmental groove on the crown portion.
7. The root is longer and in most cases slightly convex on the mesial surface. (This convexity is not, however, always present. See Fig. 10–19, specimens 6, 7, and 8.)
8. The apex of the root is usually more blunt on the second premolar.

Distal Aspect (Fig. 10–16)

This aspect of the mandibular second premolar is similar to the mesial aspect except that more of the occlusal surface may be seen. This is possible, since the distal marginal ridge is at a lower level than the mesial marginal ridge when one is posing the tooth vertically. The crowns of all posterior teeth are tipped distally to the long axes of the roots, so that when the specimen tooth is held vertically more of the occlusal surface may be seen from the distal aspect than from the mesial aspect. This is a characteristic possessed by all posterior teeth, mandibular, and maxillary. The angulation of occlusal surfaces to long axes of all posterior teeth is an important observation to remember, not only in the study of individual tooth forms but later on in the study of alignment and occlusion.

Occlusal Aspect (Figs. 10–17 and 10–20)

As mentioned before, there are two common forms of this tooth. The outline form of each type shows some variation from the occlusal aspect. The two types are similar in that portion which is buccal to the mesiobuccal and distobuccal cusp ridges.

The three-cusp type appears square lingual to the buccal cusp ridges when highly developed (Fig. 10–20, specimen 8). The round, or two-cusp, type appears round lingual to the buccal cusp ridges (Fig. 10–20, specimen 3).

The square type (specimen 8) has three cusps that are distinct; the buccal cusp is the largest, the mesiolingual cusp is next, and the distolingual cusp is the smallest.

Each cusp has well-formed triangular ridges separated by deep developmental grooves. These grooves converge in a *central pit* and form a Y on the occlusal surface. The central pit is located midway between the buccal cusp ridge and the lingual margin of the occlusal surface and slightly distal to the central point between mesial and distal marginal ridges.

Starting at the central pit, the *mesial developmental groove* travels in a mesiobuccal direction and ends in the *mesial triangular fossa* just distal to the mesial marginal ridge. The *distal developmental groove* travels in a distobuccal direction, is somewhat shorter than the mesial groove, and ends in the *distal triangular fossa* mesial to the distal marginal ridge. The lingual developmental groove extends lingually between the two lingual cusps and ends on the lingual surface of the crown just below the convergence of the lingual cusp ridges. The mesiolingual cusp is wider mesiodistally than the distolingual cusp. This arrangement places the lingual developmental groove distal to center on the crown.

Supplemental grooves and depressions are often seen, radiating from the devel-

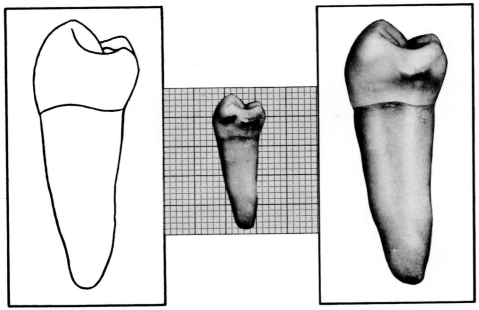

Figure 10–16. Mandibular left second premolar—distal aspect.

opmental grooves. Occasionally a groove crosses one or both of the marginal ridges. On a tooth of this type the point angles are distinct. Developmental grooves are often deep.

Specimen 8 (Fig. 10–20) is representative. Variations of this development may be seen in specimens 4, 5, 6 and 9.

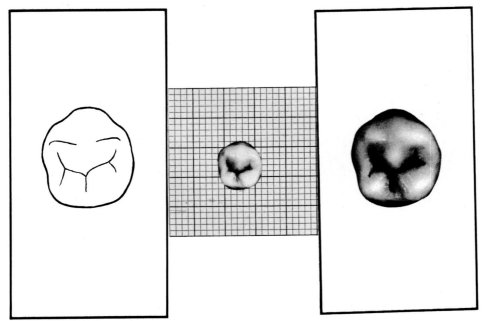

Figure 10–17. Mandibular left second premolar—occlusal aspect.

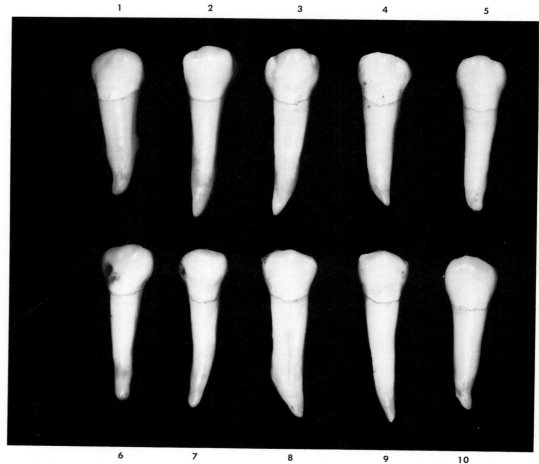

Figure 10–18.   Mandibular second premolar—ten typical specimens—buccal aspect.

The round, or two-cusp type (specimen 3) differs considerably from the three-cusp type when viewed from the occlusal aspect. Specimen 3 is a true typal form of the two-cusp type. Variations may be seen in specimens 1, 2, 7 and 10.

The *occlusal* characteristics of the two-cusp type are as follows:

1. The outline of the crown is rounded lingual to the buccal cusp ridges.

2. There is some lingual convergence of mesial and distal sides, although no more than is found in some variations of the square type.

3. The mesiolingual and distolingual line angles are rounded.

4. There is one well-developed lingual cusp directly opposite the buccal cusp in a lingual direction.

A *central developmental groove* on the occlusal surface travels in a mesiodistal direction. This groove may be straight (Fig. 10–20, specimen 3), but it is most often crescent-shaped (specimens 1, 7 and 10). The central groove has its terminals centered in *mesial* and *distal fossae,* which are roughly circular depressions having supplemental grooves and depressions radiating from the central groove and its terminals. The enamel surface inside these fossae and around their peripheries is very

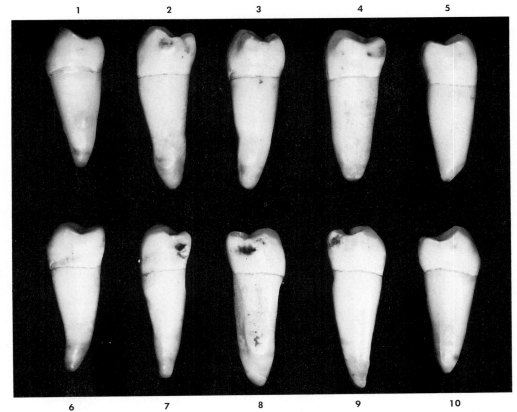

Figure 10–19. Mandibular second premolar—ten typical specimens—mesial aspect.

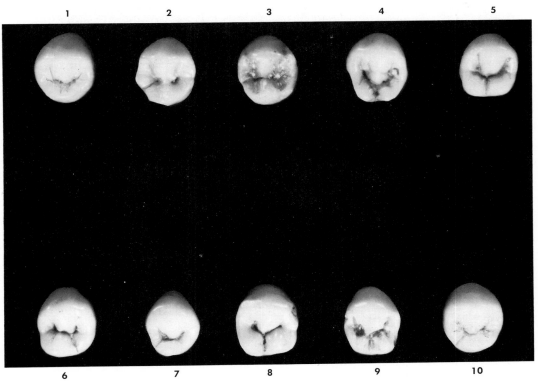

Figure 10–20. Mandibular second premolar—ten typical specimens, occlusal aspect.

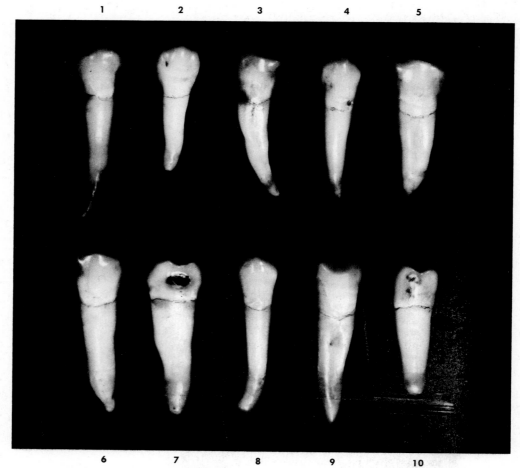

Figure 10–21.   Mandibular second premolar—ten specimens showing uncommon variations. 1, Root extremely long. 2, Root dwarfed. 3, Malformed root, developmental groove on buccal surface. 4, Contact areas on crown high and constricted. 5, Crown oversize, developmental groove buccally on root. 6, Root oversize. 7, Root malformed and of extra length. 8, Root very long with blunt apex, extreme curvature at apical third. 9, Crown and root oversize, developmental groove buccally on root. 10, Crown narrow buccolingually, very little curvature buccally and lingually.

irregular, acting as a contrast to the smoothness of cusp ridges, marginal ridges and the transverse ridge from buccal cusp to lingual cusp.

Some of these teeth show *mesial* and *distal developmental pits* centered in the mesial and distal fossae instead of an unbroken central groove (Fig. 10–20, specimen 2).

Although photographs do not demonstrate it very well, most of these two-cusp specimens show a developmental depression crossing the distolingual cusp ridge.

11

The Permanent
Maxillary Molars

The maxillary molars differ in design from any of the teeth previously described. These teeth assist the mandibular molars in performing the major portion of the work in the mastication and comminution of food. They are the largest and strongest maxillary teeth, by virtue both of their bulk and of their anchorage in the jaws. Although the crowns on the molars may be somewhat shorter than the premolars, their dimensions are greater in every respect. The root portion may be no longer than that of the premolars, but instead of one root or a root bifurcated, the maxillary molar root is broader at the base in all directions and is trifurcated into three well-developed prongs which are actually three full-sized roots emanating from a common broad base above the crown.

Generally speaking, the maxillary molars have large crowns with four well-formed cusps. They have three roots, two buccal and one lingual. The lingual root is the largest. The crowns have two buccal cusps and two lingual cusps. The outlines and curvatures of all the maxillary molars are similar. Developmental variations will be set forth under descriptions of the separate molars.

Before a detailed description of the maxillary first molar is begun, some statements must be made which are applicable to all first molars, mandibular as well as maxillary:

The permanent first molars usually appear in the oral cavity when the child is six years old. The mandibular molars precede the maxillary molars. The first permanent molar (maxillary or mandibular) erupts posterior to the second deciduous molar, taking up a position in contact with it. Therefore, the first molar is not a succedaneous tooth, since it has no predecessor. The deciduous teeth are all still in position and functioning when the first molar takes its place. Because the development of the bones of the face is downward and forward, sufficient space has been created normally at the age of six for the accommodation of this tooth.

The normal location of the first permanent molar is at the center of the fully developed adult jaw anteroposteriorly. As a consequence of the significance of their positions and the circumstances surrounding their eruption, the first molars are considered the "cornerstones" of the dental arches. A full realization of the significance of these teeth as units in the arches—their function and their positions relative to the other teeth—will be thoroughly understood when there has been an opportunity to study the arrangement of the teeth with their occlusion and the temporomandibular articulation of the jaws. Subsequent chapters cover those phases. The mandibular first molars will be described in Chapter 12.

MAXILLARY FIRST MOLAR

The crown of this tooth is wider buccolingually than mesiodistally. Usually the extra dimension buccolingually is about 1 mm. (see table). This, however, varies in individuals (see Fig. 11–17, specimens 1, 5, 7 and 9). From the occlusal aspect the inequality of the measurements in the two directions appears slight. Although the crown is relatively short, it is broad both mesiodistally and buccolingually, which gives the occlusal surface its generous dimensions.

The maxillary first molar is normally the largest tooth in the maxillary arch. It has four well-developed functioning cusps and one supplemental cusp of little practical use. The four large cusps of most physiologic significance are the mesiobuccal, the distobuccal, the mesiolingual and the distolingual. The fifth, or supplemental, cusp is called the *cusp* or *tubercle of Carabelli*. The simple term "fifth cusp" will be used here. This cusp is found lingual to the mesiolingual cusp, which is the largest of the well-developed cusps. Often the fifth cusp is so poorly developed that it is scarcely distinguishable. Usually a developmental groove is found, leaving a record of cusp development unless it has been erased by frictional wear. The fifth cusp or a developmental trace at its usual site serves to identify the maxillary first molar. A specimen of this tooth showing no trace of its typical characteristic would be rare.

There are three *roots* of generous proportions: the mesiobuccal, distobuccal and lingual. These roots are well separated and well developed, and their placement gives this tooth maximum anchorage against forces which would tend to unseat it. The roots have their greatest spread parallel to the line of greatest force brought to bear against the crown—diagonally in a buccolingual direction. The lingual root is the longest root. It is tapered and smoothly rounded. The mesiobuccal root is not so long,

Maxillary First Molar

First evidence of calcification ... At birth
Enamel completed .... 3 to 4 years
Eruption............................. 6 years
Root completed .... 9 to 10 years

Measurement Table

	Cervico-occlusal Length of Crown	Length of Root	Mesio-distal Diameter of Crown	Mesio-distal Diameter of Crown at Cervix	Labio- or Bucco-lingual Diameter of Crown	Labio- or Bucco-lingual Diameter at Cervix	Curvature of Cervical Line – Mesial	Curvature of Cervical Line – Distal
Dimensions suggested for carving technic	7.5°	b 1 12 13	10.0	8.0	11.0	10.0	1.0	0.0

°Millimeters.

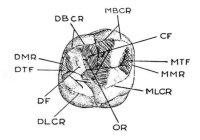

Figure 11–1. Maxillary right first molar—occlusal landmarks. *MBCR*, mesiobuccal cusp ridge; *CF*, central fossa (shaded area); *MTF*, mesial triangular fossa (shaded area); *MMR*, mesial marginal ridge; *MLCR*, mesiolingual cusp ridge; *DF*, distal fossa; *DTF*, distal triangular fossa (shaded area); *DMR*, distal marginal ridge; *DBCR*, distobuccal cusp ridge.

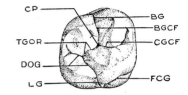

Figure 11-2. Maxillary right first molar—occlusal aspect—developmental grooves. *BG*, buccal groove; *BGCF*, buccal groove of central fossa; *CGCF*, central groove of central fossa; *FCG*, fifth cusp groove; *LG*, lingual groove; *DOG*, distal oblique groove; *TGOR*, transverse groove of oblique ridge; *CP*, central pit.

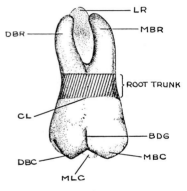

Figure 11–3. Maxillary right first molar—buccal aspect. *DBR*, distobuccal root; *LR*, lingual root; *MBR*, mesiobuccal root; *CL*, cervical line; *DBC*, distobuccal cusp; *MLC*, mesiolingual cusp; *BDG*, buccal developmental groove; *MBC*, mesiobuccal cusp.

but it is broader buccolingually and shaped (in cross section) so that its resistance to torsion is greater than that of the lingual root. The distobuccal root is the smallest of the three and smoothly rounded.

The development of maxillary first molars rarely deviates from the accepted normal.

DETAILED DESCRIPTION OF THE MAXILLARY FIRST MOLAR FROM ALL ASPECTS

Buccal Aspect (Figs. 11–4, 11–13, 11–14 and 11–15)

The crown is roughly trapezoidal, with cervical and occlusal outlines representing the uneven sides. The cervical line is the shorter of the uneven sides (Fig. 4–26, *D*).

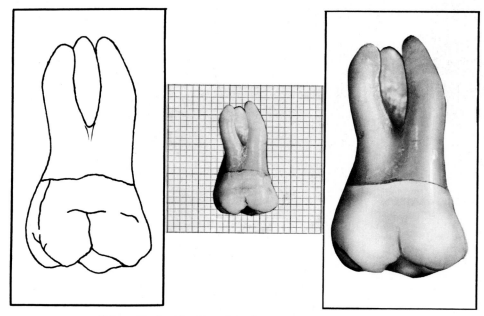

Figure 11—4. Maxillary right first molar—buccal aspect.

When looking at the buccal aspect of this tooth with the line of vision at right angles to the buccal developmental groove of the crown, one sees the distal side of the crown in perspective. This is caused by the obtuse character of the distobuccal line angle (see "Occlusal Aspect"). Parts of four cusps are seen, the mesiobuccal, distobuccal, mesiolingual and distolingual.

The mesiobuccal cusp is broader than the distobuccal cusp, and its mesial slope meets its distal slope at an obtuse angle. The mesial slope of the distobuccal cusp meets its distal slope at approximately a right angle. The distobuccal cusp is therefore sharper than the mesiobuccal cusp, and it is at least as long and often longer (Fig. 11–15, specimens 4, 6, 7, 8 and 9).

The buccal developmental groove which divides the two buccal cusps is approximately equidistant between the mesiobuccal and distolingual line angles. The groove slants occluso-apically in a line of direction parallel to the long axis of the distobuccal root. It terminates at a point approximately half the distance from its origin occlusally to the cervical line of the crown. Although the groove is not deep at any point, it becomes more shallow toward its termination, gradually fading out. Lateral to its terminus there is a dip in the enamel of the crown which is developmental in character and which extends for some distance mesially and distally.

The cervical line of the crown does not have much curvature from mesial to distal; however, it is not so smooth and regular as that found on some of the other teeth. The line is generally convex with the convexity toward the roots. ·

The mesial outline of the crown from this aspect follows a nearly straight path downward and mesially, curving occlusally as it reaches the crest of contour of the mesial surface which is the contact area. This crest is approximately two-thirds the distance from cervical line to tip of mesiobuccal cusp. The mesial outline continues downward and distally and becomes congruent with the outline of the mesial slope of the mesiobuccal cusp.

The distal outline of the crown is convex; the distal surface is spheroidal. The crest of curvature on the distal side of the crown is located at a level approximately half the distance from cervical line to tip of cusp. The distal contact area is in the middle of the middle third.

Often from this aspect a flattened area or a concave area is seen on the distal surface immediately above the distobuccal cusp at the cervical third of the crown.

All three of the roots may be seen from the buccal aspect. The axes of the roots are inclined distally. The roots are not straight, however, the buccal roots showing an inclination to curvature halfway between the point of bifurcation and the apices. The mesiobuccal root curves distally, starting at the middle third. Its axis usually is at right angles to the cervical line. The distal root is straighter, with its long axis at an acute angle distally with the cervical line. It has a tendency toward curvature mesially at its middle third.

The point of bifurcation of the two buccal roots is located approximately 4 mm. above the cervical line. This measurement varies somewhat, of course. Nevertheless, the point is much farther removed from the cervical line than in the deciduous molars. This relation is typical when all permanent molars are compared with all deciduous molars.

There is a deep developmental groove buccally on the root trunk of the maxillary first molar which starts at the bifurcation and progresses downward, becoming more shallow until it terminates in a shallow depression at the cervical line. Sometimes this depression extends slightly onto the enamel at the cervix.

The reader must keep in mind the fact that molar roots originate as a single root on the base of the crown. They then are divided into three roots, as in the maxillary molars, or into two roots, as in the mandibular molars. The common root base is called the *root trunk* (Figs. 11–3 and 11–8).

In judging the length of the roots and the direction of their axes, the part of the root trunk which is congruent with each root must be included as part of it, since it functions as an entity. Usually the lingual root is the longest and the two buccal roots are approximately equal in length. There is considerable variance in this, although the difference is a matter of a millimeter or so only in the average first molars with normal development.

From the buccal aspect, a measurement of the roots inclusively at their greatest extremities mesiodistally is less than a calibration of the diameter of the crown mesiodistally.

There is no invariable rule covering the relative length of crown and root when describing the upper first molar. On the average, the roots are about twice as long as the crown.

Lingual Aspect (Figs. 11–5, 11–6, 11–13 and 11–14)

From the lingual aspect the gross outline of the maxillary first molar is the reverse of that from the buccal aspect. Photographs or drawings show this only approximately because all teeth have breadth and thickness; consequently, perspective of two dimensions plus the human element (which enters into the technique of posing specimens and the making of drawings and photographs) are bound to result in some error in graphic interpretation.

The variation between the outline of the mesial surface and that of the distal surface is apparent. Because of the roundness of the distolingual cusp, the smooth curvature of the distal outline of the crown becoming confluent with the curvature of the cusp creates an arc which is almost a semicircle. The line which describes the lingual

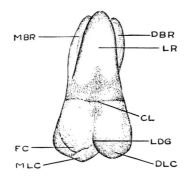

Figure 11–5. Maxillary right first molar—lingual aspect. *MBR,* mesiobuccal root; *DBR,* distobuccal root; *CL,* cervical line; *FC,* fifth cusp; *MLC,* mesiolingual cusp; *LDG,* lingual developmental groove; *DLC,* distolingual cusp.

developmental groove is also confluent with the outline of the distolingual cusp, progressing mesially and cervically and ending at a point at the approximate center of the lingual surface of the crown. A shallow depression in the surface extends from the terminus of the lingual groove to the center of the lingual surface of the lingual root at the cervical line and then continues in an apical direction on the lingual root, fading out at the middle third of the root.

The lingual cusps are the only ones to be seen from the lingual aspect. The mesiolingual cusp is much the larger, and before occlusal wear it is always the longest cusp the tooth possesses. Its mesiodistal width is about three-fifths of the mesiodistal crown diameter, the distolingual cusp making up the remaining two-fifths. The angle formed by the mesial outline of the crown and the mesial slope of the mesiolingual cusp is almost 90 degrees. An obtuse angle describes the junction of the mesial and distal slopes of this cusp.

The distolingual cusp is so spheroidal and smooth that it is difficult to describe any angulation on the mesial and distal slopes.

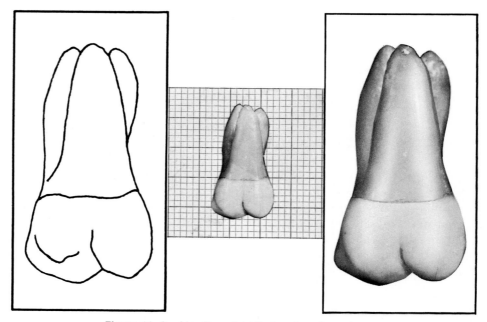

Figure 11–6. Maxillary right first molar—lingual aspect.

The lingual developmental groove starts approximately in the center of the lingual surface mesiodistally, curves sharply to the distal as it crosses between the cusps and continues on to the occlusal surface.

The fifth cusp appears attached to the mesiolingual surface of the mesiolingual cusp. It is outlined occlusally by an irregular developmental groove, which may be described as starting in a depression of the mesiolingual line angle of the crown, extending occlusally toward the point of the mesiolingual cusp, then making an obtuse angle turn toward the terminus of the lingual groove and fading out near the lingual groove terminus. If the fifth cusp is well developed, its cusp angle will be sharper and less obtuse than that of the mesiolingual cusp. The cusp ridge of the fifth cusp is approximately 2 mm. cervical to the cusp ridge of the mesiolingual cusp (Fig. 11–5).

All three of the roots are visible from the lingual aspect, the large lingual root making up most of the foreground. The lingual portion of the root trunk is continuous with the entire cervical portion of the crown lingually. The lingual root is conical, terminating in a bluntly rounded apex.

All of the mesial outline of the mesiobuccal root may be seen from this angle and part of its apex.

The distal outline of the distobuccal root is seen above its middle third, including all of its apical outline.

Mesial Aspect (Figs. 11–7, 11–8, 11–13 and 11–14)

From this aspect the increased buccolingual dimensions may be observed, as well as the cervical curvatures of the crown outlines at the cervical third buccally and lingually, and the difference in dimensions between the crown at its greatest measurement and the distance between the cusp tips in a buccolingual direction.

Starting at the cervical line buccally the outline of the crown makes a short arc buccally to its crest of curvature within the cervical third of the crown. The extent of

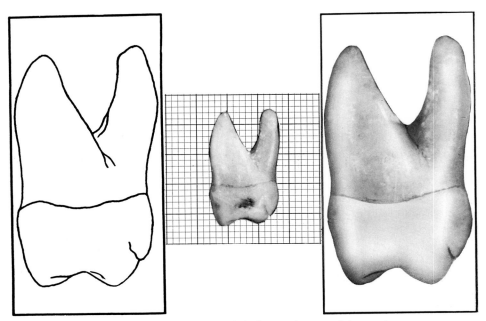

Figure 11–7. Maxillary right first molar—mesial aspect.

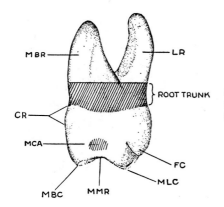

Figure 11–8. Maxillary right first molar—mesial aspect. *LR*, lingual root; *FC*, fifth cusp; *MLC*, mesiolingual cusp; *MMR*, mesial marginal ridge; *MBC*, mesiobuccal ridge; *MCA*, mesial contact area; *CR*, cervical ridge; *MBR*, mesiobuccal root.

this curvature is about 0.5 mm. (Fig. 11–13). The line of the buccal surface then describes a shallow concavity immediately occlusal to the crest of curvature (see "Buccal Aspect"). The outline then becomes slightly convex as it progresses downward and inward to circumscribe the mesiobuccal cusp, ending at the tip of the cusp well within projected outlines of the root base.

If the tooth is posed so that the line of vision is at right angles to the mesial contact area, the only cusps in sight are the mesiobuccal, the mesiolingual and the fifth cusps. The distobuccal root is hidden by the mesiobuccal root.

The lingual outline of the crown curves outward and lingually approximately to the same extent as on the buccal side. The level of the crest of curvature is near the middle third of the crown rather than a point within the cervical third, as it is buccally.

If the fifth cusp is well developed, the lingual outline dips inward to illustrate it. If it is undeveloped the lingual outline continues from the crest of curvature as a smoothly curved arc to the tip of the mesiolingual cusp. The point of the cusp is more clearly centered within projected outlines of the root base than the tip of the mesiobuccal cusp. The mesiolingual cusp is on a line with the long axis of the lingual root.

The mesial marginal ridge, which is confluent with the mesiobuccal and mesiolingual cusp ridges, is irregular, the outline curving cervically about one-fifth the crown length and centering its curvature below the center of the crown buccolingually.

The cervical line of the crown is irregular, curving occlusally, but as a rule not more than 1 mm. at any one point. If there is definite curvature it reaches its maximum immediately above the contact area.

The mesial contact area is above the marginal ridge but closer to it than to the cervical line, approximately at the junction of the middle and occlusal thirds of the crown (see Fig. 11–8). It is also somewhat buccal to the center of the crown buccolingually. A shallow concavity is usually found just above the contact area on the mesial surface of the maxillary first molar. This concavity may be continued to the mesial surface of the root trunk at its cervical third.

The mesiobuccal root is broad and flattened on its mesial surface; this flattened surface often exhibits smooth flutings for part of its length. The width of this root near the crown from the buccal surface to the point of bifurcation on the root trunk is approximately two-thirds of the crown measurement buccolingually at the cervical line. The buccal outline of the root extends upward and outward from the crown, ending at the blunt apex. The greatest projection on this root is usually buccal to the greatest projection of the crown. The lingual outline of the root is relatively straight from the bluntly rounded apex down to the bifurcation with the lingual root.

The level of the bifurcation is a little closer to the cervical line than is found between the roots buccally. A smooth depression congruent with the bifurcation extends occlusally and lingually almost to the cervical line directly above the mesiolingual line angle of the crown.

The lingual root is longer than the mesial root but is narrower from this aspect. It is banana-shaped, extending lingually with its convex outline to the lingual and its concave outline to the buccal. At its middle and apical thirds it is outside of the confines of the greatest crown projection. Although its apex is rounded, the root appears more pointed toward the end than the mesiobuccal root.

Distal Aspect (Figs. 11–10, 11–13 and 11–14)

The gross outline of this aspect is similar to that of the mesial aspect. Certain variations must be noted when the tooth is viewed from the distal aspect.

Because of the tendency of the crown to taper distally on the buccal surface, most of the buccal surface of the crown may be seen in perspective from the distal aspect. This is because the buccolingual measurement of the crown mesially is greater than the same measurement distally. All of the decrease in measurement distally is due to the slant of the buccal side of the crown.

The distal marginal ridge dips sharply in a cervical direction, exposing triangular ridges on the distal portion of the occlusal surface of the crown.

The cervical line is almost straight across from buccal to lingual. Occasionally it curves apically 0.5 mm. or so.

The distal surface of the crown is generally convex, with a smoothly rounded surface except for a small area near the distobuccal root at the cervical third. This concavity continues on to the distal surface of the distobuccal root, from the cervical line to the area of the root which is on a level with the bifurcation separating the distobuccal and lingual roots.

The distobuccal root is narrower at its base than either of the others. An outline of this root, when one views the tooth from the distal aspect, starts buccally at a point immediately above the distobuccal cusp, follows a concave path inward for a short distance, then outward in a buccal direction, completing a graceful convex arc from the concavity to the rounded apex. This line lies entirely within the confines of the outline of the mesiobuccal root. The lingual outline of the root from the apex to the bifurcation is slightly concave. There is no concavity between the bifurcation of the

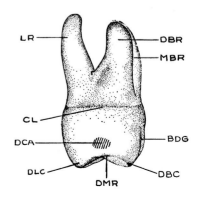

Figure 11–9. Maxillary right first molar—distal aspect. *DBR,* distobuccal root; *MBR,* mesiobuccal root; *BDG,* buccal developmental groove; *DBC,* distobuccal cusp; *DCA,* distal contact area; *CL,* cervical line; *LR,* lingual root.

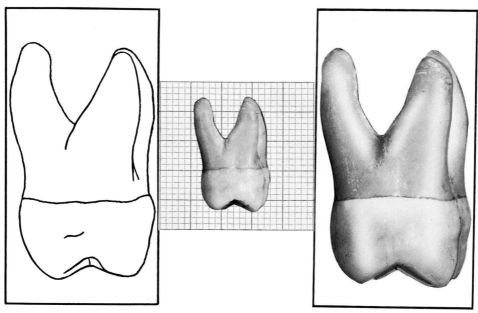

Figure 11–10. Maxillary right first molar—distal aspect.

roots and the cervical line. If anything, the surface at this point on the root trunk has a tendency toward convexity.

The bifurcation here is more apical than either of the other two areas on this tooth. The area from cervical line to bifurcation is 5 mm. or more in extent.

Occlusal Aspect (Figs. 11–1, 11–2, 11–12, 11–13, 11–14 and 11–17)

The maxillary first molar is somewhat rhomboidal from the occlusal aspect. An outline following the four major cusp ridges and the marginal ridges is especially so.

A measurement of the crown buccolingually and mesial to the buccal and lingual grooves will be greater than the measurement on that portion of the crown which is distal to these developmental grooves. Also, a measurement of the crown immediately lingual to contact areas mesiodistally is greater than the measurement immediately buccal to the contact areas. Thus it is apparent that the maxillary first molar crown is wider mesially than distally, and wider lingually than buccally.

The four major cusps are well developed, with the small minor, or fifth, cusp ap-

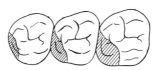

Figure 11–11. Maxillary molar primary cusp triangle. The distolingual lobe, represented by shaded areas, becomes progressively smaller on maxillary molars, starting with the first molar, which presents the greatest development of the lobe. The plain areas, roughly triangular in outline, represent the "maxillary molar primary cusp triangles."

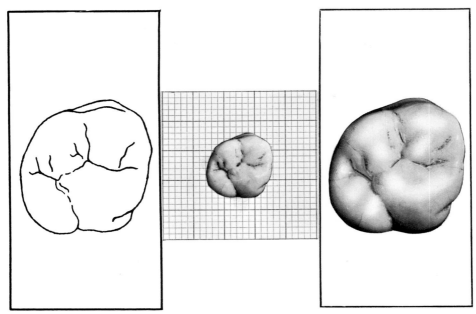

Figure 11–12. Maxillary right first molar—occlusal aspect.

pearing on the lingual surface of the mesiolingual cusp near the mesiolingual line angle of the crown. The fifth cusp may be indistinct, or all the cusp form may be absent. At this site, however, there will be nearly always traces of developmental lines in the enamel.

The mesiolingual cusp is the largest cusp; it is followed in point of size by the mesiobuccal, distolingual, distobuccal and fifth cusps.

If reduced to a geometric schematic figure, the occlusal aspect of this molar locates the various angles of the rhomboidal figure as follows: acute angles, mesiobuccal and distolingual; obtuse angles, mesiolingual and distobuccal.

An analysis of the design of occlusal surfaces of maxillary molars may be summarized as follows: Developmentally there are only three major cusps to be analyzed as primary, with the mesiolingual cusp (the most primitive), and the two buccal cusps. The distolingual cusp development common to all of the maxillary molars, and any other additional one such as the cusp of Carabelli on first molars, must be regarded as secondary.

The *maxillary molar primary cusp triangle* supposition follows the Cope-Osborn hypothesis of tooth origins. There was a tritubercular stage in human tooth development when the molar forms with only three cusps explained the background for the triangular arrangement just described.*

This primary design is also reflected in the outline of the root trunks of maxillary molars when the teeth are sectioned in those areas (see Root Sections, Chapter 13).

Another observation which bears out this theory is that the distolingual cusp becomes progressively smaller on second and third maxillary molars, often disappearing as a major cusp (Fig. 11–11).

To repeat, the triangular arrangement of the three important molar cusps is called the maxillary molar primary cusp triangle. The characteristic triangular figure, made

---

*"The Origin and Evolution of the Human Dentition." Gregory, W. K., 1922.

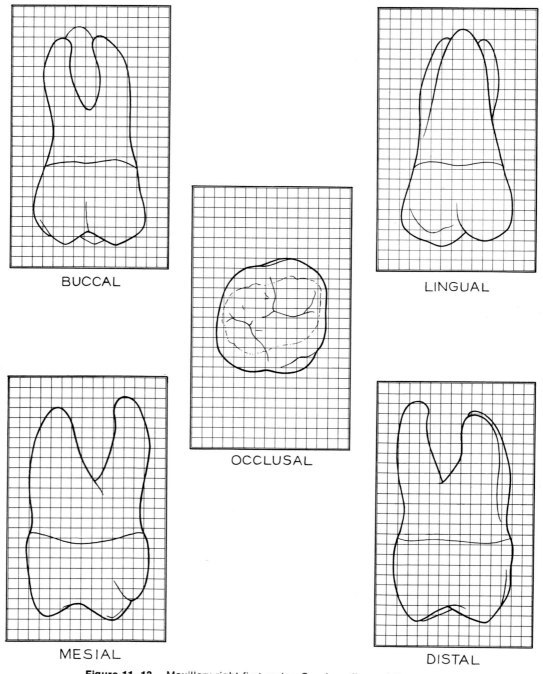

BUCCAL

LINGUAL

OCCLUSAL

MESIAL

DISTAL

Figure 11–13. Maxillary right first molar. Graph outlines of five aspects.

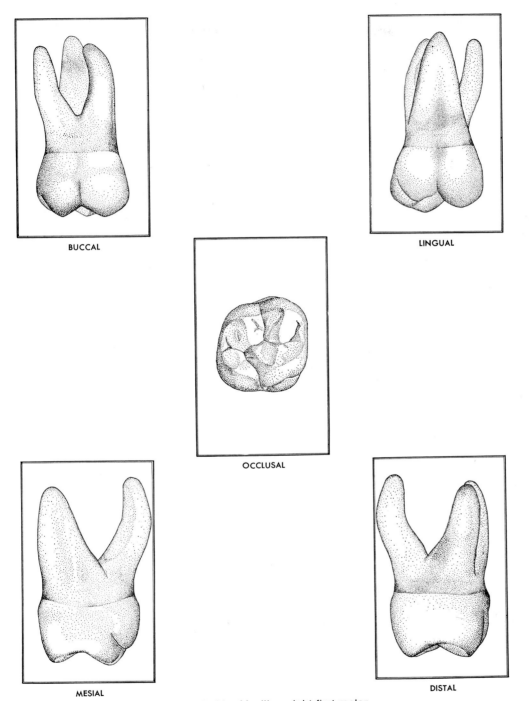

BUCCAL

LINGUAL

OCCLUSAL

MESIAL

DISTAL

Figure 11–14. Maxillary right first molar.

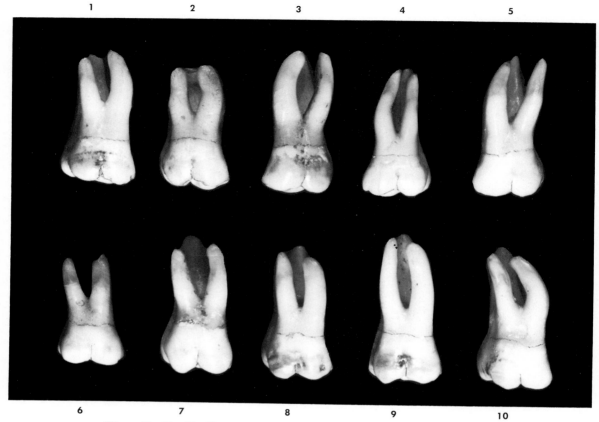

Figure 11—15.   Maxillary first molars—ten typical specimens—buccal aspect.

by tracing the cusp outlines of these cusps, the mesial marginal ridge and the oblique ridge of the occlusal surface, is representative of all maxillary molars.

The *occlusal surface* of the maxillary first molar is within the confines of the cusp ridges and marginal ridges. It may be described as follows:

There are two major fossae and two minor fossae. The major fossae are the *central fossa*, which is roughly triangular and mesial to the oblique ridge, and the *distal fossa*, which is roughly linear and distal to the oblique ridge. The two minor fossae are the *mesial triangular fossa*, immediately distal to the mesial marginal ridge, and the *distal triangular fossa*, immediately mesial to the distal marginal ridge (Fig. 11–1).

The *oblique ridge* is a triangular ridge which traverses the occlusal surface of this tooth in an oblique direction from the tip of the mesiolingual cusp to the tip of the distobuccal cusp. This ridge is reduced in height in the center of the occlusal surface, being about on a level with the marginal ridges of the occlusal surface. Sometimes it is crossed by a developmental groove which partially joins the two major fossae by means of its shallow sulcate groove.

The *mesial marginal ridge* and the *distal marginal ridge* are irregular ridges confluent with the mesial and distal cusp ridges of the mesial and distal major cusps.

The *central fossa* of the occlusal surface is a concave area bounded by the distal slope of the mesiobuccal cusp, the mesial slope of the distobuccal cusp, the crest of

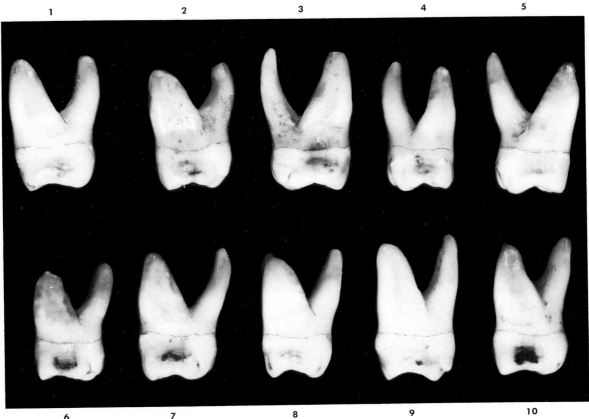

Figure 11–16.   Maxillary first molars—ten typical specimens—mesial aspect.

the oblique ridge, and the crests of the two triangular ridges of the mesiobuccal and mesiolingual cusps. The central fossa has connecting sulci within its boundaries, with developmental grooves at the deepest portions of these sulci (sulcate grooves). In addition, it contains supplemental grooves, short grooves which are disconnected, and also the central developmental pit. A worn specimen may show developmental or sulcate grooves only.

In the center of the central fossa the central developmental pit has sulcate developmental grooves, radiating from it at obtuse angles to each other. This pit is located in the approximate center of that portion of the occlusal surface which is circumscribed by cusp ridges and marginal ridges (Fig. 11–1). From this pit the *buccal developmental groove* radiates buccally at the bottom of the buccal sulcus of the central fossa, continuing on to the buccal surface of the crown between the buccal cusps.

Starting again at the central pit, the *central developmental groove* is seen to progress in a mesial direction at an obtuse angle to the buccal sulcate groove. The central groove at the bottom of the sulcus of the central fossa usually terminates at the apex of the *mesial triangular fossa.* Here it is joined by short supplemental grooves which radiate from its terminus into the triangular fossa. These supplemental grooves often appear as branches of the central groove. Occasionally one or more supplemental grooves cross the mesial marginal ridge of the crown.

The *mesial triangular fossa* is rather indistinct in outline, but it is generally trian-

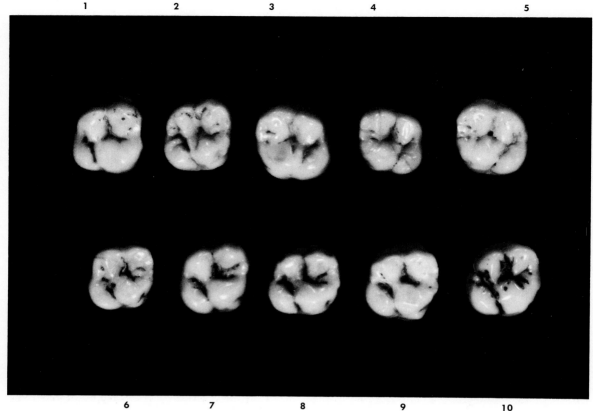

Figure 11–17. Maxillary first molars—ten typical specimens—occlusal aspect.

gular in shape with its base at the mesial marginal ridge and its apex at the point where the supplemental grooves join the central groove.

An additional short developmental groove radiates from the central pit of the central fossa at an obtuse angulation to the buccal and central developmental grooves. Usually it is considered a projection of one of these, since it is very short and usually fades out before reaching the crest of the oblique ridge. When it crosses the oblique ridge transversely, however, as it sometimes does, joining the central and distal fossae with a shallow groove, it is called the *transverse groove of the oblique ridge* (Fig. 11–17, specimens 3, 4 and 5).

The *distal fossa* of the maxillary first molar is roughly linear in form and is located immediately distal to the oblique ridge. An irregular developmental groove traverses its deepest portion. This developmental groove is called the *distal oblique groove*. It connects with the *lingual developmental groove* at the junction of the cusp ridges of the mesiolingual and distolingual cusps. These two grooves travel in the same oblique direction to the terminus of the lingual groove, which is centered below the lingual root at the approximate center of the crown lingually (Fig. 11–5, *LDG*). If the fifth cusp development is distinct, a developmental groove outlining it joins the lingual groove near its terminus. Any part of the developmental groove which outlines a fifth cusp is called the *fifth cusp groove.*

The distal oblique groove in most cases shows several supplemental grooves. Two terminal branches usually appear, forming two sides of the triangular depression immediately mesial to the distal marginal ridge. These two sides, in combination with

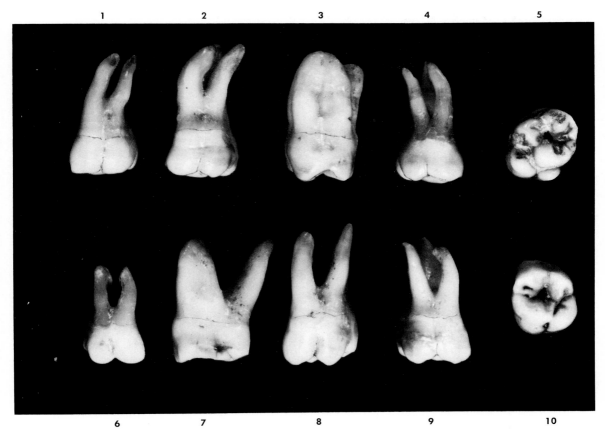

Figure 11–18. Maxillary first molars—ten specimens showing uncommon variations. 1, Unusual curvature of buccal roots. 2, Roots abnormally long with extreme curvature. 3, Lingual and distobuccal roots fused. 4, Mesiodistal measurement of root trunk smaller than usual. 5, Extreme rhomboidal development of crown, fifth cusp with maximum development. 6, Tooth well developed but much smaller than usual. 7, Extreme buccolingual measurement. 8, Extreme length, especially of the distobuccal root; buccal cusps narrow mesiodistally. 9, Well-developed crown, roots poorly developed. 10, Extreme development of lingual portion of the crown when compared with the buccal development.

the slope mesial to the distal marginal ridge, form the *distal triangular fossa*. The distal outline of the distal marginal ridge of the crown shows a slight concavity.

The distolingual cusp is smooth and rounded from the occlusal aspect, and an outline of it, from the distal concavity of the distal marginal ridge to the lingual groove of the crown, describes an arc of an ellipse.

The lingual outline of the distolingual cusp is straight with the lingual outline of the fifth cusp, unless the fifth cusp is unusually large. In the latter case the lingual outline of the fifth cusp is more prominent lingually (see specimen 9, Fig. 11–17). The cusp ridge of the distolingual cusp usually extends lingually farther than the cusp ridge of the mesiolingual cusp.

MAXILLARY SECOND MOLAR

The maxillary second molar supplements the first molar in function. In describing this tooth, direct comparisons will be made with the first molar both in form and development.

Generally speaking, the roots of this tooth are as long as, if not somewhat longer

Maxillary Second Molar

First evidence of calcification..... 2½ to 3 years
Enamel completed................... 7 to 8 years
Eruption............................... 12 to 13 years
Root completed .... 14 to 16 years

Measurement Table

	Cervico-occlusal Length of Crown	Length of Root	Mesio-distal Diam-eter of Crown	Mesio-distal Diam-eter of Crown at Cervix	Labio- or Bucco-lingual Diameter of Crown	Labio- or Bucco-lingual Diameter at Cervix	Curvature of Cervical Line — Mesial	Curvature of Cervical Line — Distal
Dimensions suggested for carving technic	7.0°	b 11 112	9.0	7.0	11.0	10.0	1.0	0.0

°Millimeters.

than, those of the first molar. The distobuccal cusp is not so large or so well developed, and the distolingual cusp is smaller. No fifth cusp is evident.

The crown of the maxillary second molar is 0.5 mm. or so shorter cervico-occlusally than that of the first molar, but the measurement of the crown bucco-lingually is about the same. *Two types* of maxillary second molars are found when one is viewing the occlusal aspect: (1) The type that is seen most has an occlusal form which resembles the first molar, although the rhomboidal outline is more extreme. This is accentuated by the lesser measurement lingually. (2) This type bears more resemblance to a typical third molar form. The distolingual cusp is poorly developed and makes the development of the other three cusps predominate. This results in a heart-shaped form from the occlusal aspect that is more typical of the maxillary *third* molar (Fig. 11–26, specimens 1 and 7).

DETAILED DESCRIPTION OF THE MAXILLARY SECOND MOLAR FROM ALL ASPECTS‘

Buccal Aspect (Figs. 11–19 and 11–24)

The crown is a little shorter cervico-occlusally and narrower mesiodistally than the maxillary first molar. The distobuccal cusp is smaller and allows part of the distal marginal ridge and part of the distolingual cusp to be seen.

The buccal roots are about the same length. These roots are more nearly parallel and are inclined distally more than those of the maxillary first molar, so that the end of the distobuccal root is slightly distal to the distal extremity of the crown. The apex of the mesiobuccal root is on a line with the buccal groove of the crown instead of the tip of the mesiobuccal cusp as was found on the first molar.

Lingual Aspect (Fig. 11–20)

Differences between the second and first molars to be noted here in addition to those mentioned before are these: (1) The distolingual cusp of the crown is smaller;

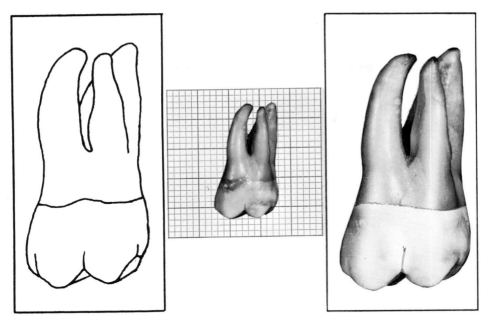

Figure 11–19. Maxillary left second molar—buccal aspect.

(2) the distobuccal cusp may be seen through the sulcus between the mesiolingual and distolingual cusp, and (3) no fifth cusp is evident.

The apex of the lingual root is in line with the distolingual cusp tip instead of the lingual groove as was found on the first molar.

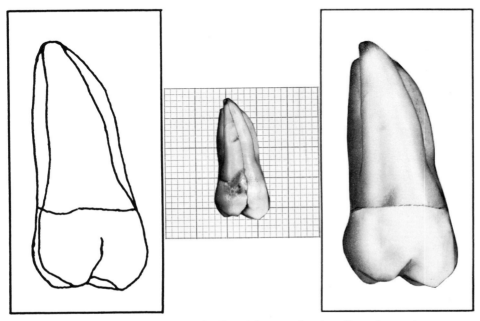

Figure 11–20. Maxillary left second molar—lingual aspect.

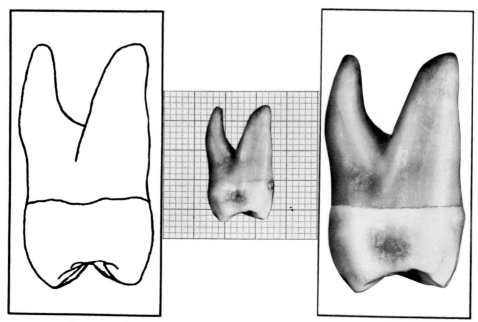

Figure 11–21. Maxillary left second molar—mesial aspect.

Mesial Aspect (Figs. 11–21 and 11–25)

The buccolingual dimension is about the same as that of the first molar, but the crown length is less. The roots do not spread so far buccolingually, being within the confines of the buccolingual crown outline.

Distal Aspect (Fig. 11–22)

Because the distobuccal cusp is smaller than in the maxillary first molar, more of the mesiobuccal cusp may be seen from this angle. The mesiolingual cusp cannot be seen. The apex of the lingual root is in line with the distolingual cusp.

Occlusal Aspect (Figs. 11–23 and 11–26)

The rhomboidal type of second maxillary molar is most frequent, although in comparison with the first molar the acute angles of the rhomboid are less and the obtuse angles greater. The buccolingual diameter of the crown is about equal, but the mesiodistal diameter is approximately 1 mm. less. The mesiobuccal and mesiolingual cusps are just as large and well developed as in the first molar, but the distobuccal and distolingual cusps are smaller and less well developed. Usually a calibration made of the crown at the greatest diameter buccally and lingually of the distal portion is considerably less than one made at the greatest diameter buccally and lingually of the mesial portion, showing more convergence distally than the maxillary first molar.

It is not uncommon to find more supplemental grooves as well as accidental grooves and pits on the occlusal surface of a maxillary second molar than are usually found on a maxillary first molar.

(*Text continued on page 260.*)

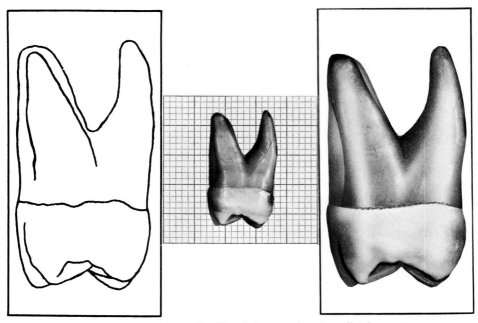

Figure 11–22.   Maxillary left second molar—distal aspect.

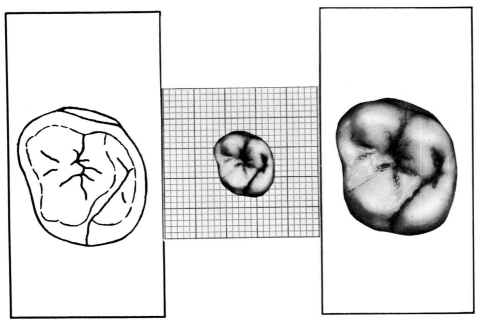

Figure 11–23.   Maxillary left second molar—occlusal aspect.

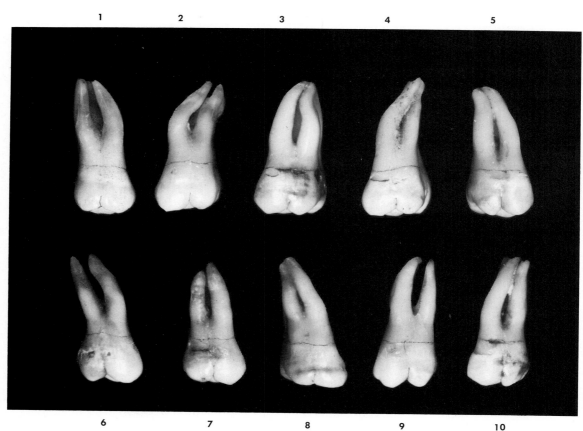

Figure 11–24.   Maxillary second molars—ten typical specimens—buccal aspect.

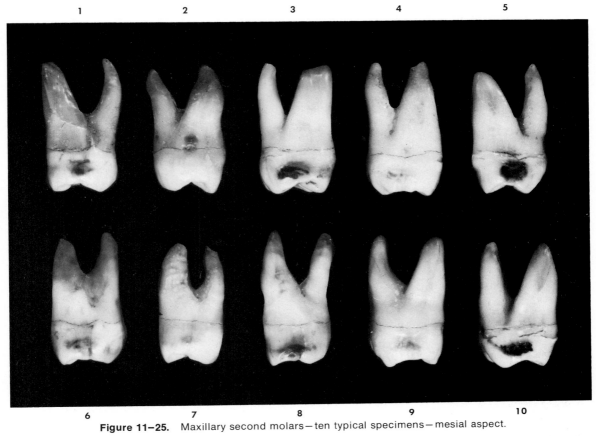

Figure 11–25. Maxillary second molars—ten typical specimens—mesial aspect.

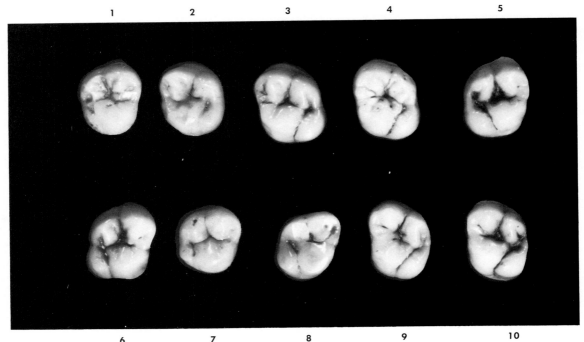

Figure 11–26. Maxillary second molars—ten typical specimens—occlusal aspect.

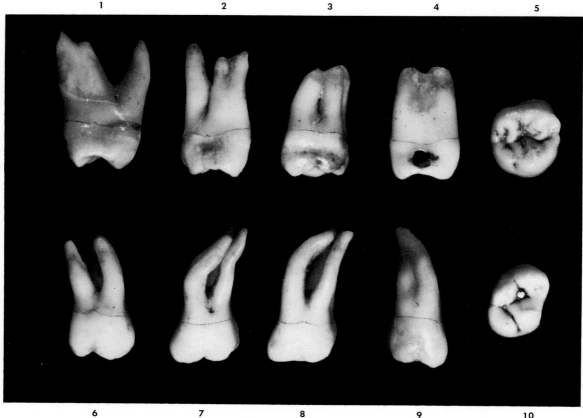

Figure 11–27. Maxillary second molars—ten specimens showing uncommon variations. 1, Roots spread similar to first molar. 2, Bifurcated mesiobuccal root. 3, Roots very short and fused. 4, Mesiobuccal and lingual roots with complete fusion. 5, Crown similar to the typical third molar form. 6, Short roots with spread similar to first molar. 7, Roots extra long with abnormal curvatures. 8, Another variation similar to specimen 7. 9, Very long roots fused. 10, Crown with extreme rhomboidal form.

MAXILLARY THIRD MOLAR

The maxillary third molar often appears as a developmental anomaly. It can vary considerably in size, contour and relative position to the other teeth. It is seldom so well developed as the maxillary second molar, to which it often bears resemblance. The third molar supplements the second molar in function, and its fundamental design is similar. The crown is smaller and the roots are, as a rule, shorter with the inclination toward fusion with the resultant anchorage of one tapered root.

The predominating third molar design, when one views the occlusal surface, is that of the heart-shaped type of second molar. The distolingual cusp is very small and poorly developed in most cases and it may be absent entirely.

All third molars, mandibular and maxillary, show more variation in development than any of the other teeth in the mouth. Occasionally they appear as anomalies bearing little or no resemblance to neighboring teeth. A few of the variations in form are shown in Figure 11–36.

For the purposes at hand it is necessary to give a short description of the third molar that is considered average in its development and one that would be in good proportion to the other maxillary molars and with an occlusal form considered normal.

Maxillary Third Molar

First evidence of calcification ...   7 to   9 years
Enamel completed .... 12 to 16 years
Eruption............................. 17 to 21 years
Root completed...................... 18 to 25 years

Measurement Table

	Cervico-occlusal Length of Crown	Length of Root	Mesio-distal Diameter of Crown	Mesio-distal Diameter of Crown at Cervix	Labio- or Bucco-lingual Diameter of Crown	Labio- or Bucco-lingual Diameter at Cervix	Curvature of Cervical Line — Mesial	Curvature of Cervical Line — Distal
Dimensions suggested for carving technic	6.5°	11.0	8.5	6.5	10.0	9.5	1.0	0.0

°Millimeters.

In describing the normal maxillary third molar, direct comparisons will be made with the maxillary second molar.

DETAILED DESCRIPTION OF THE MAXILLARY THIRD MOLAR FROM ALL ASPECTS

Buccal Aspects (Figs. 11–28 and 11–33)

The crown is shorter cervico-occlusally and narrower mesiodistally than that of the second molar. The roots are usually fused, functioning as one large root, and they

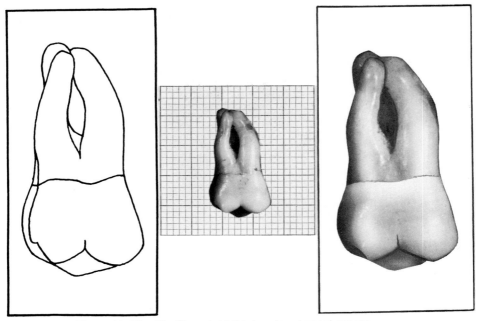

Figure 11–28.   Maxillary right third molar—buccal aspect.

are shorter cervicoapically. The fused roots end in a taper at the apex. The roots have a distinct slant to the distal, giving the apices of the fused root a more distal relation to the center of the crown.

Lingual Aspect (Fig. 11–29)

In addition to the differences mentioned above, in comparison with the maxillary second molar, there is usually just one large lingual cusp and therefore no lingual groove. However, in many cases, a third molar with the same essential features has a poorly developed distolingual cusp with a developmental groove lingually. (Fig. 11–35, specimen 2.)

Mesial Aspect (Figs. 11–30 and 11–34)

Here, aside from the differences in measurement, the main feature is the taper to the fused roots and a bifurcation, usually in the region of the apical third. (Fig. 11–30 does not show a bifurcation. See specimens 1, 2 and 3 in Fig. 11–34.) The root portion is considerably shorter in relation to the crown length. Both the crown and the root portions are inclined to be poorly developed, with irregular outlines.

Distal Aspect (Fig. 11–31)

From this aspect most of the buccal surface of the crown is in view. More of the occlusal surface may be seen than can be seen on the second molar from this aspect because of the more acute angulation of the occlusal surface in relation to the long axis of the root. The measurement from the cervical line to the marginal ridge is short.

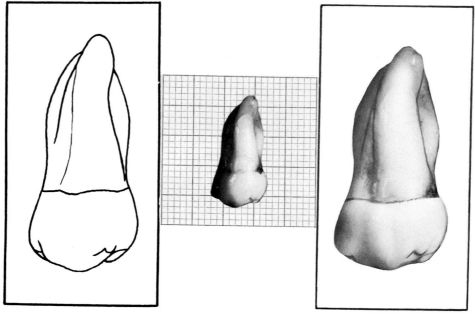

Figure 11–29.   Maxillary right third molar—lingual aspect.

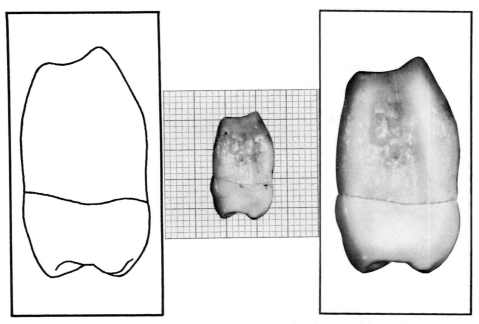

Figure 11–30.   Maxillary right third molar—mesial aspect.

Occlusal Aspect (Figs. 11–32 and 11–35)

The occlusal aspect of a typical maxillary third molar presents a heart-shaped outline. The lingual cusp is large and well developed and there is little or no distolingual cusp—which gives a semicircular outline to the tooth from one contact area

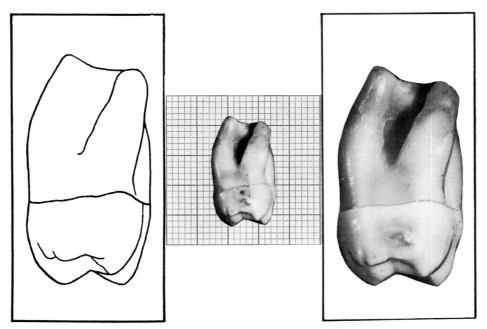

Figure 11–31.   Maxillary right third molar—distal aspect.

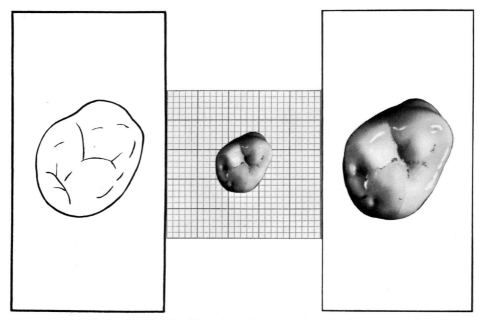

Figure 11–32.   Maxillary right third molar—occlusal aspect.

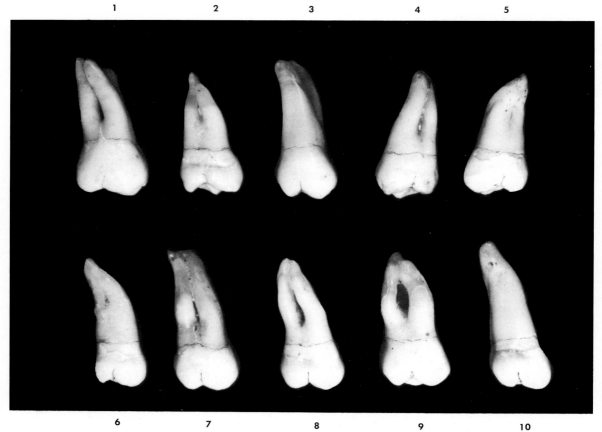

Figure 11–33.   Maxillary third molars—ten typical specimens—buccal aspect.

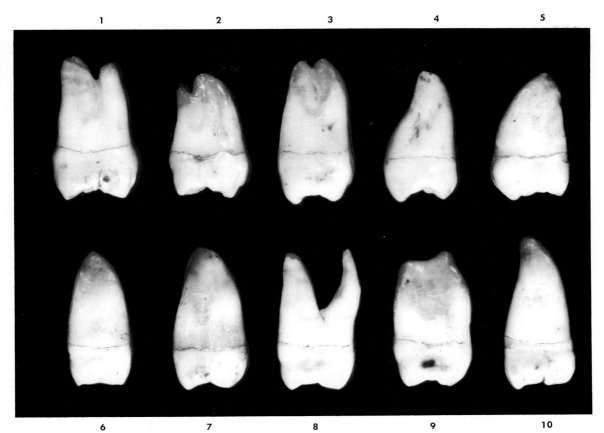

Figure 11-34.   Maxillary third molars—ten typical specimens—mesial aspect.

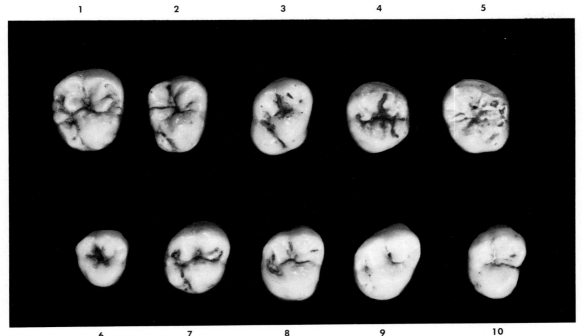

Figure 11-35.   Maxillary third molars—ten typical specimens—occlusal aspect.

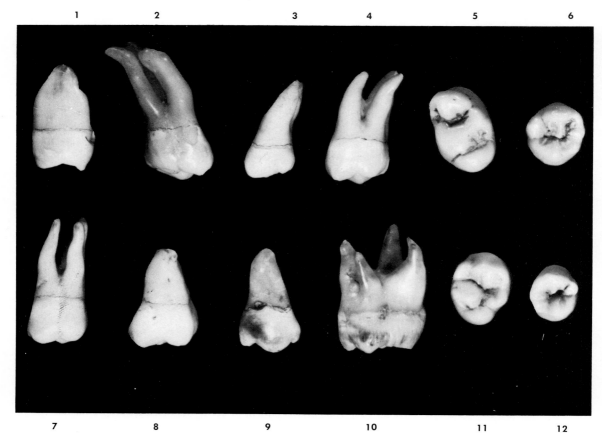

Figure 11-36. Maxillary third molars—twelve specimens showing uncommon variations. 1, Very short fused root form. 2, Extremely long roots with extreme distal angulation. 3, Complete fusion of roots with extreme distal angulation. 4, Three roots well separated, crown very wide at cervix. 5, Extreme rhomboidal outline to crown with developmental grooves oddly placed. 6, Overdeveloped mesiobuccal cusp. 7, Crown wide at cervix, with roots perpendicular. 8, Very large crown, poorly developed root form. 9, Complete absence of typical design. 10, Specimen abnormally large, with four roots well separated. 11, Five well-developed cusps, atypical in form. 12, Small specimen, atypical cusp form.

to the other. On this type of tooth there are *three* functioning cusps: two buccal and one lingual.

The occlusal aspect of this tooth usually presents many supplemental grooves and many accidental grooves unless the tooth is very much worn.

The third molar may show four distinct cusps. This type may have a strong oblique ridge, a central fossa and a distal fossa, with a lingual developmental groove similar to that of the rhomboidal type of second molar. In most instances, the crown converges more lingually from the buccal areas than the second molar does, losing its rhomboidal outline. This is not, however, always true (compare specimens 1 and 3 in Fig. 11–35).

12

The Permanent
Mandibular Molars

The mandibular molars are larger than any other mandibular teeth. They are three in number on each side of the mandible: the first, second and third mandibular molars. They resemble each other in functional form, although comparison of one with another shows variations in the number of cusps and some variation in size, occlusal design and the relative length and positions of the roots.

The crown outlines exhibit similarities of outline from all aspects, and each mandibular molar has two roots, one mesial and one distal. Third molars and some second molars may show a fusion of these roots. All mandibular molars have crowns that are roughly quadrilateral, being somewhat longer mesiodistally than buccolingually. *Maxillary* molar crowns have their widest measurement buccolingually.

The mandibular molars perform the major portion of the work of the lower jaw in mastication and in the comminution of food. They are the largest and strongest mandibular teeth, both because of their bulk and because of their anchorage.

The crowns of the molars are shorter cervico-occlusally than those of the teeth anterior to them, but their dimensions are greater in every other respect. The root portions are not so long as those of some of the other mandibular teeth, but the combined measurements of the multiple roots, with their broad bifurcated root trunks, result in superior anchorage and greater efficiency.

Usually the sum of the mesiodistal measurements of mandibular molars is equal to, or greater than, the combined mesiodistal measurements of all the teeth anterior to the first molar and up to the median line.

The crowns of these molars are wider mesiodistally than buccolingually. The opposite arrangement is true of maxillary molars.

MANDIBULAR FIRST MOLAR

Normally the mandibular first molar is the largest tooth in the mandibular arch. It has five well-developed cusps: two buccal, two lingual and a distal cusp (Fig. 12–1).

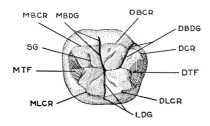

Figure 12–1.   Mandibular right first molar—occlusal aspect. *DBCR*, distobuccal cusp ridge; *DBDG*, distobuccal developmental groove; *DCR*, distal cusp ridge; *DTF*, distal triangular fossa (shaded area); *DLCR*, distolingual cusp ridge; *LDG*, lingual developmental groove; *MLCR*, mesiolingual cusp ridge; *MTF*, mesial triangular fossa (shaded area); *SG*, a supplemental groove; *MBCR*, mesiobuccal cusp ridge; *MBDG*, mesiobuccal developmental groove.

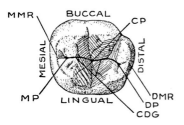

Figure 12–2.   Mandibular right first molar—occlusal aspect. Shaded area—central fossa; *CP*, central pit; *DMR*, distal marginal ridge; *DP*, distal pit; *CDG*, central developmental groove; *MP*, mesial pit; *MMR*, mesial marginal ridge.

It has two well-developed roots, one mesial and one distal, which are very broad buccolingually. These roots are widely separated at the apices.

The dimension of the crown mesiodistally is greater by about 1 mm. than the dimension buccolingually. Although the crown is relatively short cervico-occlusally, it has mesiodistal and buccolingual measurements which provide a broad occlusal form.

The mesial root is broad and curved distally, with mesial and distal fluting which provides the anchorage of two roots (Fig. 13–41). The distal root is rounder, broad at the cervical portion, and pointed in a distal direction. The formation of these roots and their positions in the mandible serve to brace efficiently the crown of the tooth against the lines of force which might be brought to bear against it.

Mandibular First Molar

First evidence of calcification..... At birth
Enamel completed................... 2½ to 3 years
Eruption............................... 6   to   7 years
Root completed 9   to 10 years

Measurement Table

	Cervico-occlusal Length of Crown	Length of Root	Mesio-distal Diam-eter of Crown	Mesio-distal Diam-eter of Crown at Cervix	Labio- or Bucco-lingual Diameter of Crown	Labio- or Bucco-lingual Diameter of Crown at Cervix	Curvature of Cervical Line— Mesial	Curvature of Cervical Line— Distal
Dimensions suggested for carving technic	7.5°	14.0	11.0	9.0	10.5	9.0	1.0	0.0

°Millimeters.

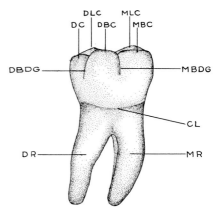

Figure 12–3. Mandibular right first molar—buccal aspect. *MBDG,* mesiobuccal developmental groove; *CL,* cervical line; *MR,* mesial root; *DR,* distal root; *DBDG,* distobuccal developmental groove; *DC,* distal cusp; *DLC,* distolingual cusp; *DBC,* distobuccal cusp; *MLC,* mesiolingual cusp; *MBC,* mesiobuccal cusp.

DETAILED DESCRIPTION OF THE MANDIBULAR FIRST MOLAR FROM ALL ASPECTS

Buccal Aspect (Figs. 12–3, 12–4, 12–12, 12–13 and 12–14)

From the buccal aspect the crown of the mandibular first molar is roughly trapezoidal, with cervical and occlusal outlines representing the uneven sides of the trapezoid. The occlusal side is the longer.

If this tooth is posed vertically, all five of its cusps are in view. The two buccal cusps and the buccal portion of the distal cusp are in the foreground, with the tips of

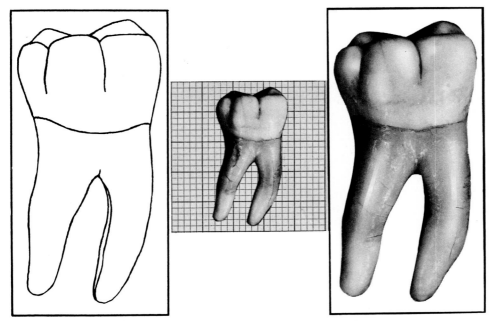

Figure 12–4.   Mandibular right first molar—buccal aspect.

the lingual cusps in the background. The lingual cusps may be seen because they are higher than the others.

Two developmental grooves appear on the crown portion. These grooves are called the *mesiobuccal developmental groove* and the *distobuccal developmental groove.* The first-named groove acts as a line of demarcation between the mesiobuccal lobe and the distobuccal lobe. The latter groove separates the distobuccal lobe from the distal lobe (Figs. 12–2 and 12–3).

The mesiobuccal, distobuccal and distal cusps are relatively flat. These cusp ridges show less curvature than those of any of the teeth described so far. The distal cusp, which is small, is more pointed than either of the buccal cusps. Flattened buccal cusps are typical of all mandibular molars. Most first molar specimens have the buccal cusps worn considerably, showing the buccal cusp ridges almost at the same level. Before they are worn, the buccal cusps and the distal cusp have curvatures that are characteristic of each one (Figs. 12–4 and 12–14, specimen 4).

The mesiobuccal cusp is usually the widest mesiodistally of the three cusps. This cusp has some curvature but is relatively flat. The distobuccal cusp is almost as wide, with a cusp ridge of somewhat greater curvature. The two buccal cusps make up the major portion of the buccal surface of the crown. The distal cusp provides a very small part of the buccal surface, since the major portion of the cusp makes up the distal portion of the crown, providing the distal contact area on the center of the distal surface of the distal cusp. The distal cusp ridge is very round occlusally, being sharper than either of the two buccal cusps.

These three cusps have the mesiobuccal and distobuccal grooves as lines of demarcation. The mesiobuccal groove is the shorter of the two, having its terminus centrally located cervico-occlusally. This groove is situated a little mesial to the root bifurcation buccally. The distobuccal groove has its terminus near the distobuccal line angle at the cervical third of the crown. It travels occlusally and somewhat mesially, parallel with the axis of the distal root.

The cervical line of the mandibular first molar is commonly regular in outline, dipping apically toward the root bifurcation.

The mesial outline of the crown is somewhat concave at the cervical third up to its junction with the convex outline of the broad contact area. The distal outline of the crown is straight above the cervical line to its junction with the convex outline of the distal contact area, which is also the outline of the distal portion of the distal cusp.

The calibration of this tooth at the cervical line is 1.5 to 2 mm. less mesiodistally than the mesiodistal measurement at the contact areas, which of course represents the greatest mesiodistal measurement of the crown.

The surface of the buccal portion of the crown is smoothly convex at the cusp portions with developmental grooves between the cusps. Approximately at the level of the ends of the developmental grooves, in the middle third, a developmental depression is noticeable. It runs in a mesiodistal direction just above the cervical ridge of the buccal surface (Fig. 12–14, specimens 6 and 8). This cervical ridge may show a smooth depression in it which progresses cervically, joining with the developmental concavity just below the cervical line which is congruent with the root bifurcation buccally.

The roots of this tooth are, in most instances, well formed and constant in development.

When the tooth is posed so that the mesiobuccal groove is directly in the line of vision, part of the distal surface of the root trunk may be seen and, in addition, one may see part of the distal area of the mesial root because the lingual portion of the root is turned distally. These areas may be seen in addition to the buccal areas of the roots and root trunk.

The mesial root is curved mesially from a point shortly below the cervical line to the middle third portion. From this point it curves distally to the tapered apex, which is located directly below the mesiobuccal cusp. The crest of curvature of the root mesially is mesial to the crown cervix. The distal outline of the mesial root is concave from the bifurcation of the root trunk to the apex.

The distal root is less curved than the mesial root, and its axis is in a distal direction from cervix to apex. The root may show some curvature at its apical third in either a mesial or a distal direction (Fig. 12–14, specimens 1 and 8). The apex is usually more pointed than that of the mesial root and is located below or distal to the distal contact area of the crown. There is considerable variation in the comparative lengths of mesial and distal roots (Fig. 12–14).

Both roots are wider mesiodistally at the buccal areas than they are lingually. Developmental depressions are present on the mesial and distal sides of both roots — a fact which lessens the mesiodistal measurement at those points. They are somewhat thicker at the lingual borders. This arrangement provides a secure anchorage for the mandibular first molar, preventing rotation. This I-beam principle increases the anchorage of each root (Chapter 13, Fig. 13–41).

The point of bifurcation of the two roots is located approximately 3 mm. below the cervical line. There is a deep developmental depression buccally on the root trunk which starts at the bifurcation and progresses cervically, becoming more shallow until it terminates at or immediately above the cervical line. This depression is smooth with no developmental groove or fold.

Lingual Aspect (Figs. 12–5, 12–6, 12–12 and 12–13)

From the lingual aspect, three cusps may be seen: two lingual cusps and the lingual portion of the distal cusp (Fig. 12–5). The two lingual cusps are pointed, and the cusp ridges are high enough to hide the two buccal cusps from view. The mesiolingual cusp is the widest mesiodistally, with its cusp tip somewhat higher than the distolingual cusp. The distolingual cusp is almost as wide mesiodistally as the mesiolingual cusp. The mesiolingual and distolingual cusp ridges are inclined at angles that are similar on both lingual cusps. These cusp ridges form obtuse angles at the cusp tips of approximately 100 degrees.

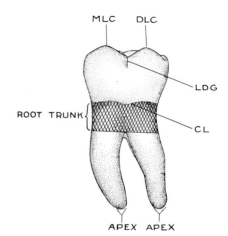

Figure 12–5. Mandibular first molar — lingual aspect. *MLC,* mesiolingual cusp; *DLC,* distolingual cusp; *LDG,* lingual developmental groove; *CL,* cervical line.

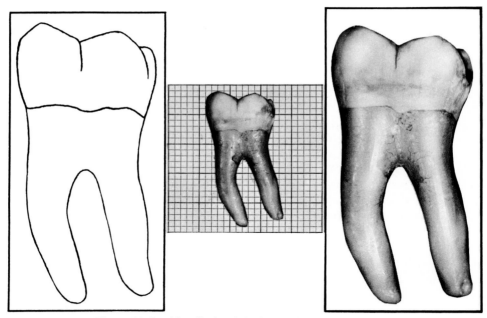

Figure 12–6. Mandibular right first molar—lingual aspect.

The *lingual developmental groove* serves as a line of demarcation between the lingual cusps, extending downward on the lingual surface of the crown for a short distance only. Some mandibular first molars show no groove on the lingual surface but show a depression lingual to the cusp ridges. The angle formed by the distolingual cusp ridge of the mesiolingual cusp and the mesiolingual cusp ridge of the distolingual cusp is more obtuse than the angulation of the cusp ridges at the tips of the lingual cusps.

The distal cusp is at a lower level than the mesiolingual cusp.

The mesial outline of the crown from this aspect is convex from the cervical line to the marginal ridge. The crest of contour mesially, which represents the contact area, is somewhat higher than the crest of contour distally.

The distal outline of the crown is straight immediately above the cervical line to a point immediately below the distal contact area; this area is represented by a convex curvature which also outlines the distal surface of the distal cusp. The junction of the distolingual cusp ridge of the distolingual cusp with the distal marginal ridge is abrupt; it gives the impression of a groove at this site from the lingual aspect. Sometimes there is a shallow developmental groove at this point (Fig. 12–10). Part of the mesial and distal surfaces of the crown and root trunk may be seen from this aspect because the mesial and distal sides converge lingually.

The cervical line lingually is irregular and tends to point sharply toward the root bifurcation and immediately above it.

The surface of the crown lingually is smooth and spheroidal on each of the lingual lobes. The surface is concave at the side of the lingual groove above the center of the crown lingually. Below this point the surface of the crown becomes almost flat as it approaches the cervical line.

The roots of the mandibular first molar appear somewhat different from the lingual aspect. They measure about 1 mm. longer lingually than buccally, but the length *seems* more extreme (Figs. 12–6 and 12–7). This impression is derived from the fact that the cusp ridges and cervical line are at a higher level (about 1 mm.). This arrangement adds a millimeter to the distance from root bifurcation to cervical line. In addition, the mesiodistal measurement of the root trunk is less toward the lingual surface than toward the buccal surface. Consequently this slenderness lingually, in addition to the added length, makes the roots appear longer than they are from the lingual aspect (Fig. 12–9).

As was mentioned, the root bifurcation lingually starts at a point approximately 4 mm. below the cervical line. This developmental depression is quite deep at this point, although it is smooth throughout and progresses cervically and becomes more shallow until it fades out entirely immediately below the cervical line. The depression is rarely reflected in the cervical line or the enamel of the lingual surface of the crown as is found in many cases on the buccal surface of this tooth.

This bifurcation groove of the root trunk is located almost in line with the lingual developmental groove of the crown.

Mesial Aspect (Figs. 12–7, 12–12, 12–13 and 12–15)

When the mandibular first molar is viewed from the mesial aspect, the specimen being held with its mesial surface at right angles to the line of vision, two cusps and one root only are to be seen: the mesiobuccal and mesiolingual cusps and the mesial root (Fig. 12–7).

The buccolingual measurement of the crown is greater at the mesial portion than it is at the distal portion. The buccolingual measurement of the mesial root is also greater than the same measurement of the distal root. Therefore, since the mesial portions of the tooth are broader and the mesial cusps are higher, the distal portions of the tooth cannot be seen from this angle.

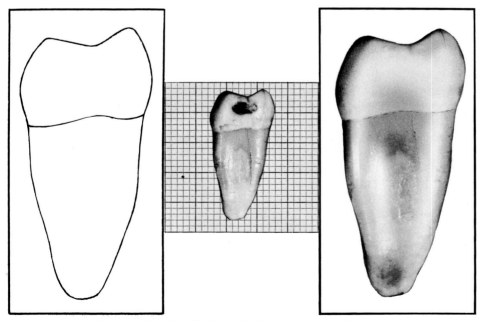

Figure 12–7.   Mandibular right first molar—mesial aspect.

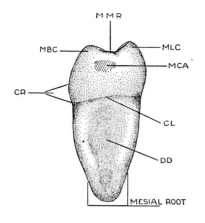

Figure 12–8. Mandibular right first molar—mesial aspect. *MMR,* mesial marginal ridge; *MLC,* mesiolingual cusp; *MCA,* mesial contact area; *CL,* cervical line; *DD,* developmental depression; *CR,* cervical ridge; *MBC,* mesiobuccal cusp.

As mentioned before, all of the posterior mandibular teeth have crown outlines from the mesial aspect which show a characteristic relation between crown and root. The crown from the mesial or distal aspect is roughly rhomboidal and the entire crown has a lingual tilt in relation to the root axis. It should be remembered that the crowns of maxillary posterior teeth have the center of the occlusal surfaces between the cusps in line with the root axes (Fig. 4–26 *E, F*).

It is interesting to note the difference between the *outline form of the mandibular first molar and the mandibular second premolar from the mesial aspect* (See Chapter 10). The first molar compares as follows:

1. The crown is a fraction of a millimeter to a millimeter shorter in the first molar.
2. The root is usually that much shorter also.
3. The buccolingual measurement of crown and root of the molar is 2 mm. or more greater.
4. The lingual cusp is longer than the buccal cusp. (The opposite is true of the second premolar.)

Regardless of these differences, *the two teeth have the same functional form except for the added reinforcement given to the molar lingually.* Because of the added root width buccolingually, the buccal cusps of the first molar do not approach the center axis of the root as does the second premolar, and the lingual cusp tips are within the lingual outline of the roots instead of being on a line with them.

From the mesial aspect, the buccal outline of the crown of the mandibular first molar is convex immediately above the cervical line. Before occlusal wear has shortened the buccal cusps, this curvature is over the cervical third of the crown buccally, outlining the *buccal cervical ridge* (Fig. 12–8). This ridge is more prominent on some first molars than on others (Fig. 12–15). Just as on mandibular premolars, this ridge curvature does not exceed similar contours on other teeth as a rule when the mandibular first molar is posed in the position it assumes in the mandibular arch (Fig. 12–7 and Fig. 12–15, specimens 1 and 2).

Above the buccal cervical ridge, the outline of the buccal contour may be slightly concave on some specimens (Fig. 12–15, specimens 1 and 2); or the outline may just be less convex or even rather flat as it continues occlusally outlining the contour of the mesiobuccal cusp. The mesiobuccal cusp is located directly above the buccal third of the mesial root.

The lingual outline of the crown is straight in a lingual direction, starting at the cervical line and joining the lingual curvature at the middle third, the lingual curvature being pronounced between this point and the tip of the mesiolingual cusp. The crest of the lingual contour is located at the center of the middle third of the crown. The tip of the mesiolingual cusp is in a position directly above the lingual third of the mesial root.

The mesial marginal ridge is confluent with the mesial ridges of the mesiobuccal and mesiolingual cusps. The marginal ridge is placed about 1 mm. below the level of the cusp tips.

The cervical line mesially is rather irregular and tends to curve occlusally about 1 mm. toward the center of the mesial surface of the tooth (Fig. 12–15, specimens 1, 4, 9 and 10). The cervical line may assume a relatively straight line buccolingually (speciments 3, 6 and 8).

In all instances the cervical line is at a higher level lingually than buccally, usually about 1 mm. higher. The difference in level may be greater. This relation depends upon the assumption that the tooth is posed vertically. When the first molar is in its normal position in the lower jaw, leaning to the lingual, the cervical line is nearly level buccolingually.

The surface of the crown is convex and smooth over the mesial contours of the mesiolingual and mesiobuccal lobes. A flattened or slightly concave area exists at the cervical line immediately above the center of the mesial root. This area is right below the contact area and joins the concavity of the central portion of the root at the cervix. The contact area is almost centered buccolingually in the mesial surface of the crown, and it is placed below the crest of the marginal ridge about one third the distance from marginal ridge to cervical line. (See stained contact area on specimen, Fig. 12–9. Before contact wear has occurred, the contact area is not so broad. Refer also to Fig. 12–4.)

The buccal outline of the mesial root drops straight down from the cervical line buccally to a point near the junction of cervical and middle thirds of the root. There is a gentle curve lingually from this point to the apex, which is located directly below the mesiobuccal cusp.

The lingual outline of the mesial root is slanted in a buccal direction, although the outline is nearly straight from the cervical line lingually to the point of junction of middle and apical thirds of the root. From this point the curvature is sharply buccal to the bluntly tapered apex. On those specimens which show a short bifurcation at the mesial root end, the curvature at the apical third lingually is slight (Fig. 12–15, specimens 2 and 10).

The mesial surface of the mesial root is convex at the buccal and lingual borders, with a broad concavity between these convexities the full length of the root from cervical line to apex. If a specimen tooth is held in front of a strong light so that one may see the distal side of the mesial root from the apical aspect, it is noted that the same contours exist on the root distally as are found mesially, and the root is very thin where the concavities are superimposed. The root form appears to be two narrow roots fused together with thin hard tissue between.

The mesial surface of the distal root is smooth, with no deep developmental depressions.

Distal Aspect (Figs. 12–10, 12–12 and 12–13)

Since the gross outline of the distal aspect of crown and root of the mandibular first molar is similar to the mesial aspect, the description of outline form will not be repeated. When considering this aspect from the standpoint of a three-dimensional figure, however, one sees more of the tooth from the distal aspect because the crown

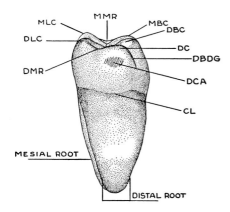

Figure 12–9. Mandibular right first molar—distal aspect. *MMR*, mesial marginal ridge; *MBC*, mesiobuccal cusp; *DBC*, distobuccal cusp; *DC*, distal cusp; *DBDG*, distobuccal developmental groove; *DCA*, distal contact area; *CL*, cervical line; *DMR*, distal marginal ridge; *DLC*, distolingual cusp; *MLC*, mesiolingual cusp.

is shorter distally than mesially, and the buccal and lingual surfaces of the crown converge distally. The buccal surface shows more convergence than the lingual surface. The distal root is narrower buccolingually than the mesial root.

If a specimen of the first molar is held with the distal surface of the crown at right angles to the line of vision, a great part of the occlusal surface may be seen and some part of each of the five cusps also comparing favorably with the mandibular second premolar. This is caused in part by the placement of the crown on the roots with a distal inclination to the long axes. The slight variation in crown length distally does not provide this view of the occlusal surface (Figs. 12–9 and 12–10).

From the distal aspect, the distal cusp is in the foreground on the crown portion. The distal cusp is placed a little buccal to center buccolingually, the distal contact area appearing on its distal contour.

The distal contact area is placed just below the distal cusp ridge of the distal cusp and at a slightly higher level above the cervical line than was found mesially when comparing the location of the mesial contact area.

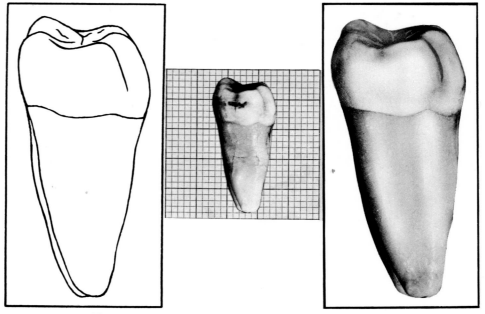

Figure 12–10. Mandibular right first molar—distal aspect.

The distal marginal ridge is short and is made up of the distal cusp ridge of the distal cusp and the distolingual cusp ridge of the distolingual cusp. These cusp ridges dip sharply in a cervical direction, meeting at an obtuse angle. Often a developmental groove or depression is found crossing the marginal ridge at this point. The point of this angle is above the lingual third of the distal root instead of being centered over the root as is true of the center of the mesial marginal ridge.

The distal contact area is centered over the distal root, which arrangement places it buccal to the center point of the distal marginal ridge.

The surface of the distal portion of the crown is convex on the distal cusp and the distolingual cusp. Contact wear may produce a flattened area at the point of contact on the distal surface of the distal cusp. Just above the cervical line, the enamel surface is flat where it joins the flattened surface of the root trunk distally.

The cervical line distally usually extends straight across buccolingually. It may be irregular, dipping root-wise just below the distal contact area (Fig. 12–10).

The end of the distobuccal developmental groove is located on the distal surface and forms a concavity at the cervical portion of the distobuccal line angle of the crown. The distal portion of the crown extends out over the root trunk distally at quite an angle (Fig. 12–4). The smooth flat surface below the contact area remains fairly constant to the apical third of the distal root. Sometimes a developmental depression is found here. The apical third portion of the root is more rounded as it tapers to a sharper apex than is found on the mesial root.

The lingual border of the mesial root may be seen from the distal aspect.

Occlusal Aspect (Figs. 12–1, 12–2, 12–11, 12–12, 12–13 and 12–16)

The mandibular first molar is somewhat hexagonal from the occlusal aspect (Fig. 12–2). The crown measurement is 1 mm. or more greater mesiodistally than buc-

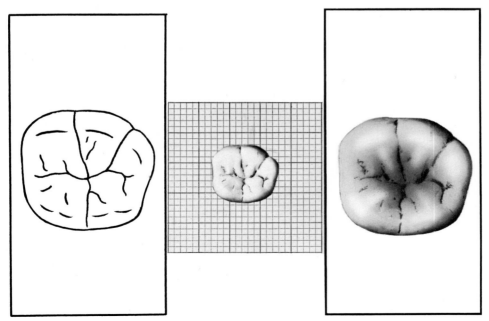

Figure 12–11.   Mandibular right first molar—occlusal aspect.

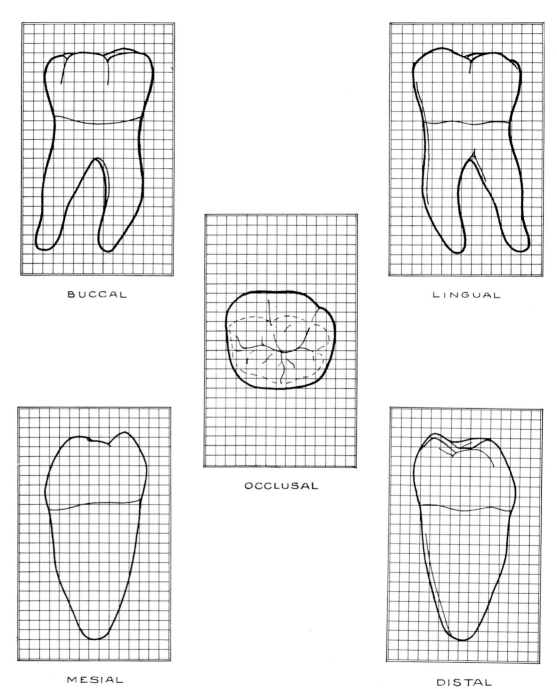

BUCCAL

LINGUAL

OCCLUSAL

MESIAL

DISTAL

Figure 12–12.   Mandibular right first molar. Graph outlines form five aspects.

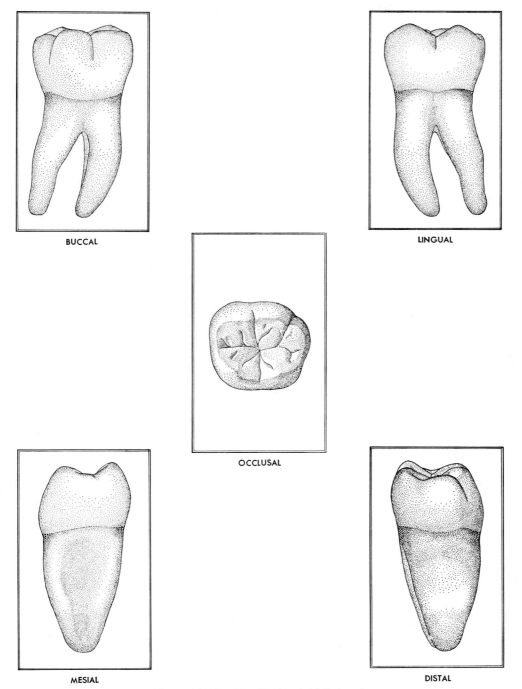

BUCCAL

LINGUAL

OCCLUSAL

MESIAL

DISTAL

Figure 12–13. Mandibular right first molar.

1   2   3   4   5

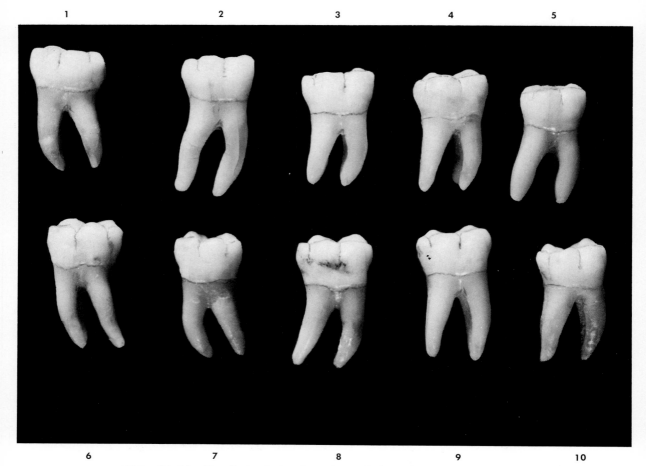

6   7   8   9   10

Figure 12–14.   Mandibular first molars—ten typical specimens—buccal aspect.

colingually. It must be remembered that the opposite arrangement is true of the maxillary first molar.

The buccolingual measurement of the crown is greater on the mesial than on the distal. Also, a measurement of the crown at the contact areas, which includes the two buccal cusps and the distal cusp, shows greater measurement than the mesiodistal measurement of the two lingual cusps. In other words, the crown converges lingually from the contact areas. This convergence varies in individual specimens (Fig. 12–16, specimens 1 and 4).

It is interesting to note the degree of development of the individual cusps from the occlusal aspect. The mesiobuccal cusp is slightly larger than either of the two lingual cusps, which are almost equal to each other in size; the distobuccal cusp is smaller than any one of the other three mentioned, and the distal cusp is in most cases much the smallest of all.

There is more variance in the development of the distobuccal and distal lobes than in any of the others (Fig. 12–16, specimens 1, 7 and 10).

When the tooth is posed so that the line of vision is parallel with the long axis, a great part of the buccal surface may be seen, whereas only a small portion of the lingual surface may be seen lingual to the lingual cusp ridges. No part of the mesial

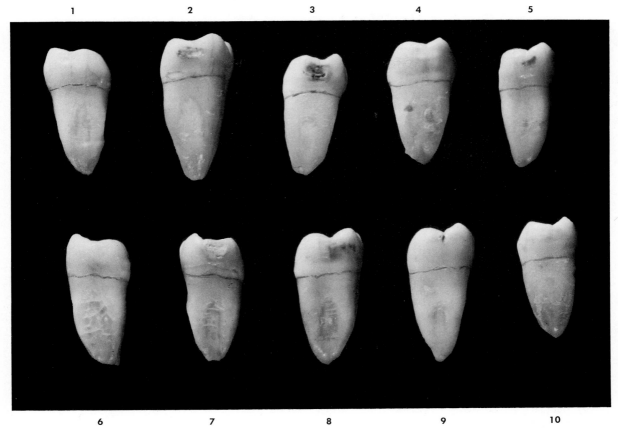

Figure 12–15.   Mandibular first molars—ten typical specimens—mesial aspect.

or distal surfaces is in view below the outline of the mesial and distal marginal ridges. (Compare tooth outlines from the other aspects.)

All mandibular molars, including the first molar, are essentially quadrilateral in form. The mandibular first molar, in most instances, has a functioning distal cusp, although this is small in comparison with the other cusps. Occasionally four-cusp first molars are found, and more often one discovers first molars with distobuccal and distal cusps showing fusion with little or no trace of a distobuccal developmental groove between them (Fig. 12–16, specimen 1; Fig. 12–17, specimens 4 and 5). *From a developmental viewpoint all mandibular molars have four major cusps, whereas maxillary molars have only three major cusps* (Fig. 11–11).

The *occlusal* surface of the mandibular first molar may be described as follows: There is a major fossa and there are two minor fossae. The major fossa is the *central fossa* (Fig. 12–2). It is roughly circular, and it is centrally placed on the occlusal surface between buccal and lingual cusp ridges. The two minor fossae are the *mesial triangular fossa,* immediately distal to the mesial marginal ridge, and the *distal triangular fossa,* placed immediately mesial to the distal marginal ridge (Fig. 12–1).

The developmental grooves on the occlusal surface are the *central developmental groove,* the *mesiobuccal developmental groove,* the *distobuccal developmental groove* and the *lingual developmental groove.* Supplemental grooves, accidental short grooves and developmental pits are also found. Most of the

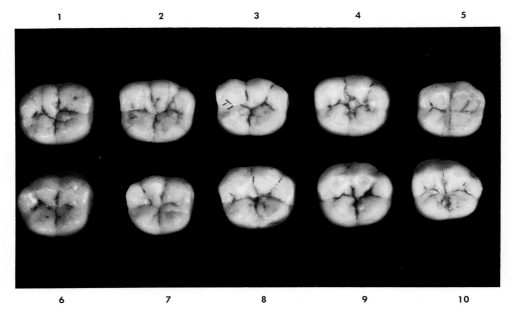

Figure 12–16.   Mandibular first molars—ten typical specimens—occlusal aspect.

supplemental grooves are tributary to the developmental grooves within the bounds of cusp ridges.

The *central fossa* of the occlusal surface is a concave area bounded by the distal slope of the mesiobuccal cusp, both mesial and distal slopes of the distobuccal cusp, the mesial slope of the distal cusp, the distal slope of the mesiolingual cusp and the mesial slope of the distolingual cusp (Fig. 12–2).

All of the developmental grooves converge in the center of the central fossa at the *central pit.*

The *mesial triangular fossa* of the occlusal surface is a smaller concave area than the central fossa, and it is bounded by the mesial slope of the mesiobuccal cusp, the mesial marginal ridge and the mesial slope of the mesiolingual cusp. The mesial portion of the central developmental groove terminates in this fossa. Usually a buccal and a lingual supplemental groove join it at a *mesial pit* within the boundary of the mesial marginal ridge. Sometimes a supplemental groove crosses the mesial marginal ridge lingual to the contact area (Fig. 12–16, specimens 2, 8, 9 and 10).

The *distal triangular fossa* is in most instances less distinct than the mesial fossa. It is bounded by the distal slope of the distal cusp, the distal marginal ridge and the distal slope of the distolingual cusp. The central groove has its other terminal in this fossa. Buccal and lingual supplemental grooves are less common here. An extension of the central groove quite often crosses the distal marginal ridge, however, lingual to the distal contact area.

Starting at the central pit in the central fossa, the central developmental groove travels an irregular course mesially, terminating in the mesial triangular fossa. A short distance mesially from the central pit, it joins the mesiobuccal developmental groove. The latter groove courses in a mesiobuccal direction at the bottom of a sulcate groove separating the mesiobuccal and distobuccal cusps. At the junction of the cusp ridges of those cusps, the mesiobuccal groove of the occlusal surface is confluent with the mesiobuccal groove of the buccal surface of the crown. The lingual developmental groove of the occlusal surface is an irregular groove coursing in a lingual direction at

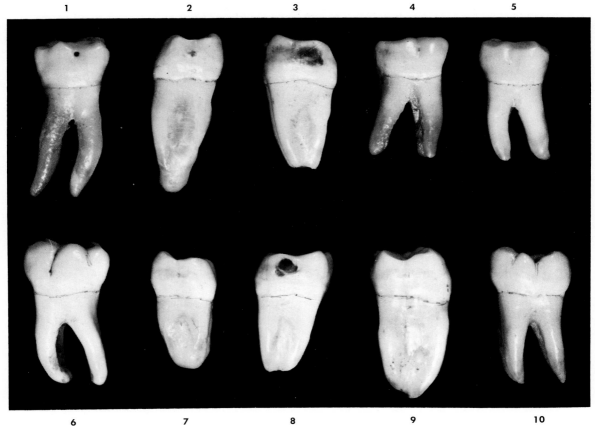

Figure 12-17. Mandibular first molars—ten specimens showing uncommon variations. 1, Root extremely long, crown small. 2, Mesial root longer than average with rounded apex. 3, Crown very wide buccolingually, roots short. 4, Roots short. 5, Crown has no buccal developmental grooves. 6, Crown and roots poorly formed. 7, Roots dwarfed. 8, Short roots, crown wide buccolingually. 9, Crown and root oversize buccolingually. 10, Extra tubercle or cusp attached to mesiolingual lobe.

the bottom of the lingual sulcate groove to the junction of lingual cusp ridges, where it is confluent with the lingual extension of the same groove. Again starting at the central pit, the central groove may be followed in a distobuccal direction to a point where it is joined by the distobuccal developmental groove of the occlusal surface. From this point the central groove courses in a distolingual direction, terminating in the distal triangular fossa. The distobuccal groove passes from its junction with the central groove in a distobuccal course, joining its buccal extension on the buccal surface of the crown at the junction of the cusp ridges of the distobuccal and distal cusps.

The central developmental groove seems to be centrally located in relation to the buccolingual crown dimension. This arrangement makes the triangular ridges of lingual cusps longer than the triangular ridges of buccal cusps.

Note the relative position and relative size of the distal cusp from the occlusal aspect. The distal portion of it joins the distal contact area of the crown.

MANDIBULAR SECOND MOLAR

The mandibular second molar supplements the first molar in function. Its anatomy differs in some details.

Mandibular Second Molar

First evidence of calcification..... 2½ to 3 years
Enamel completed................... 7 to 8 years
Eruption .... 11 to 13 years
Root completed .... 14 to 15 years

Measurement Table

	Cervico-occlusal Length of Crown	Length of Root	Mesio-distal Diam-eter of Crown	Mesio-distal Diam-eter of Crown at Cervix	Labio- or Bucco-lingual Diameter of Crown	Labio- or Bucco-lingual Diameter of Crown at Cervix	Curvature of Cervical Line — Mesial	Curvature of Cervical Line — Distal
Dimensions suggested for carving technic	7.0°	13.0	10.5	8.0	10.0	9.0	1.0	0.0

°Millimeters.

Normally, the second molar is smaller than the first molar by a fraction of a millimeter in all dimensions. It does not, however, run true to form. It is not uncommon to find mandibular second molar crowns somewhat larger than first molars, and although the roots are not so well formed, they may be longer.

The crown has four well-developed cusps: two buccal and two lingual, of nearly equal development. There is neither a distal nor a fifth cusp, but the distobuccal cusp is larger than that found on the first molar.

The tooth has two well-developed roots, one mesial and one distal. These roots are broad buccolingually, but they are not so broad as those of the first molar, nor are they so widely separated.

DETAILED DESCRIPTION OF THE MANDIBULAR SECOND MOLAR FROM ALL ASPECTS

In describing this tooth, direct comparisons will be made with the first mandibular molar.

Buccal Aspect (Figs. 12–18 and 12–23)

The crown is somewhat shorter cervico-occlusally and narrower mesiodistally than in the first molar. The crown and root show a tendency toward greater over-all length, but are not always longer (Fig. 12–23, specimens 4, 7 and 9).

There is but one developmental groove buccally, the *buccal developmental groove*. This groove acts as a line of demarcation between the mesiobuccal and the distobuccal cusps, which are about equal in their mesiodistal measurements.

The cervical line buccally in many instances points sharply toward the root bifurcation (Fig. 12–23, specimens 1, 2, 3, 5 and 9).

The roots may be shorter than those of the first molar, but they vary considerably in this as well as in their development generally. The roots are usually closer together, and their axes are nearly parallel. They may spread as much as those of the first molar (Fig. 12–23, specimen 5), or they may be fused for all or part of their length (specimens 8 and 9).

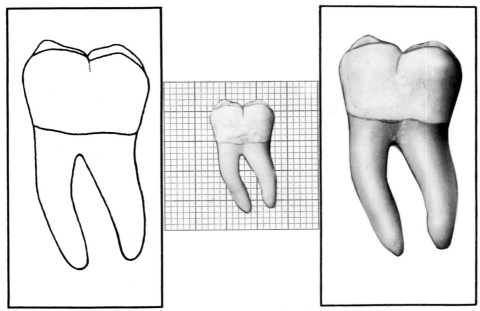

Figure 12–18.   Mandibular left second molar—buccal aspect.

The roots are inclined distally in relation to the occlusal plane of the crown, their axes forming more of an acute angle with the occlusal plane than is found on the first molar. When one compares all of the mandibular molars, it may seem that the first molar shows one angulation of roots to occlusal plane, the second molar a more acute angle and the third molar an angle which is more acute still. (See Chapter 16 on Occlusion.)

Lingual Aspect (Fig. 12–19)

Differences in detail between the mandibular second molar and the mandibular first molar, to be noted from the lingual aspect, are these:

1. The crown and root of the mandibular second molar converge lingually but to a slight degree; little of the mesial or distal surfaces may therefore be seen from this aspect.

2. The mesiodistal calibration at the cervix lingually is always greater accordingly than that of the first molar.

3. The curvatures mesially and distally on the crown which describe the contact areas are more noticeable from the lingual aspect. They prove to be at a slightly lower level, especially in the distal area, than those of the first molar.

Mesial Aspect (Figs. 12–20 and 12–24)

Except for the differences in measurement from the mesial aspect, the second molar differs little from the first molar.

The cervical ridge buccally on the crown portion is in most instances less pronounced, and the occlusal surface may be more constricted buccolingually (Fig. 12–24, specimens 2, 8 and 10).

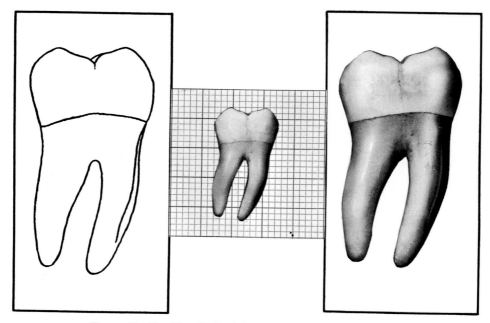

Figure 12–19.   Mandibular left second molar—lingual aspect.

The cervical line shows less curvature, being straight and regular in outline buc-colingually.

The mesial root is somewhat pointed apically. If part of the distal root is in sight it is seen buccally. In the first molar, when the distal root is in sight from the mesial aspect, it is in view lingually.

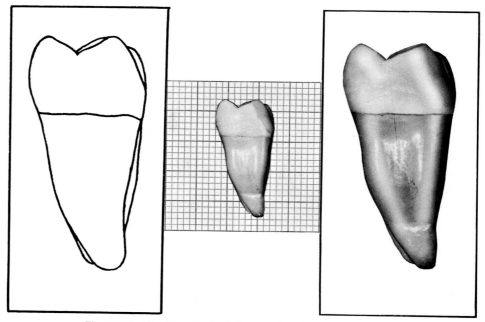

Figure 12–20.   Mandibular left second molar—mesial aspect.

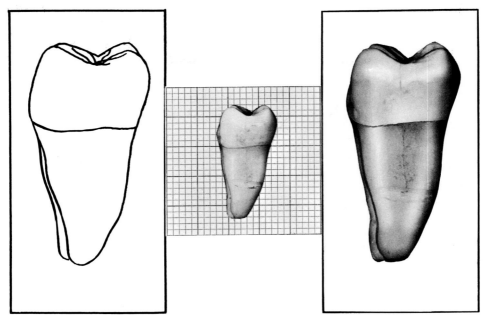

Figure 12–21.   Mandibular left second molar—distal aspect.

Distal Aspect (Fig. 12–21)

From the distal aspect, the second molar is similar in form to the first molar except for the absence of a distal cusp and a distobuccal groove. The contact area is centered on the distal surface buccolingually and is placed equidistant from cervical line and marginal ridge.

Occlusal Aspect (Figs. 12–22 and 12–25)

The occlusal aspect of the mandibular second molar differs considerably from the first molar. These variations serve as marks of identity. The small distal cusp of the first molar is not present, and the distobuccal lobe development is just as pronounced, and sometimes more so, than that of the mesiobuccal lobe. There is no distobuccal developmental groove occlusally or buccally. The buccal and lingual developmental grooves meet the central developmental groove at right angles at the central pit on the occlusal surface. These grooves form a cross, dividing the occlusal portion of the crown into four parts which are nearly equal.

In general, the cusp slopes on the occlusal surface are not so smooth as those found on first molars, since they are roughened by many supplemental grooves radiating from the developmental grooves.

The following characteristics of mandibular second molars from the occlusal aspect should be observed and noted:

1. Many of them are rectangular from the occlusal aspect (Fig. 12–25, specimens 7 and 9).

2. Many show considerable prominence cervically on the mesiobuccal lobe only (Fig. 12–25, specimens 1, 3 and 6).

3. Most second molars exhibit more curvature of the outline of the crown distally

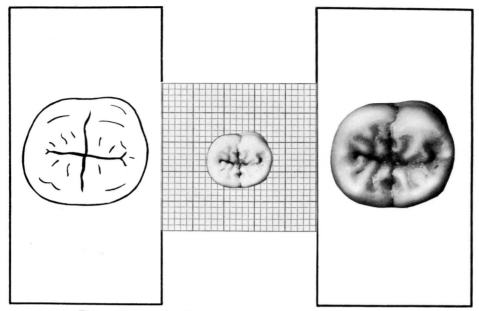

Figure 12–22. Mandibular left second molar—occlusal aspect.

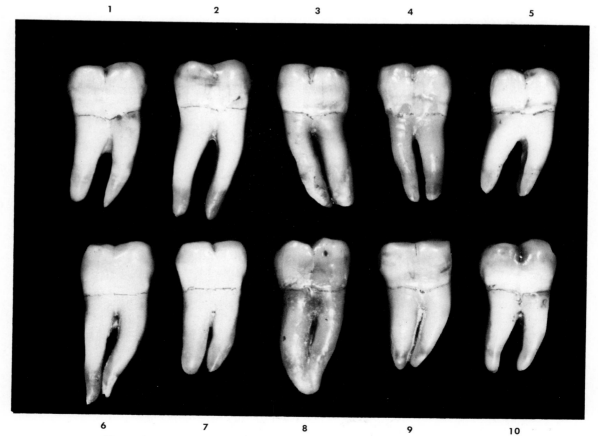

Figure 12–23. Mandibular second molars—ten typical specimens—buccal aspect.

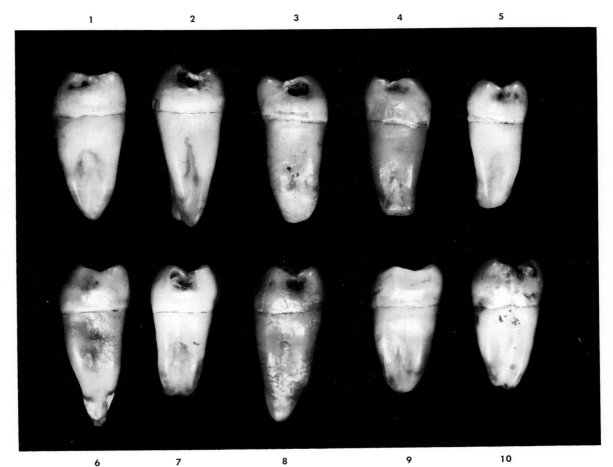

Figure 12–24.   Mandibular second molars — ten typical specimens — mesial aspect.

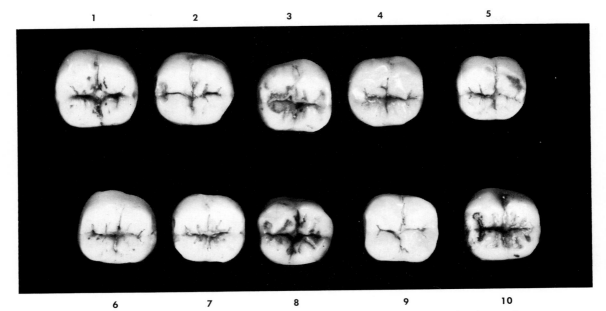

Figure 12–25.   Mandibular second molars — ten typical specimens — occlusal aspect.

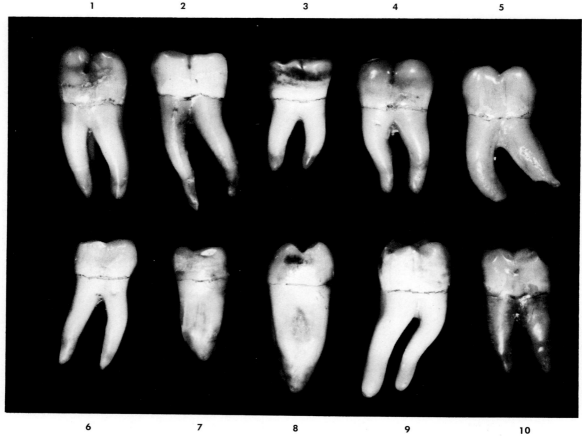

Figure 12–26. Mandibular second molars — ten specimens showing uncommon variations. 1, Mesio-distal measurements at contact areas and cervix almost equal. 2, Roots twisted and of extra length. 3, Very small specimen, short roots. 4, Roots short for such a large crown. 5, Roots thick and malformed generally. 6, Dwarfed crown, roots extra long. 7, Mesial aspect, protective curvature buccally and lingually is absent. 8, Roots of extra size, occlusal surface constricted buccolingually. 9, Roots malformed. 10, Crown wide mesiodistally at the cervix, roots short.

than mesially, showing a semicircular outline to the disto-occlusal surface in comparison with a square outline mesially.

4. The cusp ridge of the distobuccal cusp lies buccal to the cusp ridge of the mesiobuccal cusp (Fig. 12–25, specimens 2, 3, 8 and 10; Fig. 12–22).

MANDIBULAR THIRD MOLAR

The mandibular third molar varies considerably in different individuals and presents many anomalies both in form and in position. It supplements the second molar in function, although the tooth is seldom so well developed, the average mandibular third molar showing irregular development of the crown portion, with under-sized roots, more or less malformed. Generally speaking, however, its design conforms to the general plan of all mandibular molars, conforming more closely to that of the second mandibular molar in the number of cusps and occlusal design than it does to the mandibular first molar. Occasionally, mandibular third molars are seen that are well formed and comparable in size and development to the mandibular first molar.

Many instances of mandibular third molars with five or more cusps are found,

Mandibular Third Molar

First evidence of calcification ... 8 to 10 years
Enamel completed .... 12 to 16 years
Eruption............................. 17 to 21 years
Root completed..................... 18 to 25 years

Measurement Table

	Cervico-occlusal Length of Crown	Length of Root	Mesio-distal Diameter of Crown	Mesio-distal Diameter of Crown at Cervix	Labio- or Bucco-lingual Diameter of Crown	Labio- or Bucco-lingual Diameter of Crown at Cervix	Curvature of Cervical Line – Mesial	Curvature of Cervical Line – Distal
Dimensions suggested for carving technic	7.0°	11.0	10.0	7.5	9.5	9.0	1.0	0.0

°Millimeters.

with the crown portions larger than those of the second molar. In these cases the alignment and occlusion with other teeth is not normal, because insufficient room is available in the alveolar process of the mandible for the accommodation of such a large tooth and the occlusal form is too variable.

Although it is possible to find dwarfed specimens of mandibular third molars (Fig. 12–35, specimen 2), most of them which are not normal in size are larger than normal in the crown portion particularly. Roots of these oversize third molars may be short and poorly formed.

The opposite situation is likely in maxillary third molars. Most of the anomalies are undersized. Mandibular third molars are the most likely to be impacted, wholly or partially, in the jaw. The lack of space accommodation is the chief cause.

DETAILED DESCRIPTION OF THE MANDIBULAR THIRD MOLAR FROM ALL ASPECTS

Buccal Aspects (Figs. 12–27 and 12–32)

From the buccal aspect, mandibular third molars vary considerably in outline. At the same time, they all have certain characteristics in common.

The outline of the crowns from this aspect is in a general way that of all mandibular molars. The crown is wider at contact areas mesiodistally than at the cervix, the buccal cusps are short and rounded, and the crest of contour mesially and distally is located a little more than half the distance from cervical line to tips of cusps. The type of third molar which is more likely to be in fair alignment and in good occlusion with other teeth is the four-cusp type; this is smaller and shows two buccal cusps only from this aspect (Fig. 12–32, specimens 1, 4, 5, 8, 9, and 10).

The average third molar also shows two roots, one mesial and one distal. These roots are usually shorter, with a poorer development generally, than the roots of first or second molars, and their distal inclination in relation to the occlusal plane of the crown is greater. The roots may be separated with a definite point of bifurcation, or they may be fused for all or part of their length (Fig. 12–32).

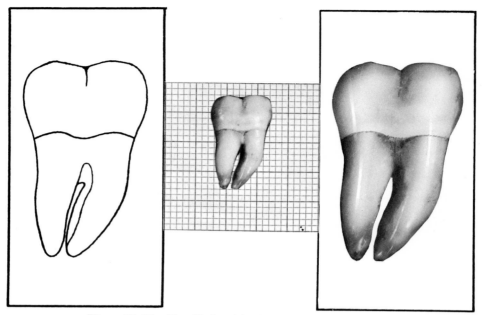

Figure 12–27.   Mandibular right third molar—buccal aspect.

Lingual Aspect (Fig. 12–28)

Observations from the lingual aspect add little to those already made from the buccal aspect. The mandibular third molar, when well developed, corresponds closely to the form of the second molar except for size and root development.

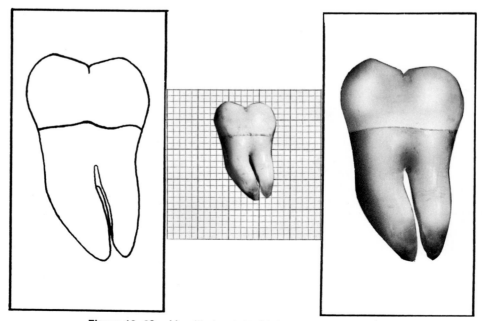

Figure 12–28.   Mandibular right third molar—lingual aspect.

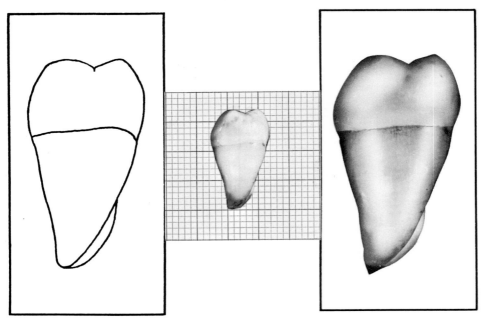

Figure 12–29. Mandibular right third molar—mesial aspect.

Mesial Aspect (Figs. 12–29 and 12–33)

From the mesial aspect, this tooth resembles the mandibular second molar except in dimensions. The roots, of course, are shorter, with the mesial root tapering more from cervix to apex. The apex of the mesial root is usually more pointed.

Distal Aspect (Fig. 12–30)

The anatomic appearance of the distal portion of this tooth is much like that of the second molar except for size.

Those specimens which have oversize crown portions are much more spheroidal above the cervical line. The distal root appears small, both in length and in buccolingual measurement, when compared with the large crown portion.

Occlusal Aspect (Figs. 12–31 and 12–34)

The occlusal aspect is quite similar to that of the second mandibular molar when the development is such as to facilitate good alignment and occlusion (Fig. 12–34, specimens 2, 3, 4, 6, 7, 8 and 9).

The tendency is toward a more rounded outline and a smaller buccolingual measurement distally. See following pages for Figures 12–30 through 12–35.

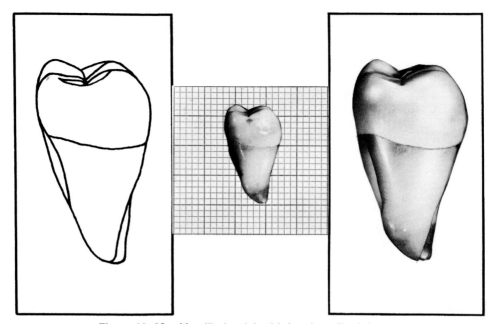

Figure 12–30.   Mandibular right third molar—distal aspect.

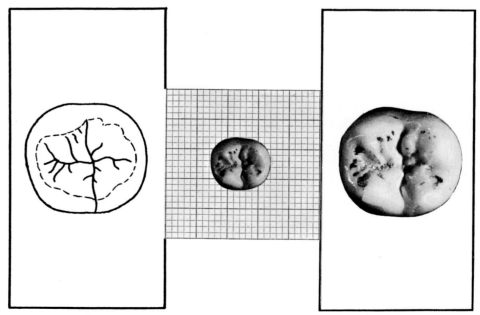

Figure 12–31.   Mandibular right third molar—occlusal aspect.

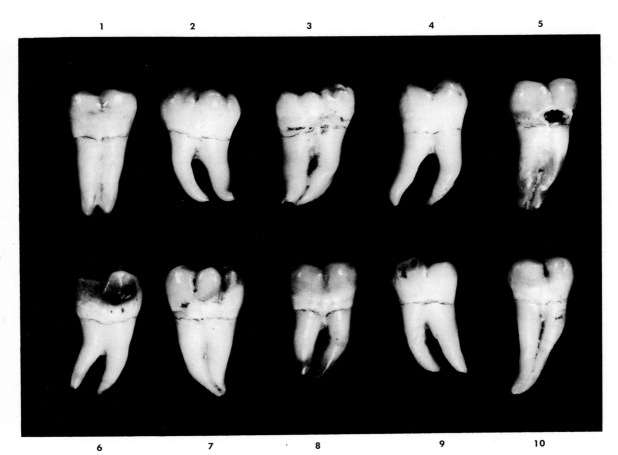

Figure 12–32.   Mandibular third molars—ten typical specimens—buccal aspect.

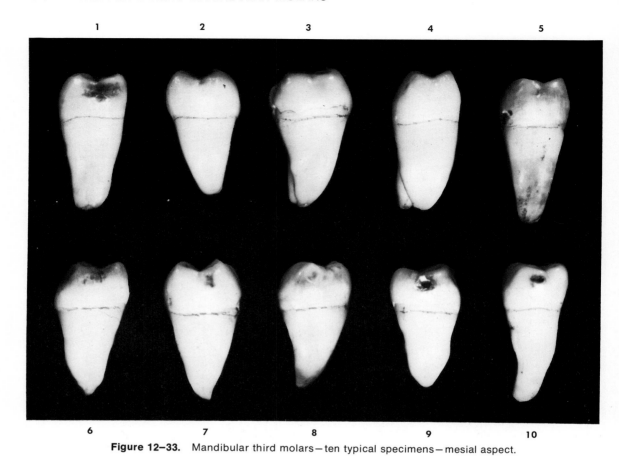

Figure 12–33. Mandibular third molars—ten typical specimens—mesial aspect.

Figure 12–34. Mandibular third molars—ten typical specimens—occlusal aspect.

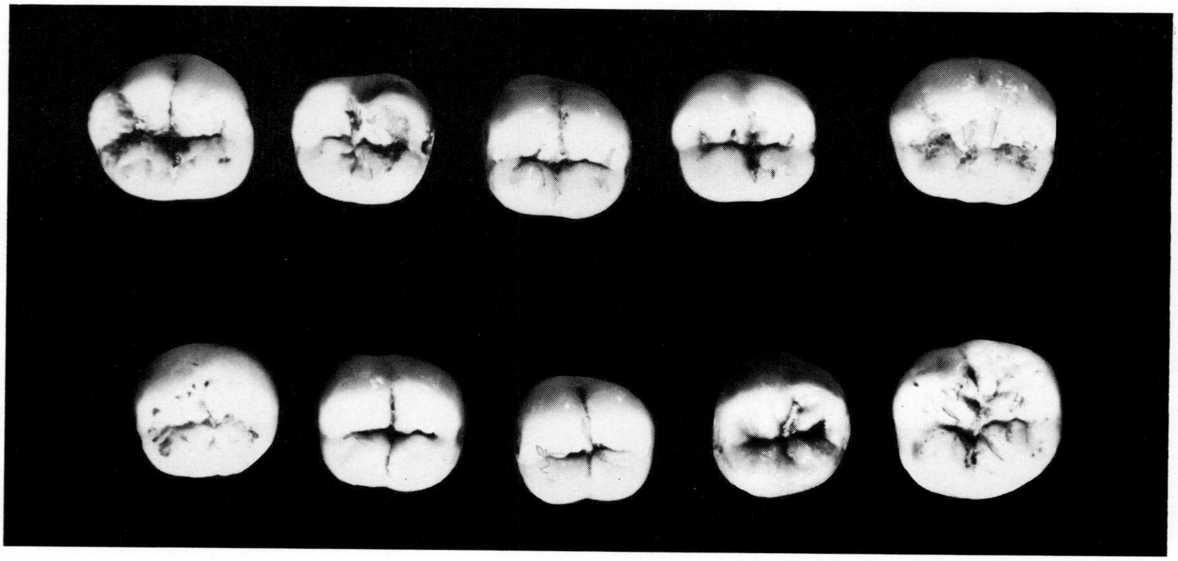

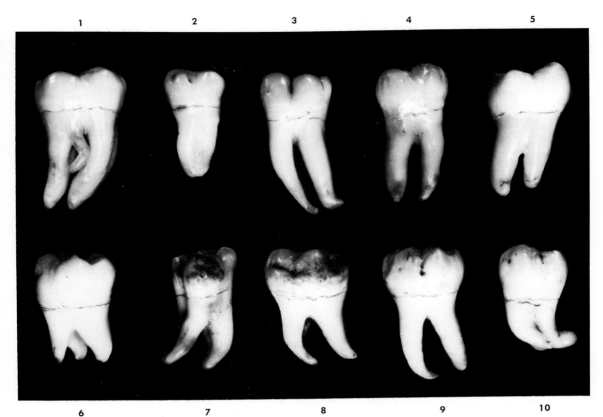

Figure 12–35.   Mandibular third molars—ten specimens showing uncommon variations. 1, Oversize generally, extra root lingually. 2, Dwarfed specimen, odd extra cusp, fused roots. 3, Crown resembling first molar, long slender roots. 4, Formation closely resembling second molar. 5, Large crown, malformed roots. 6, Multicusp crown, dwarfed roots. 7, No resemblance to typical functional form. 8, Large crown, dwarfed roots. 9, Odd crown form and root form. 10, Crown long cervico-occlusally, roots fused and malformed.

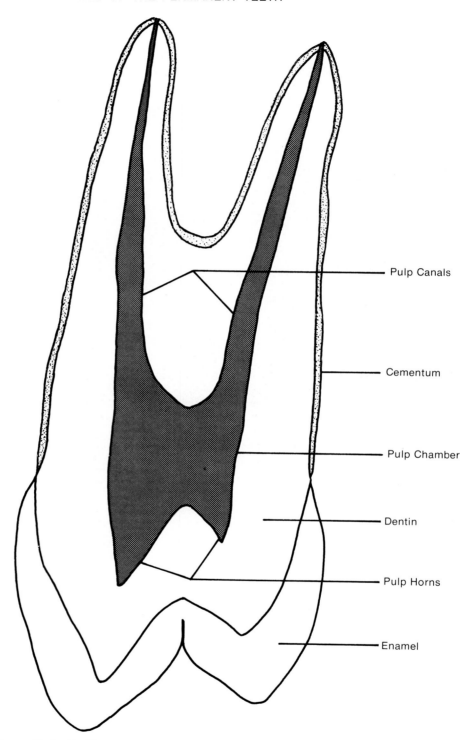

Figure 13–1. Profile of a young maxillary premolar in buccolingual cross section. This drawing was copied from an enlarged photomicrograph of an actual specimen.* The silhouette of the pulp tissue represents the entire pulp cavity, which is divided into a pulp chamber with branching pulp canals. Pulp horns would be this prominent in a very young person only.

*After Permar, Oral Embryology and Microscopic Anatomy, Lea & Febiger, 4th Ed.

13

The Pulp Cavities of the Permanent Teeth

The dental pulp is the soft tissue component of the tooth. It is a connective tissue originating from the *mesenchyme* of the *dental papilla* and it performs multiple functions throughout life. It is the formative organ of the dentin and it is the source of nutrition and maintenance of the dentin. One of the pulp's most important functions is sensory and defensive; if the tooth is exposed to any irritation which the pulp detects, it will produce a very definite defense reaction which could serve as a warning of the approach of trouble.

The pulp is located in the center of the main body of the tooth, which is dentin. The anatomical outline of the pulp, viewed mesiodistally or faciolingually, will reflect roughly the form of the dentin body. The macroscopic anatomy of pulp cavities in turn will reflect the outer form of the pulp tissue which reposed in the pulp chambers and pulp canals of the teeth in vitro.

Because the primary purpose of this book is to present studies in *macroscopic* anatomy, there will be no attempt to compete with excellent books already covering the subjects of Oral Histology and Embryology. Those books treat thoroughly the development and function of pulp tissue. The formation and function of pulp tissue will be mentioned here only as they affect the anatomy of the pulp cavities as portrayed in the *macroscopic* approach to the study.

There are two fields in dentistry that must pay particular attention to pulp cavity anatomy; these are operative dentistry and endodontics. Cavity preparation and the preparation of crown portions in crown or fixed appliance techniques will presuppose a thorough knowledge of pulp chamber size and shape. A pulp cavity may be large, as in young individuals, or it may be shrunken and constricted by excessive formation of secondary dentin; or there may be calcification within the pulp tissue itself. The operator should make a thorough diagnosis of the situation before beginning any treatment procedure.

For study of the anatomy of pulp cavities in teeth, longitudinal sections of each tooth, labio- or buccolingually and also mesiodistally should be made. In addition, transverse sections should be prepared with cuts through the crowns or roots at various levels. These dissections expose to view a central cavity with an outline corresponding in general to that of the dentin body. This space is called the *pulp cavity*, and in life it contained the dental pulp (Fig. 13–1). That portion of the pulp cavity found mainly within the coronal portion of the tooth is called the *pulp chamber*, while the remainder, found within the root, is called the *pulp canal*. The constricted opening of the pulp canal at the root end is called the *apical foramen*. It is possible for any tooth root to have more than one foramen; in such cases, the canals have two or more branches which make their exits at or near the apical end of the root. These may be called *multiple foramina* or *supplementary canals* (Figs. 13–5 and 13–6).

The *pulp chamber* is centered in the crown and is always a single cavity. The pulp canals of roots are continuous with this cavity. Many roots are found with more than one canal. The mesial root of the mandibular first molar, for instance, usually contains two pulp canals; these two canals, however, may end in a common foramen (Fig. 13–43, A, 1, 6).

The shape of the pulp chamber varies with the shape of the crown. Also, when the roots are much wider in one direction than in another, the pulp canal forms will vary accordingly. Since the crowns of the teeth are wider in all measurements than the root forms, and the roots taper from the root trunk to the apices, the pulp cavities of the teeth follow the same design. The pulp cavities taper from their largest measurement within the crown to a final constriction at the apical foramen. Sometimes the canals are so constricted as they approach the apical foramen that it is very difficult to avoid obliterating them in making cross sections.

The size of the pulp cavity is influenced by the age of the tooth, its functional activity and its history. The dental pulp decreases in size gradually as the tooth ages. The youngest teeth are provided, therefore, with the largest, most open pulp cavities (Fig. 13–7, 1, 2).

Throughout its life the *dental pulp* retains its ability to deposit what is called *secondary dentin*, a deposit which reduces the pulp cavity in size. Sometimes in old age or as a result of pathologic changes, the pulp cavity may become partially or entirely obliterated (Fig. 13–2).

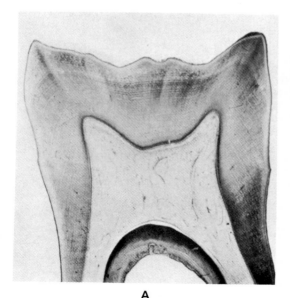 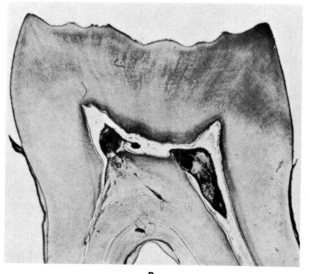

A   B

Figure 13–2.   Comparison in size of the pulps of two intact lower first permanent molars at different ages. *A*, eight years. The pulp chamber is large. Magnification × 8. *B*, Age, fifty-five years. The pulp is greatly reduced in size, and pulp stones (denticles) are present. Magnification × 8. (Dental Histology and Comparative Dental Anatomy. Kronfeld, Lea and Febiger, 1937.)

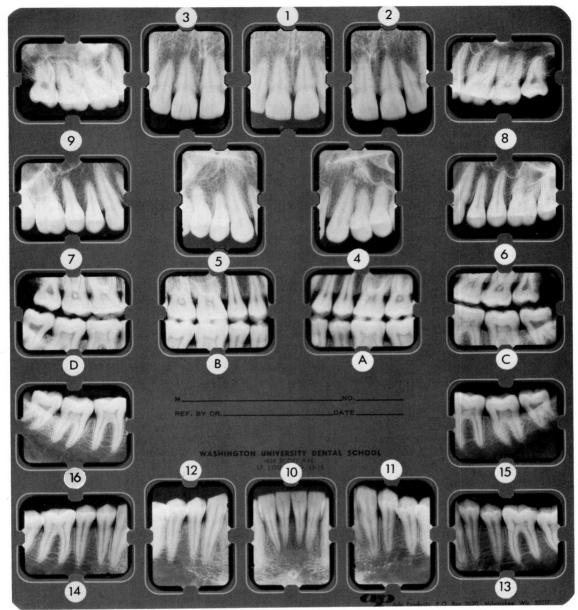

Figure 13-3. *Complete Dental Radiograph Examination.**

Maxillary Teeth
1. Central incisors
2. Right central and lateral incisors
3. Left central and lateral incisors
4. Right canine and premolars
5. Left canine and premolars
6. Right premolars and first molar
7. Left premolars and first molar
8. Right molars
9. Left molars

Mandibular Teeth
10. Central and lateral incisors
11. Right canine and premolars
12. Left canine and premolars
13. Right premolars and first molar
14. Left premolars and first molar
15. Right molars
16. Left molars

Bite Wing Radiographs

A. Right premolars, first and second molars
B. Left premolars, first and second molars

C. Right molars
D. Left molars

*Courtesy of Dr. William Koch, Washington University School of Dentistry, St. Louis, Mo.

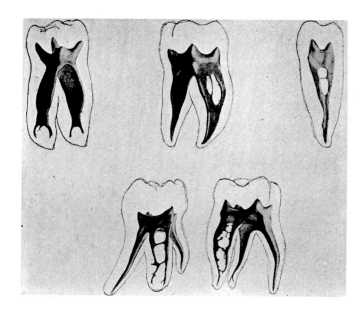

Figure 13–4. Molar pulp canal filling. Note the formation in the pulp chambers of the original pulp horns. (Prepared by Dr. Richard H. Riethmuller.)

During the period of root development the diameter of the root canal is greatest at the free, or apical end of the root, at which level it presents a funnel-shaped opening (Fig. 13–7, 1). As the root continues to develop, this funnel-shaped opening is reduced in size, and finally, as the formative process nears completion, the opening becomes more constricted until the apex of the root is mature, with a small apical foramen, or with multiple foramina (Fig. 13–7, 4).

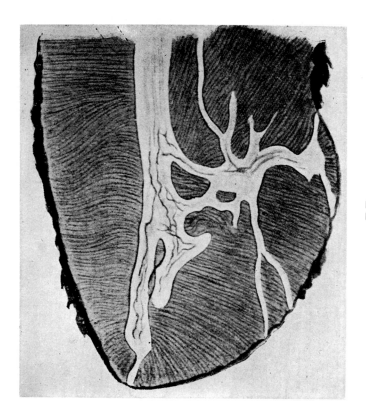

Figure 13–5. Apical end on root showing branching pulp canals. (Prepared by Dr. Richard H. Riethmuller.)

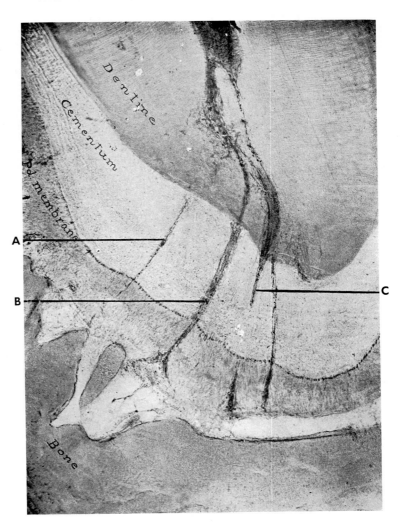

Figure 13-6. A section through the apex of a root showing three foramina, *A, B,* and *C* (Talbot).

There are prolongations or domes in the roof of the pulp chamber that correspond to the various cusps of the crown. The projections of pulp tissue occupying these spaces are called *pulp horns* (Fig. 13–4). If the cusp form of the crown of a tooth is well developed, the horns of the pulp chamber will correspond; but if the cusps are small, the pulp horns will be short or missing entirely. Posterior teeth have well-accented pulp horns. When anterior teeth, in young persons, have well-marked developmental lobes, accented pulp horns may be expected, especially in the labial portion, as extensions into the three labial lobes. These are always most marked in young teeth and they become smaller or disappear as age advances (Fig. 13–8, B, 5, 6).

The entire pulp cavity tends to become smaller with age, owing to the development of a secondary deposit. Several things may contribute to this activity, malocclusion, thermal shock, occlusal trauma, abrasion, etc. Cross sections of teeth with substantial deposits of secondary dentin are easy to obtain. Often it is possible, when studying such sections, to see the original outline of the pulp chamber because of the translucency and color variation between the secondary dentin and the primary dentin.

When studying teeth in cross section it is important to observe the labio- or buccolingual sections, for it is in these cuts that the pulp cavities show the greatest

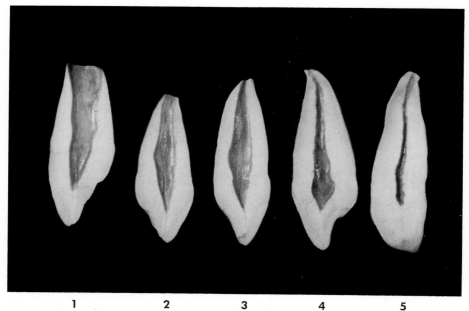

Figure 13–7. Labiolingual sections showing various stages of development of the maxillary canine. 1, Crown complete, root partially completed with large pulp cavity, wide open at the apical end. 2, Tooth almost complete except for lack of constriction of apical foramen. 3, Canine of young individual with large pulp cavity and complete root tip with generous foramen. 4, Typical average canine in adult stage with constricted apical foramen. 5, Canine of an old individual with constricted pulp chamber and canal; it will be noted that this specimen has lost its original crown form through wear and erosion.

number of variations. Students and even practitioners are apt to be less familiar with the root canal anatomy from the mesial and distal aspects. *Routine radiographs of the teeth show the cross-sectional anatomy well from the labial and buccal aspects only (Fig. 13–3). The outlines of the pulp cavities vary little from those aspects, since they tend to conform generally to the crown and root outlines. Because of technical difficulties it is impossible to get good radiographs of the teeth in situ showing the cross-sectional anatomy from the mesial or distal aspect.* Often single-rooted teeth will have more than one canal, or those teeth which are usually single-rooted may show bifurcation or multiple roots without their being discovered through radiographs. The practitioner must be aware of these variations, and he must be continuously on the alert when making a diagnosis, even though he has complete mouth radiographs to assist him. The radiographic examination may not tell him all he needs to know.

THE PULP CAVITIES OF MAXILLARY TEETH

MAXILLARY CENTRAL INCISORS (FIRST INCISORS) (Fig. 13–8, A, B, C, D)

Labiolingual Cross Section (A)

The pulp cavity follows the general outline of the dentin body. The pulp chamber is pointed toward the incisal then swells with the increase in crown dimen-

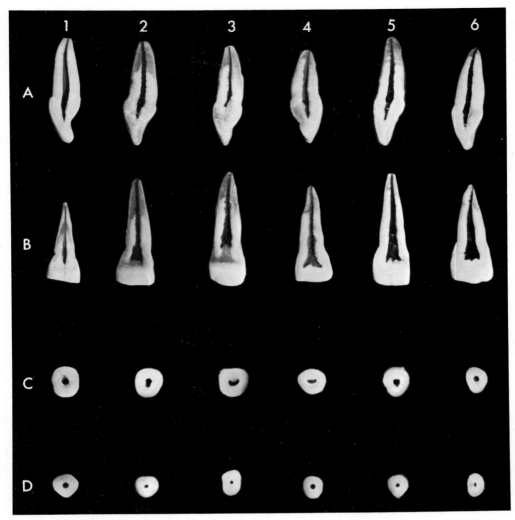

Figure 13–8. *Maxillary central incisor—cross sections of natural specimens.*

A, 1 to 6, Labiolingual sections. This aspect does not show in radiographs.
B, 1 to 6, Mesiodistal sections.
C, 1 to 6, Cervical sections of root.
D, 1 to 6, Mid-root sections.

sions. From the cervical level of the crown it tapers gradually as it traverses the root, ending in a constriction at the apex. From this angle it may be noted that the pulp chamber portion is narrow and pointed, as mentioned previously.

Mesiodistal Cross Section (B)

The pulp chamber is wider from this view, conforming in general to the shape of the dentin body. It is not unusual to find definite vestigial indications of pulp horns in the incisal portion (Fig. 13–8, B, 4, 5 and 6). The root canal tapers rather evenly along with the root toward its apex. As a rule the mesiodistal width of the root canal is somewhat greater than the labiolingual dimension. Ordinarily the maxillary central incisor pulp cavity is not constricted; therefore, the penetration of root canal instruments is rarely difficult. The uniformity of the cavity makes it readily accessible, unless an unusual secondary deposit of dentin, which may include pulp stones, exists. However, a radiographic examination will expose the problem in that case (Fig. 13–8, B, 1, 2 and 3).

Cervical Cross Section (C)

The cervical cross section is produced by cutting through the tooth at the cementoenamel junction, where the root and crown are joined. Usually this will expose the pulp chamber at its widest dimension and show the location of the root canal or canals.

This section of the maxillary central incisor shows the pulp chamber rather perfectly centered (Fig. 13–8, C, 1–6). In young individuals the chamber and canal will be "roundly triangular" in outline, which in this instance reflects the root outline most typical of the tooth. In older individuals the pulp cavity at this level becomes round or crescent shaped, and influenced by secondary dentinal deposit as age advances (section C, 4 and 6). Although the typical cervical cross section of this tooth will be triangular with rounded corners, some maxillary central incisors present a different picture. They will look rectangular generally or angular with rounded corners (section C, 2 and 5). The calibration will be generous all around. This bulk provides the crown with a substantial base.

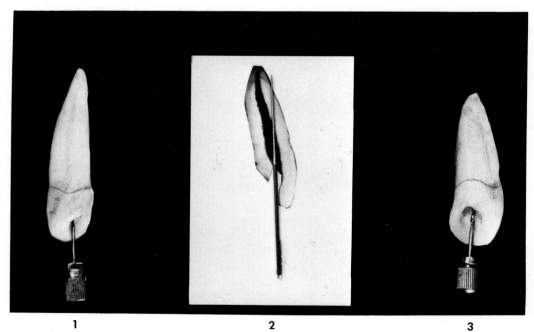

| 1 | 2 | 3 |

Figure 13–9. 1. Maxillary canine opened to allow easy entry of canal instruments in the general direction of the pulp canal. 2. Photo of a labiolingual section of a maxillary central incisor. A straight probe is placed over a simulated lingual opening showing the necessity for instrument flexibility in order to follow the path of the pulp canal. 3. A canal reamer placed in a natural central incisor. The instrument is tight up against the linguoincisal portion of the lingual opening in the attempt to follow the root canal.

MAXILLARY LATERAL INCISOR (SECOND INCISOR) (FIG. 13–10, A, B, C, D)

Labiolingual Cross Section (A)

The anatomical form of the pulp cavity of the maxillary lateral incisor resembles that of the central incisor because the functional form of the two teeth is similar. Dimensionally the lateral incisor is smaller except for root length. Sometimes the root of the lateral will prove to be the longer of the two. The description of the maxillary central incisor pulp cavity, when viewing this cross section, also may be applied to that of the lateral incisor.

Mesiodistal Cross Section (B)

The pulp cavity displayed by this section conforms generally to the outline of the dentin body of the tooth. It will be narrower over all than that found in the maxillary

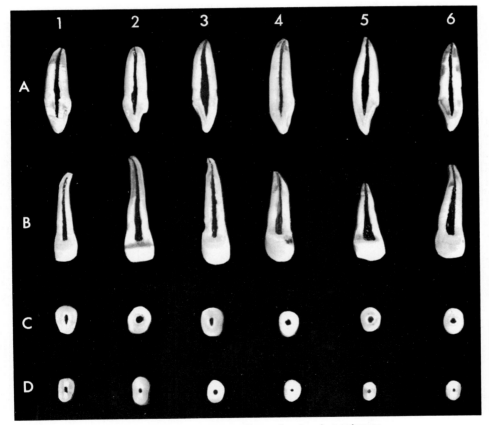

Figure 13–10. *Maxillary lateral incisor—cross sections of natural specimens.*

A, 1 to 6, Labiolingual sections. This aspect does not show in radiographs.
    B, 1 to 6, Mesiodistal sections.
    C, 1 to 6, Cervical sections of root.
    D, 1 to 6, Mid-root sections.

central incisor, because of the smaller dimensions of the lateral incisor. However, the root canal is not constricted as a rule, allowing ease of root treatment. There is one distinction when comparing this tooth to the central incisor; the pulp chamber of the lateral will usually show a rounded form incisally, seldom showing evidences of a design to accommodate pulp horns.

Cervical Cross Section (C)

The cervical cross section shows the pulp chamber and single canal well centered. The root form of the lateral incisor shows considerable variation so the shape of the canal will vary accordingly (See *Lateral Incisor*, Chapter 6.). Two of the sections displayed in Figure 13–10 show considerable secondary dentin deposit (D, 4, 6).

(Text continued on page 312.)

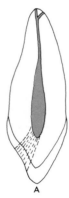
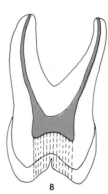

A   B

Figure 13–11.   *A,* Drawing of a labiolingual cross section of a maxillary canine. Dotted lines represent the opening suggested for the approach to the pulp chamber. *B,* Drawing of a buccolingual cross section of a maxillary molar. Dotted lines represent the opening suggested for the approach to the roof of the pulp chamber.

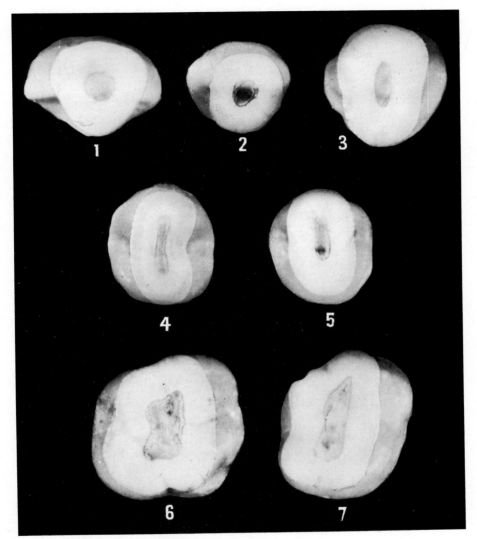

Figure 13–12.   *Maxillary permanent teeth.*

1, Central incisor.
2, Lateral incisor.
3, Canine.
4, First premolar.
5, Second premolar.
6, First molar.
7, Second molar.

Interesting photographs of natural teeth made by a process of double exposure. Tooth specimens were sawed through at the cervical line, an exposure was made with the sections placed together and an exposure made of occlusal and incisal views. Then the crown was removed and another exposure made of the cross section at the cervix on the same film.

The result is shown above, and the proportion of crown outline to cervical outline is accurately portrayed. The angulation of the field when such small specimens were exposed, and the possibility of movement, made standardization too difficult; consequently, some of the pictures do not have the crown and cervices centered in line with the long axis. Nevertheless, from an operative point of view, a comparison of the above photos makes an interesting study. (Made and submitted by Dr. John T. Bird, Washington University School of Dentistry.)

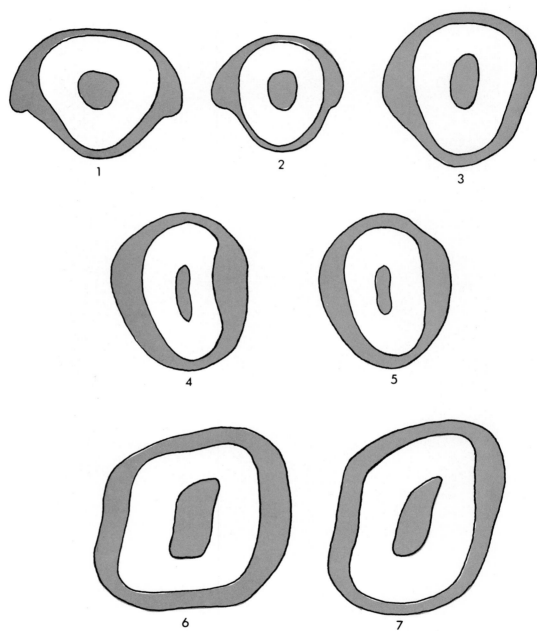

Figure 13–13.   Tracings of crown outlines and root trunk outlines from Figure 13–12 placed in proper relation to each other. The photos of crowns and roots were correct in showing relative sizes, but the difficulties experienced in making double exposures prevented correct alignment at times.

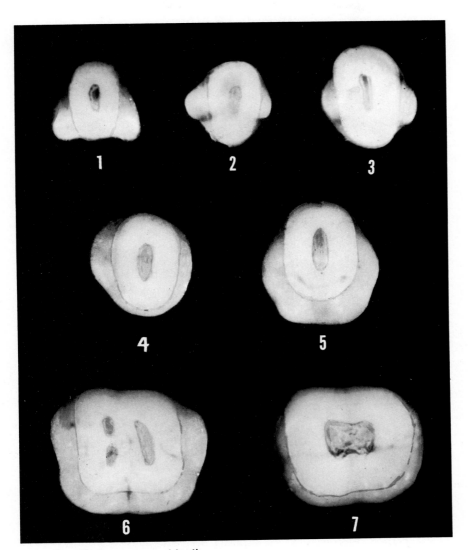

Figure 13-14. *Mandibular permanent teeth.*

1, Central incisor.
2, Lateral incisor.
3, Canine.
4, First premolar.
5, Second premolar.
6, First molar.
7, Second molar.
Double exposure photos of mandibular teeth to be compared with Figure 13-12.

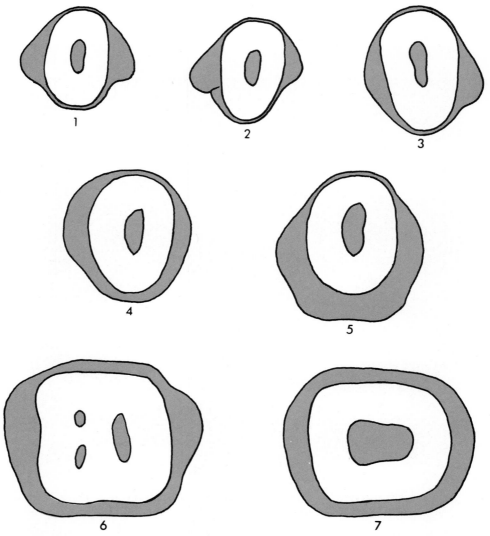

Figure 13–15. Tracings of crown outlines and root trunk outlines from Figure 13–14, placed in proper relation to each other. The photos of crowns and roots were correct in showing relative sizes, but the difficulties experienced in making double exposures prevented correct alignment at times.

MAXILLARY CANINE (FIG. 13–16, A, B, C, D, E)

Labiolingual Cross Section (A, D)

The labiolingual measurement of the maxillary canine root registers the largest root calibration of width of any tooth in the mouth. Therefore the pulp cavity will be very generous in size labiolingually (A, D). Ordinarily, the extra width to accommodate a bulk of pulp tissue will be shown in most of these canines in the half of the root closest to the crown, because the canal at that point is continuous with the pulp chamber of the crown. The apical half of the pulp canal will narrow down to average width on its way to the apical end of the root. Many exceptions will be found to the typical form of pulp cavity just mentioned. Those that do not conform will usually show a generous labiolingual measurement for all the root length (Fig. 13–16, A, 3, 7,

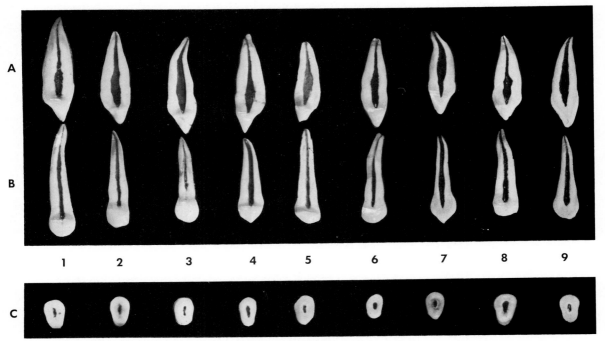

Figure 13–16.   *Maxillary Canine.*

A. Labiolingual cross section, exposing the mesial or distal aspect of the pulp cavity. This aspect does not show in dental radiographs.
B. Mesiodistal cross section, exposing the labial or lingual aspect of the pulp cavity.
C. Cervical cross section. A transverse cut at the cementoenamel junction exposing the pulp chamber. These are the openings to root canals that will be seen in the floor of the pulp chamber.
D. Labiolingual cross section, exposing the mesial or distal aspect of the pulp cavity.
E. Mesiodistal cross section, exposing the labial or lingual aspect of the pulp cavity.

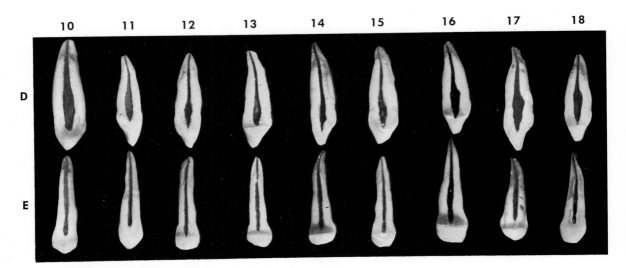

9, 10). The problems of root treatment may be multiplied by the anatomy of the pulp cavity, as it is positioned in a labiolingual direction in the maxillary canine. It must be emphasized again that a standard technique in radiography will not give a true picture in this instance. A diagnosis of the local condition must be made clinically.

Mesiodistal Cross Scetion (B, E)

The pulp cavity seems much narrower when viewing this section. The shape of it would compare favorably with the other maxillary anteriors except for the length. It must be remembered that the maxillary canine possesses the longest root in the dentition.

Since the mesiodistal measurement of the root is less than the labiolingual measurement, it follows that the pulp canal in this section will be narrower also. If constriction of the canal is discovered in one of these teeth, very likely the constriction is in a mesiodistal direction (B, 3; E, 13). The shape of the root canal is elliptical rather than round, with the long calibration labiolingually.

Cervical Cross Section (C)

The pulp cavity typically is centered in the root of the tooth. In general the outline of the periphery of the cavity will duplicate the root form in miniature. The root of the maxillary canine is wider labially than it is lingually, so the greater width labially is reflected in the calibration of the width of the root canal labially. Also, since the root is narrower mesiodistally than labiolingually, the pulp chamber and root canal adapt to this form. As mentioned before, constriction of the canal would likely be in a mesiodistal direction (C, 1, 3).

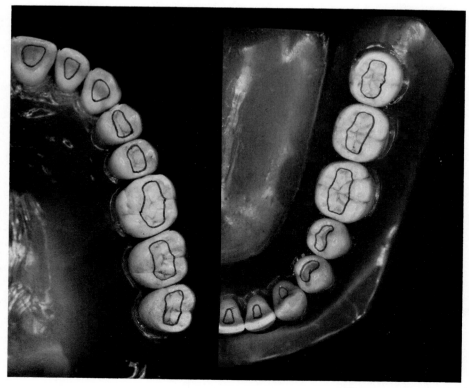

(See opposite page for legend.)

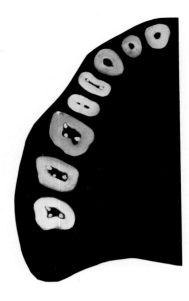

Figure 13–18. Cut-outs of photos of cervical cross sections of maxillary teeth. The cut-outs were carefully executed and placed in proper alignment on black background. Note the alignment and the relative shapes of pulp chambers. White dots point to the approximate location of root canal openings in the pulp chambers of teeth expected to have more than one canal.

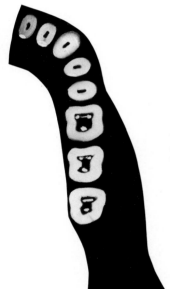

Figure 13–19. Cut-outs of photos of cervical cross sections of mandibular teeth. The cut-outs were placed in alignment to conform to one-half of the mandibular dental arch. Note the alignment and the shapes of pulp chambers. White dots point to the probable location of root canals in the molars. Multiple canals are to be expected in mandibular molars only.

Figure 13–17. This illustration shows the occlusal aspects of posterior teeth and the lingual aspects of anterior teeth in upper and lower jaws from the median line posteriorly to include the third molars.

The outline markings represent the extent and locations of openings thought to be necessary for the approach to pulp chambers for endodontic procedure. Posterior teeth are to be opened as wide as consistent with good finish in final restoration. The more generous opening allows better reflection of light with the mouth mirror, thereby assisting the operator to locate pulp chambers and canals. Needless to say, the wider openings are required also in order to direct properly various points and instruments during treatment.

The pulp chambers of anterior teeth are approached from the lingual. The incisal margin of the opening must be extended incisally as far as possible without undermining the incisal edge of the tooth. Because the incisal edge is in line generally with the pulp canal, instruments should be inserted as nearly in line with the pulp canal as possible; therefore, the suggested approach to the incisal edge. See Fig. 13–9.

MAXILLARY FIRST PREMOLAR (FIG. 13-20, A, B, C, D, E)

Buccolingual Cross Section (A, D)

The maxillary first premolar may have two well-developed, fully formed roots, or, as is more often the case, two root projections from the middle third of the root portion. It is not uncommon though for this tooth to have one broad root for its entire length. *Rarely, however, does it have less than two fully formed root canals* (A, 4, 6). This cross section will display a broad pulp chamber buccolingually with accommodations for well-developed pulp horns in the roof of the chamber. Only when secondary deposit is extensive will this form be absent. Those teeth with the most distinct separate root development will have relatively large pulp chambers (A, 1, 2, 9). Characteristically, all root canals in this tooth, regardless of root form, will have smooth, funnel-like openings leading into the canals from the pulp chamber floor.

A comparison of pulp chambers in this tooth is interesting. The teeth with the least root separation will usually have the deepest pulp chambers (A, 4, 8; D, 13, 18). The age of the patient and the comparison of root length must be considered also in these cases.

The pulp chamber floor will be below the level of the cementoenamel junction where cervical cross sections are made. This design puts the floor considerably below the normal gum line in vitro.

The root canals taper evenly from the floor of the pulp chamber to the end of the root form. The lingual root canal tends to be larger, regardless of the root form. The teeth with the least root spread will have the straightest pulp canals, with a tendency to parallelism in those with a more complete fusion. (Compare A2 with A6)

Mesiodistal Cross Section (B, E)

The shape of the pulp cavity of the maxillary first premolar, when viewing a mesiodistal cross section, shows a cavity similar to the maxillary canine; it is relatively narrow with an even taper from pulp chamber to root end. Since the root is shorter and since the measurement over all is less than the canine, the pulp cavity will vary accordingly.

Pulp stones and secondary dentin deposit may cause some difficulty in endodontic procedure (B, 4, 8; C, 7; E, 14).

Cervical Cross Section (C)

The cross section at the cervical line made transversely through the root at the cementoenamel junction demonstrates the outline form of the root trunk as it joins the crown of the tooth. The maxillary first premolar has a characteristic root outline at this level. Usually it is kidney shaped. This form is assisted by a deep indentation mesially that is part of a developmental depression which extends up into the cervical third of the crown mesially, before the cervical cut is made (Fig. 9–1). The root form cervically is wider buccolingually than mesiodistally, with a constricted kidney-shaped pulp chamber centered in it.

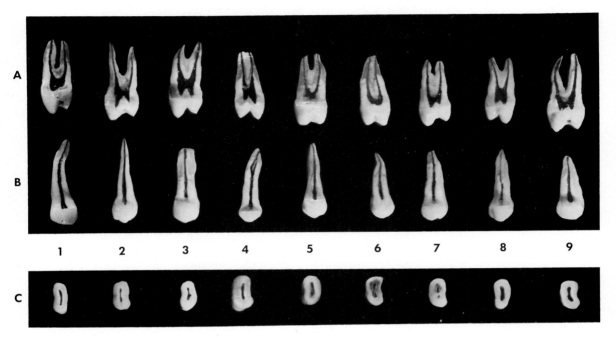

Figure 13–20 *Maxillary First Premolar*

A. Buccolingual cross section, exposing the mesial or distal aspect of the pulp cavity. This aspect does not show on dental radiographs.
B. Mesiodistal cross section, exposing the buccal or lingual aspect of the pulp cavity.
C. Cervical cross section. A transverse cut at the cementoenamel junction exposing the pulp chamber. These are the openings to root canals that will be seen in the floor of the pulp chamber.
D. Buccolingual cross section, exposing the mesial or distal aspect of the pulp cavity.
E. Mesiodistal cross section, exposing the buccal or lingual aspect of the pulp cavity.

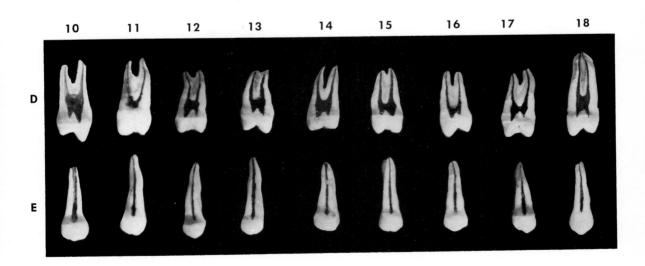

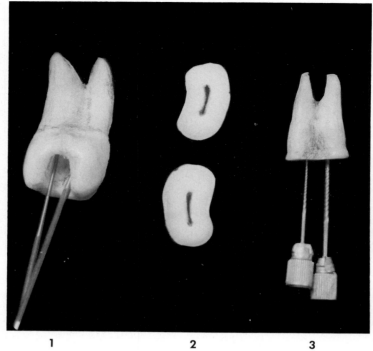

Figure 13–21.   Maxillary first premolar. 1, Odd angle view of the maxillary first premolar showing the approach to the root canals with instruments as they are placed within a generous opening made in the occlusal surface of the crown. Some bifurcation of the roots with two distinct canals is characteristic of this tooth. 2, Cervical sections of two of these teeth, one right and one left. At this point the root form is noticeably kidney shaped, with the mesial surface curved in toward the pulp chamber. This developmental depression, reflected also in the cervical third of the mesial surface of the crown, is characteristic of this tooth alone. (See Figure 9–1.) 3, Instruments are placed in the two canals with the crown cut away as an added demonstration. Note the depression showing cervically on the root.

MAXILLARY SECOND PREMOLAR (FIG. 13–22, A, B, C, D, E)

Buccolingual Cross Section (A, D)

A comparison of maxillary premolar pulp cavities in buccolingual cross section brings out some interesting points. The two maxillary premolars are not alike. They cannot be compared in the same manner, for instance, as were the mandibular central and lateral incisors. It is rare to find bifurcated roots in this tooth, although it is not uncommon to find two pulp canals, one buccal and one lingual. This aspect shows one feature common to the first premolars, and that is the shape of the roof of the pulp chamber, which accommodates two well-developed pulp horns, one for each cusp, buccal and lingual. The rest of the pulp cavity of the second premolar is not comparable. From this aspect, the average pulp cavity is very broad at its junction with the pulp chamber, and then it narrows very gradually remaining quite wide until it reaches mid-root or beyond. There it constricts rapidly, becoming a typical root canal in diameter as it approaches the apical third of the root (A, 1, 6, 8, etc.). In most cases, the canal is accessible apically; sometimes the apical foramen seems quite open. This is a departure from the situation in the maxillary first premolar (A, 2, 7, D, 12, 17, 18). It is not a rare occasion to find the pulp canal branching into accessory canals near the apical end (D, 10, 16). Endodontists will be interested in another characteristic found among the maxillary second premolars when a study is made of their pulp cavities and

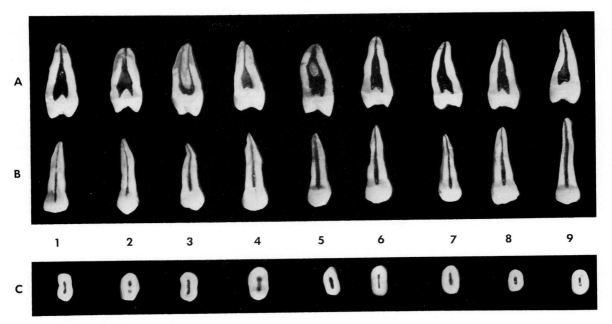

1 2 3 4 5 6 7 8 9

Figure 13–22. *Maxillary Second Premolar.*

A. Buccolingual cross section, exposing the mesial or distal aspect of the pulp cavity. This aspect does not show on dental radiographs.
B. Mesiodistal cross section, exposing the buccal or lingual aspect of the pulp cavity.
C. Cervical cross section. A transverse cut at the cementoenamel junction exposing the pulp chamber. These are the openings to root canals that will be seen in the floor of the pulp chamber.
D. Buccolingual cross section, exposing the mesial or distal aspect of the pulp cavity.
E. Mesiodistal cross section, exposing the buccal or lingual aspect of the pulp cavity.

10   11   12   13   14   15   16   17   18

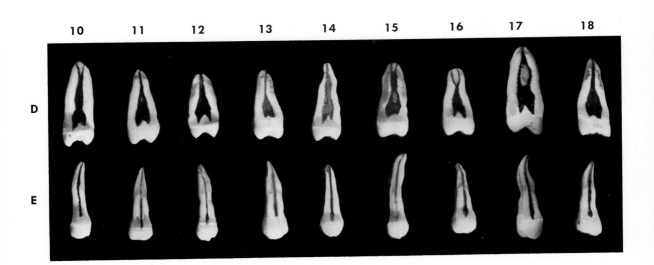

root formations. Buccolingual cross sections will be found with the single broad pulp canal divided at mid-root into two canals by a dentin "island" (A, 5; D, 15, 17). Then moving apically, the two canals join up again and become one as the apical third of the root is approached. This explains why at times a root canal instrument working through the crown of the tooth seems to penetrate one time and then seems obstructed the next. Deliberate manipulation will coax the instrument to by-pass the obstruction. The buccolingual cross section is produced by cutting one half of the tooth away; therefore, what appears as an "island" is actually a bar of dentin connecting the two halves. An instrument must by-pass the bar on both the buccal and lingual sides.

Mesiodistal Cross Section (B, E)

There seems to be no variation in the appearance of the pulp cavity in the mesiodistal section of the second maxillary premolar as distinguished from the maxillary first premolar. The cavity appears slender, becoming even narrower as it approaches the root end. Any difficulty encountered in penetrating root canals in this tooth because of constriction can usually be attributed to the form of the canals as seen from this aspect (B, 2, 7; E, 11, 12, 15).

Cervical Cross Section (C)

The cervical cross section of the maxillary second premolar generally will demonstrate a root trunk that is smoothly oval in shape (C, 2, 4, 7, etc.). A few will show a crimp in the side of the root mesial or distal, but none will approach the kidney shape of the maxillary first premolar (C, 1, 3). The pulp chamber will be centered in the root and will repeat the outline of the root in miniature.

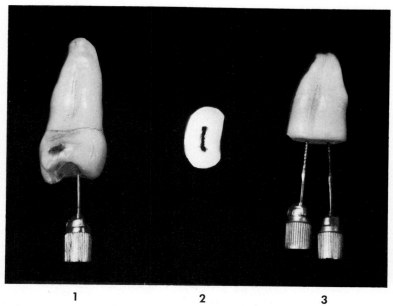

| 1 | 2 | 3 |

Figure 13–23. Maxillary second premolar. 1, Position of instrument as it enters single broad canal through a comparatively wide occlusal opening buccolingually. Sometimes the broad canal buccolingually will branch as it progresses apically. (See No. 16, Figure 13–22.) 2, Cross section of root at cemento-enamel junction. It is slightly kidney shaped with elongated pulp chamber, but it is less extreme in this respect than the maxillary first premolar. 3, Two root canal instruments placed partially parallel in the broad canal with the crown removed for clarity of observation.

MAXILLARY FIRST MOLAR (FIG. 13–24, A, B, C, D, E)

Buccolingual Cross Section (A, D)

The buccolingual cross section of the maxillary first molar as a rule presents a view of the pulp chamber and the pulp canals of the lingual root and the mesiobuccal root. These roots were chosen for dissection because anatomically they were more

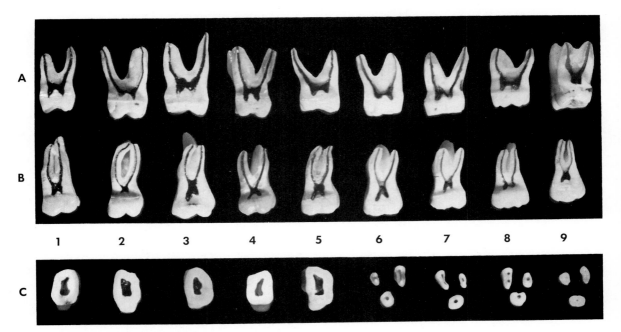

Figure 13–24. *Maxillary First Molar.*

A. Buccolingual cross section, exposing the mesial or distal aspect of the pulp cavity. This aspect will not show on dental radiographs.

B. Mesiodistal cross section, exposing the buccal or lingual aspect of the pulp cavity.

C. Five transverse cross sections at cervical line and four transverse sections at midroot.

D. Buccolingual cross section, exposing the mesial or distal aspect of the pulp cavity.

E. Mesiodistal cross section, exposing the buccal aspect of the pulp cavity.

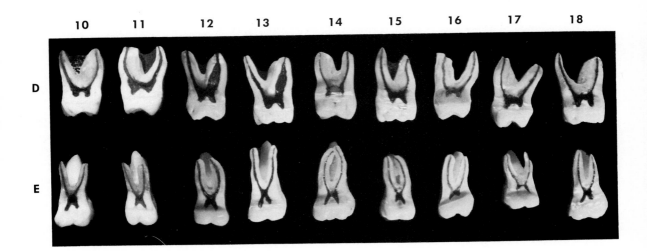

representative of this tooth. The distobuccal root, although small in cross section, is straighter, with fewer variations in the form of the root canal. The root canal of the mesiobuccal root of the maxillary first molar stands out as a distinct anatomic variant. It is always questionable, during endodontic procedure, whether instrumentation will be entirely successful in removing tissue or in the enlargement process before filling (Figs. 13–4 and 13–5). If any canal will allow ease of access it will be the lingual root canal. Normally this canal is rather straight and the most open of the three root canals. The canal will be the deepest of the three because the lingual root is the longest one. The pulp chamber shows a pronounced formation structured to accommodate pulp horns. This must be remembered when opening the crown through the occlusal surface. If any section of the roof of the pulp chamber remains as an undercut, endodontic treatment may be jeopardized (Fig. 13–11).

Mesiodistal Cross Section (B, E)

The mesiodistal cross section of the maxillary first molar includes the distobuccal root, which was not included in the buccolingual cross section. In this view it will be noted that the root canals are thin in cross section. The mesiobuccal root is more inclined to curvature than the distobuccal root. Files and reamers used in attempting enlargement have to be carefully manipulated in order to follow curvatures smoothly (B, 2, 5; E, 12, 14, 15). The distobuccal root canal can be curved, but usually it is rather straight. Although narrow, if it is not blocked, the smallest files will follow the canal as it traverses the relatively straight root; then larger ones, graduated, may follow (B, 3, 4; E, 10, 11, 16). The pulp chamber from this view is somewhat narrow when compared to the appearance of the chamber in the buccolingual cross section. Nevertheless, it shows distinctive peaked spaces for the accommodation of pulp horns.

Cervical Cross Section and Mid-Root Sections (C)

The cervical cross section of the maxillary first molar can be described as somewhat rhomboidal in character, with the corners rounded. The pulp chamber will be centered and its outline form will be similar to that of the cervical section, but in miniature. The angles of the cervical cross section of this tooth may be described as follows: the mesiobuccal angle is acute, and the distobuccal angle is obtuse, with both lingual angles conforming in general to right angles. The form just described is a reflection of the functional form of the maxillary first molar when sighted from directly above the occlusal surface of the crown. The root canals have the following relation to the pulp chamber floor: the lingual canal, which is largest, will be centered lingually; the distobuccal canal will be near the obtuse angle of the pulp chamber; and last, but far from least, because the location is difficult, the mesiobuccal root canal will be buccal and mesial to the distobuccal canal, in what seems an extreme corner position, resting within the acute angle of the pulp chamber.

The **Mid-Root Sections** are added to molar descriptions because some molars are multi-rooted; others with two roots only may have more than one canal in one or more roots. The root forms are not identical, therefore a comparison of pulp canals at mid-root is in order. At mid-root the cross sections and root canals of the maxillary first molar may be described as follows: the lingual root, which is largest, is rather round, with an open round canal centered in it; the mesiobuccal canal is banana shaped at this point, showing two separate tiny canals or, as in most cases, a curved flat canal difficult to deal with endodontically. The distobuccal mid-section is quite a bit smaller than the other two roots but is also consistently rounder. A tiny root canal is centered

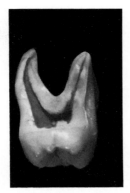

Figure 13–25.   A cross section of a maxillary molar exposing the *distobuccal* root canal, in addition to the lingual root canal in a buccolingual section. After making a few of these sections it was decided not to demonstrate this cut in the records of cross sections of maxillary molars.

The mesial roots of all maxillary molars are the complicated ones, whereas the distobuccal canal, although inclined toward constriction, is shorter, single, and nearly always quite straight. Also, it shows up quite well in the mesiodistal cross section. Exposing the single lingual canal from the distal instead of the mesial was of no consequence.

at this point but, strange as it may seem, dental operators will often find this canal penetrable when the mesiobuccal canal is not (C, 6, 7, 8). Of course, occasionally one will find all the roots of this tooth filled with secondary dentin deposit so dense that any one root may be partially or even entirely closed (C, 9).

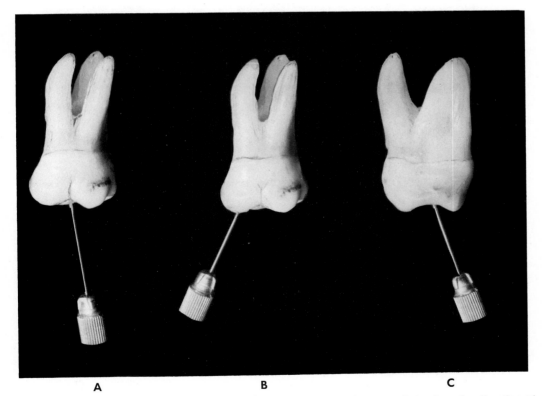

A   B   C

Figure 13–26.   Maxillary first molar. Pulp canal files placed in three canals to show the direction of the canals in relation to the crown of the tooth. *A,* Root canal instrument placed in the mesiobuccal root of a specimen tooth, showing the direction of entry in relation to the clinical crown. *B,* In distobuccal root—note the extreme angle. *C,* In lingual root, also extreme in another direction.

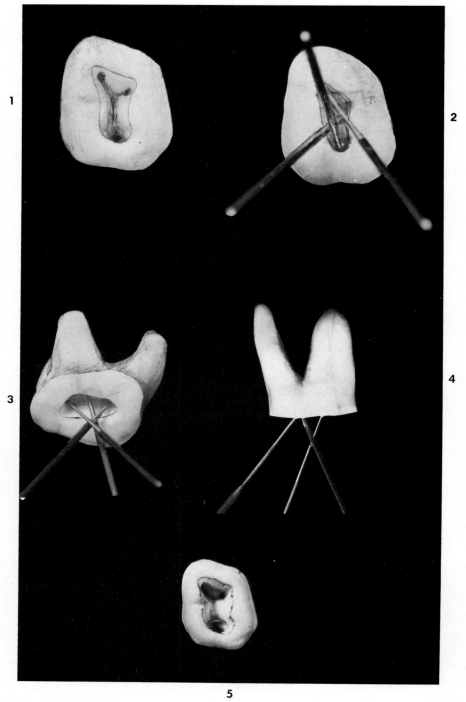

Figure 13–27. Maxillary first molar. 1, The exposed pulp chamber as it looks somewhat enlarged with the crown removed at the cementoenamel junction. Note the relative location of the entrances to pulp canals. The distobuccal and the lingual canal openings are in line buccolingually, but the mesiobuccal canal opening is in a rather extreme mesiobuccal direction toward the mesiobuccal line angle of the tooth crown. 2, The same subject with probes in the canals, demonstrating the varied directions traveled. 3, The same subject as 2, with the tooth over on its side, presenting a different perspective. 4, The same specimen as 3, providing still another view for comparison. 5, An unretouched photograph of another specimen of maxillary first molar showing rather graphically the open pulp chamber with its entrances to pulp canals.

MAXILLARY SECOND MOLAR (FIG. 13-28, A, B, C, D, E)

Buccolingual Cross Section (A, D)

The form of any pulp cavity will be affected by the shape of the tooth. Therefore, in order to describe the cavity as presented by the buccolingual cross section of the

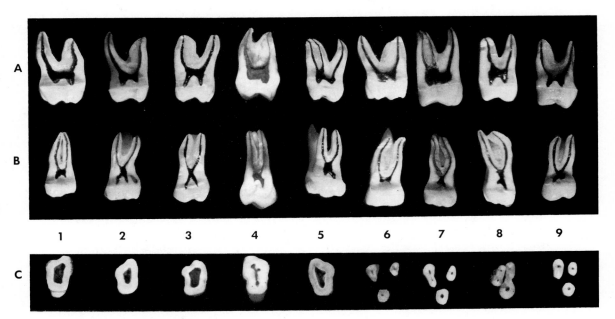

Figure 13–28.   *Maxillary Second Molar.*

A. Buccolingual cross section, exposing the mesial or distal aspect of the pulp cavity. This aspect does not show in dental radiographs.
B. Mesiodistal cross section, exposing the buccal or lingual aspect of the pulp cavity.
C. Five transverse cross sections at cervical line and four transverse sections at midroot.
D. Buccolingual cross section, exposing the mesial or distal aspect of the pulp cavity.
E. Mesiodistal cross section, exposing the buccal or lingual aspect of the pulp cavity.

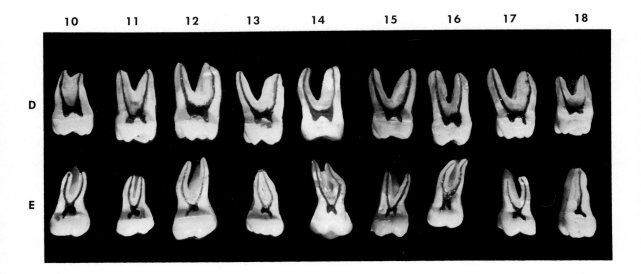

maxillary second molar, a review of the tooth form is required. The review is simplified by comparing the second molar with the maxillary first molar. Biologically, the first molars serve as model patterns for the remaining molars, maxillary or mandibular. When well formed, the buccal roots of maxillary second molars are straighter and closer together than those of the maxillary first molars. There is more of a tendency toward fusion of roots, but most second molars will possess a lingual root entirely separate and well developed (Fig. 13–28, A, 1, 2, 6, etc.). The second molar has a crown at least as wide buccolingually as the first molar, therefore the pulp chamber will be of generous proportions buccolingually also. The buccolingual cross section shows the mesiobuccal root canal as being less complicated than that of the first molar and therefore will be more favorable for endodontic treatment. As a rule, the mesiobuccal root of the maxillary second molar will house only one root canal. Anomalies are found, however (A, 5, 7). The pulp chamber roof from this angle exhibits the form that was necessary to enclose the pulp horns when all was live tissue.

Mesiodistal Cross Section (B, E)

It may be noted in the illustration of mesiodistal cross sections of maxillary second molars that the design of pulp chamber and root canals compares favorably with those of the maxillary first molars. The buccal roots may not spread apart as much, and there may be more tendency for the fusion of roots. The pulp chamber is much more constricted from this angle but pulp horn formation is still much in evidence.

Cervical Cross Section and Mid-Root Sections (C)

The cervical cross section of the maxillary second molar will reflect the more extreme angulation of the second molar crown form when compared with the maxillary first molar. The mesiobuccal line angle is more acute, and the distobuccal line angle is more obtuse. The outline of the pulp chamber will reflect this form. The location of pulp canals will be noted as follows. The mesiobuccal canal will seem far buccal, as well as mesial, following the form of the acute mesiobuccal angulation (C, 4, 5). The distobuccal canal more nearly approaches the midpoint distally in the floor of the pulp chamber between the mesiobuccal canal and the lingual canal. The latter assumes the typical locale.

The Mid-Root Sections

Although the roots of the maxillary second molar seem less well developed than those of the first molar, in most cases they are reasonably well formed and separated (C, 6, 7, 9). The mid-root sections will show small openings of root canals at this point; nevertheless, these are distinct openings. If the mesiobuccal root happens to be broad and flat like that of the first molar, it may have two canals (C, 8). This specimen shows maxillary second molar roots that were developed close together, with some fusion having taken place also.

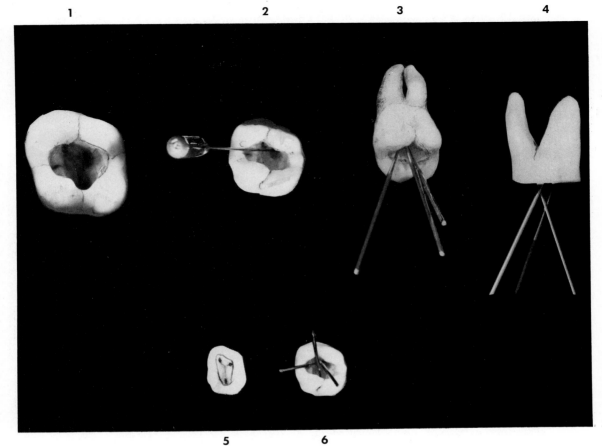

Figure 13–29. Maxillary second molar. 1, Occlusal opening necessary to expose pulp chamber and canals. 2, Extreme angle at which instrument enters distobuccal canal. 3, All three canals have been entered by probes; this photo and 4 will emphasize the variation in the angulation of root canals in this tooth. Five and 6 are photos of the pulp chamber with canal locations shown in a cervical cross section, and an occlusal view of probe angulations as they enter canals.

MAXILLARY THIRD MOLAR (FIG. 13–30, A, B, C, D, E)

Maxillary third molars vary so much in development that there will be no thought here of trying to describe the usual cross sections in detail. Nevertheless, a sample of cross sections displayed in the same manner and number in order to compare them with the cross sections of neighboring maxillary molars is indicated. These can be studied in Fig. 13–30. When the development and eruption of the maxillary third

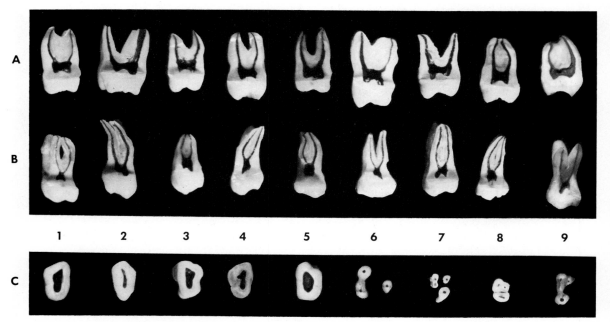

Figure 13–30. *Maxillary Third Molar.*

A. Buccolingual cross section, exposing the mesial or distal aspect of the pulp cavity. This aspect
   will not show on dental radiographs.
B. Mesiodistal cross section, exposing the buccal or lingual aspect of the pulp cavity.
C. Five transverse cross sections at cervical line and four transverse sections at midroot.
D. Buccolingual cross section, exposing the mesial or distal aspect of the pulp cavity.
E. Mesiodistal cross section, exposing the buccal or lingual aspect of the pulp cavity.

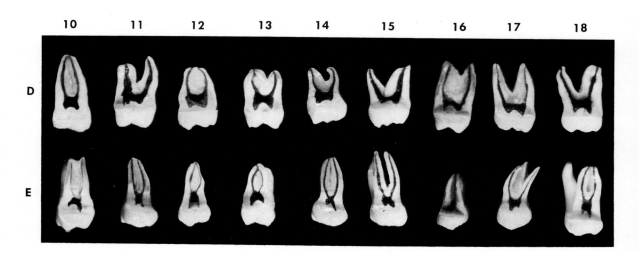

molar can be compared to the other maxillary molars, it will give the appearance of being a smaller and weaker maxillary second molar. The crown will be triangular rather than quadrilateral and the roots will be shorter than those of the second molar, more curved, and they will show a tendency toward fusion into the equivalent of one tapered root (Fig. 13–30, B, 3, 5; E, 11, 12, 16, etc.). This description includes the most normally developed maxillary third molar, but to say it included the greatest number to be seen might be an erroneous statement. To the endodontist, biologically it has one fact in its favor; it is eight or nine years younger than the first molar. Normally the pulp chambers and root canals of the third molar submit to treatment more readily as a consequence. However, this does not take into consideration the likelihood of having to deal with malformations so often found during the clinical examination. Many maxillary third molars will depart from the normal in crown and root formation. In these teeth, naturally, the pulp cavities will depart from the normal also (A, 2, 6; B, 2, 7; D, 14; E, 16, etc.). Although third molars as a class have been condemned generally by both the dental profession and the laity, they must not be condemned without "trial and investigation." Many a third molar, properly nurtured, has been an asset much appreciated by all concerned, and especially so by the host later on in life.

MANDIBULAR CENTRAL INCISOR (FIRST INCISOR)
(FIG. 13–31, A, B, C, D, E)

Labiolingual Cross Section (A, D)

Although the mandibular central incisor is the smallest tooth in the mouth, it may be noted from this aspect that the labiolingual measurement of crown and root is quite substantial. In fact, the mandibular central incisor along with the mandibular lateral incisor, is comparable in dimension in this respect with the *maxillary* lateral incisor. The pulp cavity looks generous in size, and the spacing appears quite broad, conforming to the crown and root outline of the labiolingual cross section. This design should be anticipated; however, an immediate comparison must be made with the mesiodistal design of the pulp chamber and root canal. This view, which appears in dental radiographs, shows the cavity to be quite thin in a mesiodistal direction.

Mesiodistal Cross Section (B, E)

Although from this angle the cross section of the mandibular central incisor demonstrates the narrowness of the pulp cavity, the fact remains that ordinarily the root canal can be penetrated by the smallest root canal files, probably with the assistance of the broader measurement labiolingually. Occasionally, of course, secondary deposit will interfere with treatment (B, 7; D, 16, 18; E–13, 18).

Cervical Cross Section (C)

This aspect gives the viewer the proportions of the root trunk of this tooth. Even though the mesiodistal calibration is small, the labiolingual measurement is large enough to support the tooth when resisting the forces of occlusion. Those forces are applied against the tooth mainly in a labiolingual direction during protrusive and retrusive movements of the jaw. It will be noted in the study of Fig. 13–31 that there is some variation in the size of mandibular central incisors (lateral incisors included) in different persons. Examination of series C will show also that the root design may vary.

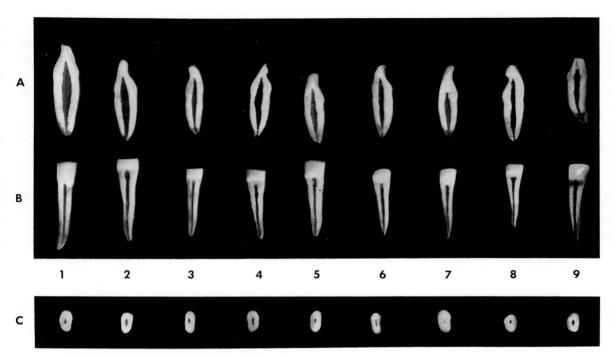

Figure 13–31. *Mandibular Central Incisor (First incisor).*

A. Labiolingual cross section, exposing the mesial or distal aspect of the pulp cavity. This aspect will not show on dental radiographs.

B. Mesiodistal cross section, exposing the labial or lingual aspect of the pulp cavity.

C. Cervical cross section. A transverse cut at the cementoenamel junction exposing the pulp chamber. These are the openings to root canals that will be seen in the floor of the pulp chamber.

D. Labiolingual cross section, exposing the mesial or distal aspect of the pulp cavity.

E. Mesiodistal cross section, exposing the labial or lingual aspect of the pulp cavity.

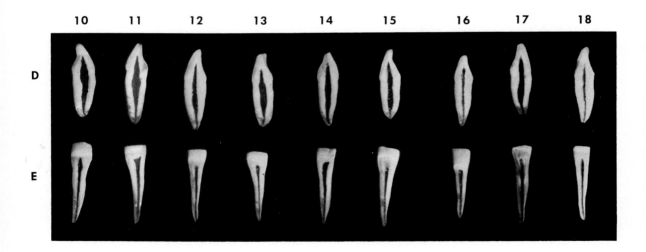

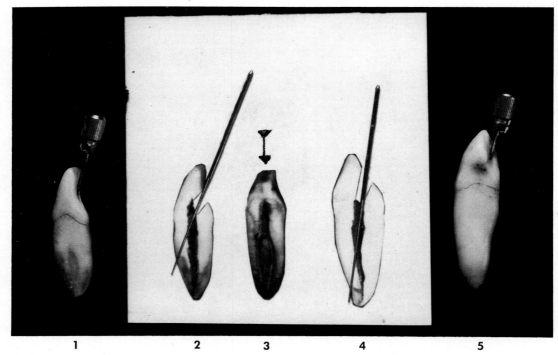

Figure 13–32. *Mandibular Central Incisor and Canine.*

1, *Mandibular central incisor* with a canal instrument placed in the canal through a lingual opening designed to save the incisal portion of the tooth. Note the angle of the instrument. 2, Photo of labiolingual section of this tooth. A straight probe is placed over a simulated lingual opening, showing the necessity for instrument flexibility in order to follow the pulp canal. 3, Photo of labiolingual cross section of another central incisor that had lost its incisal portion through abrasion. Note the "island" dividing the canal into a labial and lingual portion. This situation is common but cannot be diagnosed from a radiograph taken with standard technique. A practical approach to the abraided type would be to enter the tooth through an opening in the incisal portion (note arrow). 4, Labiolingual section of a *mandibular canine.* The added dimensions of this tooth allow more freedom in probing the canal through a lingual opening. 5, A *mandibular canine* showing the position and angulation of a root canal instrument when placed through a lingual opening in the crown.

MANDIBULAR LATERAL INCISOR (SECOND INCISOR) (FIG. 13–33, A, B, C, D, E)

Labiolingual Cross Section (A, D)

The mandibular lateral incisor tends to be a trifle larger in all dimensions than the mandibular central incisor; therefore, its pulp cavity will vary in size proportionately, but the essential design is the same. The labiolingual cross section will bear this out. (Compare Fig. 13–33 with Fig. 13–31.) As mentioned before in this book, the function of the two teeth is almost identical; therefore, the form and dimensions will be similar, conforming to their duplicate needs. Since the pulp cavity in the mandibular lateral incisor is a little more generous in size, it may prove to be a little more amenable to endodontic treatment.

Mesiodistal Cross Section (B, E)

The pulp chamber and canal in this section will demonstrate a slender cavity with even, straight walls the entire length. It resembles the mandibular *central* incisor in this respect, but it may appear a little wider and more open. Narrow constrictions and canal blockages would be likely to show up in this cross section (E, 12, 14, 18).

Cervical Cross Section (C)

The cervical cross section of the mandibular lateral incisor will show the pulp canal as centered in the root. A comparison of several of these sections bears out an earlier statement that the mandibular lateral incisor is not only somewhat larger than the mandibular central, but that there is considerable variation in the form of the root trunk. Actually, some sections of the larger teeth will resemble the cervical sections of small mandibular canines (C, 2, 3, 4)

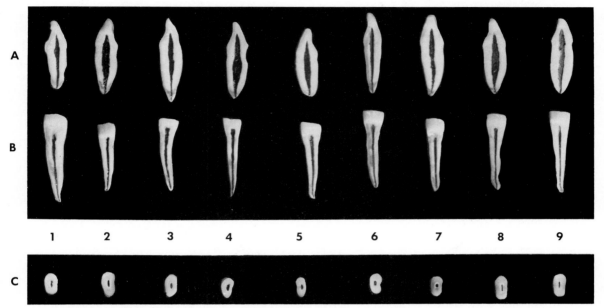

Figure 13–33. *Mandibular Lateral Incisor (Second incisor).*

A. Labiolingual cross section, exposing the mesial or distal aspect of the pulp cavity. This aspect will not show on the dental radiograph.
B. Mesiodistal cross section, exposing the labial or lingual aspect of the pulp cavity.
C. Cervical cross section. A transverse cut at the cementoenamel junction, exposing the pulp chamber. These are the openings to root canals that will be seen in the floor of the pulp chamber.
D. Labiolingual cross section, exposing the mesial or distal aspect of the pulp cavity.
E. Mesiodistal cross section, exposing the labial or lingual aspect of the pulp cavity.

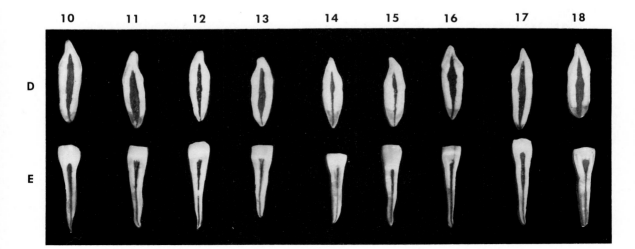

MANDIBULAR CANINE (FIG. 13–34, A, B, C, D, E)

Labiolingual Cross Section (A, D)

The pulp cavity in this cross section of the mandibular canine compares favorably in size and shape with that of the maxillary canine. This might be expected because the dimensions of the two teeth labiolingually are comparable. The pulp chamber is pointed incisally, and sometimes appears with a rounded roof later in life; the pulp canal is quite wide labiolingually in the upper portion of the root, narrowing down at about the half way point in the root as it approaches the apex (A, 1, 5, 6, etc.). Other teeth will show the constriction to straight sides in the apical third only (A, 3, 7, 10; E, 11, 14). In all broad-rooted teeth (including the canines), one may find an "island" in the center of the broadest portion. This form creates a "double" canal on each side of the obstruction until the canal becomes single again as it approaches the apex of the root (A, 4). Some canines are quite large and long, whereas others are smaller than average. Mandibular canines tend to run shorter than maxillary canines. However, this may prove to be only in those individuals with slender mandibles. Although it is not the rule, the mandibular canine can be longer than the maxillary canine. Pulp cavities would vary accordingly.

There is one outstanding anatomic variation in the mandibular canine; it is not uncommon to find that this tooth has two roots, or at least a fused root with two canals in the root portion, one labial and one lingual. The pulp cavity in a tooth of this kind would vary accordingly if a labiolingual cross section could be examined (Fig. 8–24, specimens 1, 2, 5, 6). These anomalies do not show always on radiographs; consequently, great care must be observed in searching for the possibility of two root canals when the mandibular canine is under treatment.

Mesiodistal Cross Section (B, E)

Generally speaking, when viewing the mesiodistal cross section of the mandibular canines, it is immediately apparent that from this aspect this tooth is similar to the maxillary canine. The cross section will be a little narrower mesiodistally, but the root will appear quite long and may show some curvature at the apical portion. The curvature can be either in a mesial or a distal direction. Oddly enough, the curvature will be in a mesial direction most often.

The root canal from this aspect appears narrow with rather straight sides for the full length of the root until it becomes more constricted as it approaches its terminal end.

Cervical Cross Section (C)

The cervical cross section of the mandibular canine shows some variation in size and shape of the root when comparing several of the cross sections. The root canal is centered as usual and takes on the general shape, much diminished of course, of the root outline from this aspect. Some roots will be smoothly oblong, with the greatest measurement labiolingually; others will show proportions more akin to the maxillary canine, with calibration of the lingual portion appearing less than that of the labial portion of the root (C, 2, 3, 9). Usually the pulp cavity of the mandibular canine will be readily accessible in endodontic treatment. Exceptions may always be found, of course. (C, 5; E, 14).

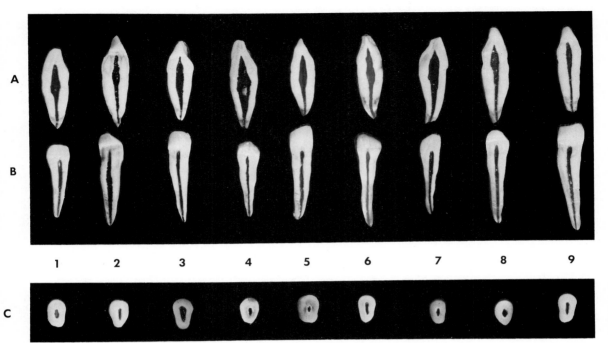

Figure 13–34. *Mandibular Canine.*

A. Labiolingual cross section, exposing the mesial or distal aspect of the pulp cavity. This aspect will
   not show on dental radiographs.
B. Mesiodistal cross section, exposing the labial or lingual aspect of the pulp cavity.
C. Cervical cross section. A transverse cut at the cementoenamel junction, exposing the pulp chamber.
   These are the openings to root canals that will be seen in the floor of the pulp chamber.
D. Labiolingual cross section, exposing the mesial or distal aspect of the pulp cavity.
E. Mesiodistal cross section, exposing the labial or lingual aspect of the pulp cavity.

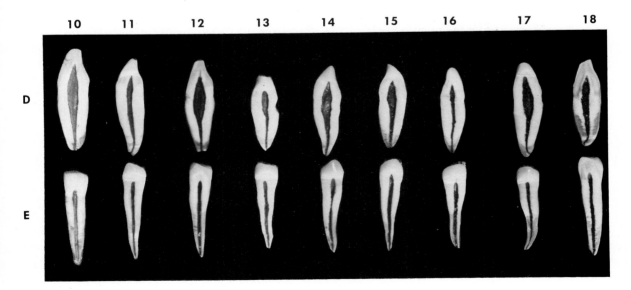

MANDIBULAR FIRST PREMOLAR (FIG. 13–35, A, B, C, D, E)

Buccolingual Cross Section (A, D)

The mandibular first premolar looks like a small mandibular canine with a dwarfed lingual cusp that is nonfunctional. Therefore, one would expect to find a pulp cavity which might be compared to that of the canine. This is the situation, except for the smaller dimensions of the pulp cavity in the premolar tooth. The buccolingual cross section of the mandibular first premolar has a pointed pulp chamber to accommodate a generous pulp horn which pointed formerly toward the tip of the large and well-formed buccal cusp of the crown. A pulp horn formation associated with the small lingual cusp will be missing or insignificant (D, 15, 16).

Like the canine, this section indicates a broad root canal the width of the pulp chamber that tapers as it progresses apically. The average premolar pulp canal will become more constricted at the half way point of the root length (A, 3, 4; D, 10, 11). Some mandibular first premolars, like the mandibular canine, will have pulp canals that are quite broad buccolingually until the final approach to the apical end of the root (A, 8; D, 14, 15).

Mesiodistal Cross Section (B, E)

The mesiodistal cross section of the mandibular first premolar displays the typical form of pulp cavity seen in this section of all premolars. The pulp chamber and canal are narrower from this angle, tapering evenly until a constricted apical foramen is reached. The pulp canal usually affords easy penetration in endodontic treatment. If there is difficulty it will be caused, more than likely, by a constriction in a mesiodistal direction (B, 3; E, 11, 12, 17).

Cervical Cross Section (C)

All premolars may vary considerably in crown size in different persons. The larger teeth will have crowns and roots that are in proportion. The mandibular first premolar may appear small when compared to other teeth in the same mouth. Therefore, the cervical cross sections of this tooth will show size variations (C, 8, 9). The overall design of the root from this angle will be that of a small mandibular canine, wider facially than lingually. The pulp canal is, of course, usually wider buccolingually than mesiodistally.

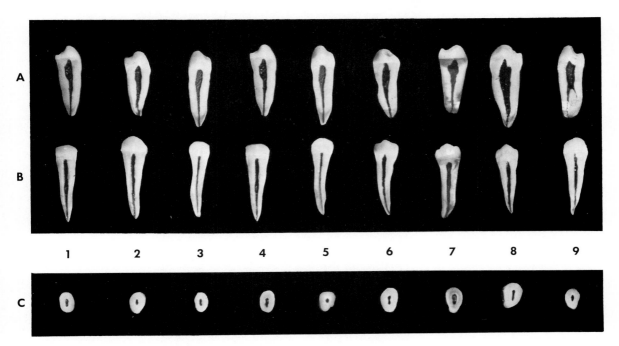

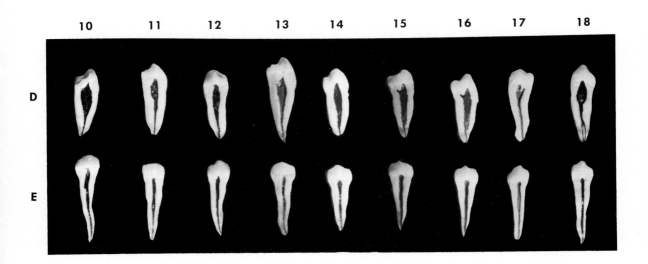

Figure 13–35. *Mandibular First Premolar.*

A. Buccolingual cross section, exposing the mesial or distal aspect of the pulp cavity. This aspect will
   not show in a dental radiograph.
B. Mesiodistal cross section, exposing the buccal or lingual aspect of the pulp cavity.
C. Cervical cross section. A transverse cut at the cementoenamel junction, exposing the pulp chamber.
   These are the openings to root canals that will be seen in the floor of the pulp chamber.
D. Buccolingual cross section, exposing the mesial or distal aspect of the pulp cavity.
E. Mesiodistal cross section, exposing the buccal or lingual aspect of the pulp cavity.

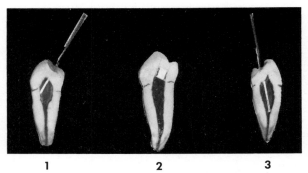

Figure 13–36. Mandibular first premolar. Compare this figure with Fig. 13–37. 1, A small opening made in the central groove of the occlusal surface will not allow access to the root canal because of the angulation of the occlusal surface with long axis of the root. 2, A cut-out that indicates the minimum of occlusal access permissible. 3, Even with the generous opening into the occlusal surface, care will be required in approaching the apical third of the root.

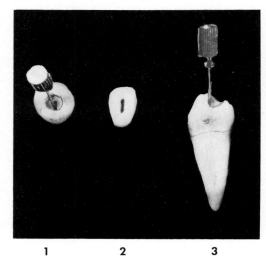

Figure 13–37. Mandibular first premolar. 1, Occlusal view of occlusal opening necessary to facilitate entrance of root canal instruments. 2, The root outline and pulp chamber opening to be found at the level of cementoenamel junction. 3, Profile view buccolingually, showing relationship of the alignment of the instrument to the opening in the crown. The cusp of the mandibular first premolar leans lingually so that it is almost centered over the root. The occlusal opening must approach the cusp tip in order to allow easy access to instruments. In this respect this tooth is similar to the mandibular canine.

MANDIBULAR SECOND PREMOLAR (FIG. 13–38, A, B, C, D, E)

Buccolingual Cross Section (A, D)

In line with the added size of crown and root, the buccolingual cross section of the mandibular second premolar will reflect the added size when comparison is made with that of the mandibular first premolar. Except for this differentiation, a description of the second premolar pulp cavity will come close to being a repetition of the description of the pulp cavity of the mandibular first premolar. Two details that differ when viewing the buccolingual cross section can be noted. One is that from this angle the pulp chamber and wide canal are confined in most cases to the crown and upper part of the root. The pulp canal then constricts to a consistent narrow path on the way to the root apex (A, 4, 5, 7, etc.). Some, of course, do not conform to the average. The second anatomical detail that differs in a second premolar as distinguished from a first mandibular premolar is this: the roofs of pulp chambers are pointed to accommodate more than one pulp horn in most cases (A, 1; D, 10, 13). This

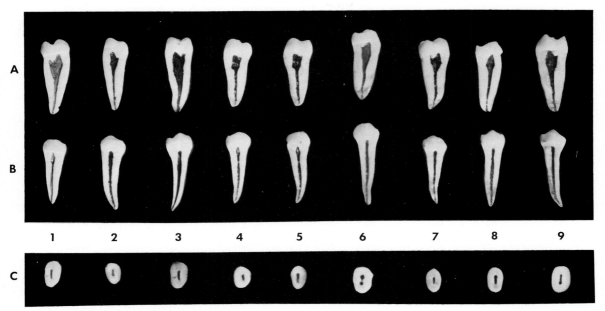

Figure 13–38. *Mandibular Second Premolar.*

A. Buccolingual cross section, exposing the mesial or distal aspect of the pulp cavity. This aspect will not show in a dental radiograph.
B. Mesiodistal cross section, exposing the buccal or lingual aspect of the pulp cavity.
C. Cervical cross section. A transverse cut at the cementoenamel junction, exposing the pulp chamber. These are the openings to root canals that will be seen in the floor of the pulp chamber.
D. Buccolingual cross section, exposing the mesial or distal aspect of the pulp cavity.
E. Mesiodistal cross section, exposing the buccal or lingual aspect of the pulp cavity.

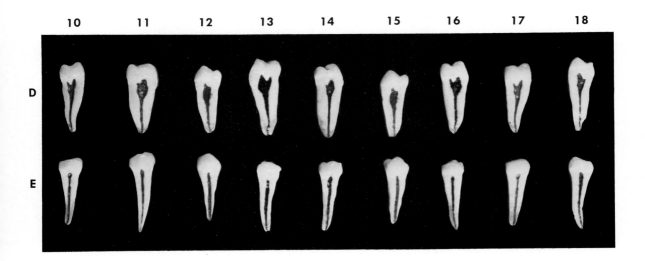

design coincides with the generous cusp development buccally and lingually in the second mandibular premolar; it is especially noticeable when making comparisons of lingual cusps of the two premolars.

Mesiodistal Cross Sections (B, E)

Except for added root size and length and the obvious effect on pulp cavity measurements it would bring about, the description will be identical to the mandibular first premolar (and the mandibular canine) when describing the mesiodistal cross section of the mandibular second premolar. The root is often quite long and curved at the apical third. Although it may curve mesially or distally, it favors a distal direction.

Cervical Cross Section (C)

The root base is substantial in mandibular second premolars, which of course is reflected in the cross sections at the cementoenamel junction. Many of these specimens will resemble those of the mandibular canine even in overall dimensions. The calibrations are greater buccolingually than mesiodistally. The shape of the pulp chambers and root canals of these teeth resembles the outline of the root, but in miniature. Some of the roots are "roundly rectangular" but most of them are "roundly triangular." (Compare Fig. C, 8 with C, 3.)

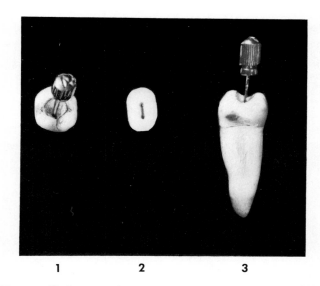

1   2   3

Figure 13–39. The mandibular second premolar. 1, Occlusal view of canal instrument entering the root canal occlusally. Note the size of the opening necessary to properly approach the pulp chamber. 2, Cross section of this tooth at the cervical line that exposes the pulp chamber. 3, Profile view buccolingually, showing the angle at which the instrument enters the root canal. Compare this picture with its counterpart showing the mandibular first premolar (Fig. 13–37).

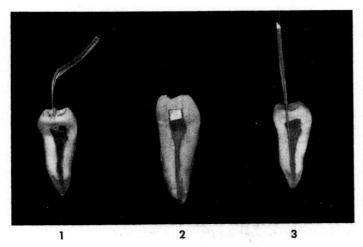

Figure 13–40.   Mandibular second premolar. Actual cross sections. 1, A small opening in the center of the occlusal surface will leave undercuts in the pulp chamber roof. 2, A window in the side of the specimen indicates the width of opening necessary to obliterate undercuts. 3, A probe placed over the photo to show the straight approach possible when dealing with the mandibular second premolar. Nevertheless, it must be noted that the lingual wall only is in line with the center of the occlusal surface.

MANDIBULAR FIRST MOLAR (FIG. 13–41, A, B, C, D, E)

Buccolingual Cross Sections (Fig. 13–41, A, D)

As mentioned heretofore, the first molars biologically are forerunners of the other molars in the same jaw, and thereby serve as models in the formation of the latter teeth. A thorough study of the cross sections of the mandibular first molar, therefore, will give considerable insight into what may be expected when the mandibular second and third molars are to be studied.

The buccolingual cross section of the mandibular first molar will demonstrate a generous pulp chamber with accommodations for prominent pulp horns. Some of these pulp chambers are quite deep, the floor extending well down into the root formation (A, 1, 2; D, 16, 18). The mesial root has the more complicated root canal arrangement of the two roots, thus the cross section under consideration will show some variation in root canal design. Some teeth will have a single broad canal (very thin though, mesiodistally) which remains quite wide buccolingually until it approaches the apical end of the root, when it narrows down to a pointed apical foramen (A, 3, 5, 8, etc.). More than likely, most of the mandibular first molars will present two separate canals in the mesial root and many will join in a common opening apically (A, 1, 2; D, 11, 14). Others will have the two canals separated all the way from the floor of the pulp chamber to the apical end of the root, keeping two separate apical foramina (A, 4, 7, 9; D, 10, 12, 16).

Mesiodistal Cross Section (B, E)

The mesiodistal cross sections of the mandibular first molar present few variables in the form of pulp chamber or pulp canal. The pulp chamber will seem generous enough with the usual pulp horn formation, and the dual root formation will have the root canals centered throughout the root form. The mesial root will show considerable curvature in most cases, the distal root appearing shorter and quite straight. Unfortunately, the longer curved mesial root contains the most constricted canal mesiodistally. (See buccolingual cross section above.) The distal root usually presents a shorter, rounder and more open canal (B, 1, 3; E, 13, etc.).

Cervical Cross Section (C, 1, 2, 3, 4, 5)

The cervical cross section of the mandibular first molar is generally quadrilateral in form. Distally it tapers a little from the wider buccolingual measurement mesially. The pulp chamber outline reflects this formation in miniature. The pulp chamber floor has two small funnel shaped openings into the mesial root of this tooth, one buccal and one lingual. A single opening which is less constricted is centered distally in the pulp chamber leading into the distal root.

Mid-Root Cross Sections (C, 6, 7, 8, 9)

The mid-root formation of the mandibular first molar is consistent with the major form of this tooth. Usually the mesial root will appear at mid-form somewhat kidney shaped, with two separate canals (C, 6). It may show one narrow flat canal, the shape of the root remaining somewhat the same. The distal root is rounder and should present one round root canal only (C, 7, 9). Occasionally two narrow canals will be discovered in the distal root (C, 6).

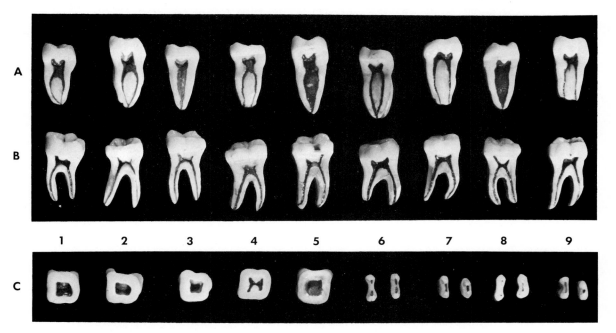

Figure 13–41. *Mandibular First Molar.*

A. Buccolingual cross section, exposing the mesial or distal aspect of the pulp cavity. This aspect will not show in a dental radiograph.
B. Mesiodistal cross section, exposing the buccal or lingual aspect of the pulp cavity.
C. Five transverse cross sections at cervical line and four transverse sections at midroot.
D. Buccolingual cross section, exposing the mesial or distal aspect of the pulp cavity.
E. Mesiodistal cross section, exposing the buccal or lingual aspect of the pulp cavity.

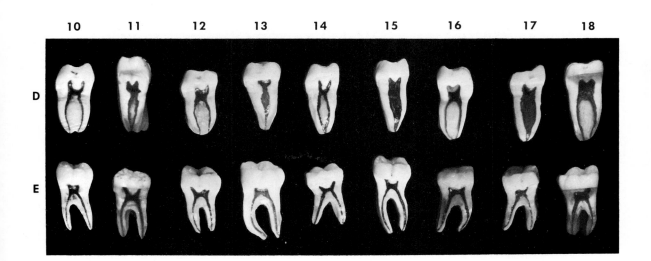

344

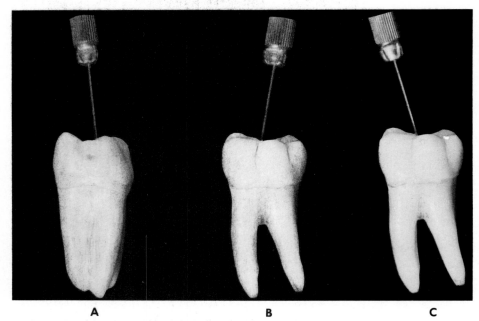

Figure 13–42. Mandibular first molar. Pulp canal files placed in canals to show the direction of canals in relation to the crown of the tooth. *A*, The canal instrument is fairly straight when viewed from the mesial as it enters the buccal portion of the mesial canals. *B*, Same as 1 but viewed from the buccal. The instrument leans considerably toward the distal. *C*, The instrument leans forward considerably as it enters the distal root canal.

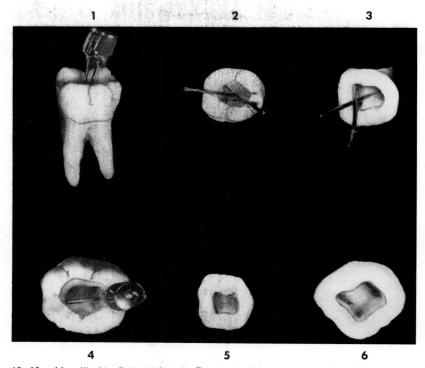

Figure 13–43. Mandibular first molar. 1, Root canal instruments placed in two mesial canals. Note the angulation and the parallelism. 2, An occlusal view showing the extent of opening necessary for convenience in approaching the root canals in the pulp chamber. Three probes in place indicate the variation in the directions the canals traverse. 3, The same illustration with the crown portion of the tooth removed and the image enlarged somewhat. 4. Occlusal view of the occlusal opening. Note the extreme angle of the instrument entering the distal root canal. A narrower occlusal opening would not permit ease of access. 5, 6, Two views, one enlarged, show the design of the pulp chamber with canal entrances at a cervical cross section of the mandibular first molar. Usually there are two canals or their equivalent in the mesial root, while the distal root normally contains one broad canal.

MANDIBULAR SECOND MOLAR (FIG. 13–44, A, B, C, D, E)

Buccolingual Cross Section (A, D)

Anatomically, the mandibular second molar differs little from the mandibular first molar. The proportions of crown and root are much the same. Therefore, the pulp cav-

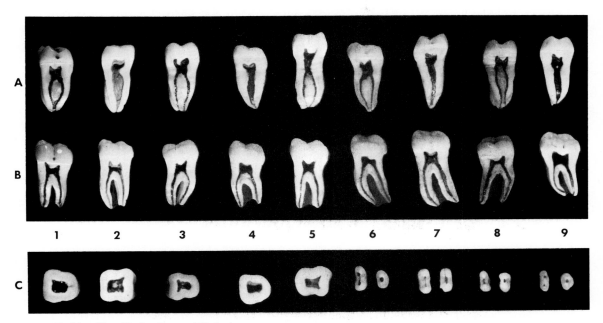

Figure 13–44. *Mandibular Second Molar.*

A. Buccolingual cross section, exposing the mesial or distal aspect of the pulp cavity. This aspect does not show on the dental radiograph.
B. Mesiodistal cross section, exposing the buccal or lingual aspect of the pulp cavity.
C. Five transverse cross sections at cervical line and four transverse sections at midroot.
D. Buccolingual cross section, exposing the mesial or distal aspect of the pulp cavity.
E. Mesiodistal cross section, exposing the buccal aspect of the pulp cavity.

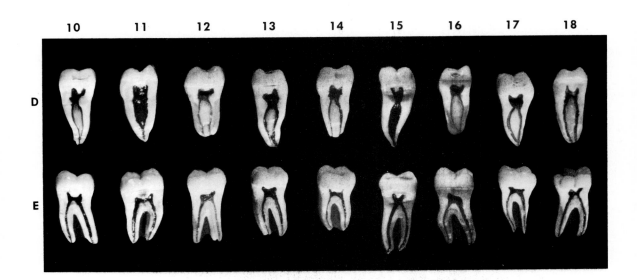

ities viewed in cross section will show similarity. Roots of second molars may be straighter, with less spread than first molars; some may have shorter roots, but there is no assurance that any of these differences will be manifest in any one case. However, good radiographs of lower molars are easily obtained; these will portray a nearly perfect picture of the way a mesiodistal cross section of the tooth in question would look (B, E). The length and shape of the roots with pulp chamber and root canals will show nicely.

The buccolingual cross section which is being discussed at present shows the pulp chamber and pulp canals to be more variable and thus more complicated in form. The pulp chamber and pulp canals are, however, quite similar in most ways to the pulp cavities of mandibular first molars. A generous pulp chamber that accommodates spaces for well-developed pointed pulp horns, both buccally and lingually, will be evident. Most mandibular second molars will have two canals in the mesial root; some will join in a common apical foramen, whereas some will present one wide flat canal pointing to a single opening at root end. (Compare Fig. 13–44, A, 1, with A, 2, etc.). Other well-formed mandibular second molars will have two separate canals in the mesial root that keep divided the full length of the root, and with two separate foramina (A, 3, 8; D, 12, 14).

Mesiodistal Cross Section (B, E)

There will be little to add to the discussion under this heading for the mandibular second molar because of some coverage under the previous heading. Except for the tendency to straighter roots, closer together in some mouths, the mesiodistal cross sections of the second molar look very much like the identical cross sections of mandibular first molars. Mesial roots will have narrow, curved root canals usually, with shorter, straighter and more open canals in distal roots.

From the endodontic point of view distal roots with a single, more open canal are usually accessible and penetrable but mesial root canals present more of a problem; therefore, each mandibular second molar must be approached as a likely variation from the one treated previously.

Cervical Cross Section (C, 1, 2, 3, 4, 5)

The cervical cross section of the mandibular second molar is similar to the mandibular first molar. It is not as "square" because the distal portion tapers more. Therefore, the pulp chamber shows more taper distally also. The floor of the pulp chamber may have two openings mesially leading into buccal and lingual root canals in the mesial root and one opening centered distally leading into the single root canal in the distal root.

Mid-Root Cross Sections (C, 6, 7, 8, 9)

Mid-root cross sections of the mandibular second molar show little variation. The mesial root will be kidney shaped; broad buccolingually and narrow mesiodistally. It will present two separate root canals or one canal that is narrow mesiodistally and wide buccolingually. The distal root will be "rounder" than the mesial root; some distal roots may be quite round (C, 6, 9). It might be well here to remind those who are endodontically inclined that since people vary genetically, their teeth will vary too. The endodontist must consider the variations in form and size when making a clinical diagnosis. The form and dimensions of a tooth will have a real bearing on its pulp cavity design.

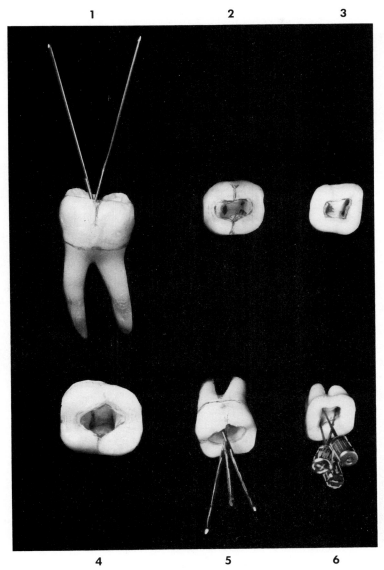

Figure 13–45.   Mandibular second molar. 1, Buccal view of the mandibular second molar with probes in canals showing the direction of insertion. The picture continues to prove the lack of parallelism existing in multirooted posterior teeth by the directions traversed by pulp canals. Also, root canals seldom follow a course at right angles to the occlusal surfaces of crowns. 2, Occlusal opening of the left second molar showing easy access to the pulp chamber. 3, A cervical cross section of this molar, which shows graphically in an actual photograph of a natural specimen the shape and location of the canal openings and an anatomically correct outline of the pulp chamber. 4, A close-up of the occlusal opening in the second molar and the approach to the pulp canals. 5, An odd angle of the whole tooth showing the direction taken by probes in the three canals. 6, Instruments placed in the canals with the crown portion of the tooth removed to permit a closer survey of the situation.

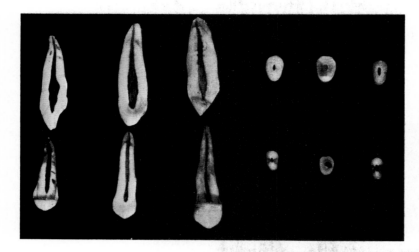

Figure 13–46. Variations in size and shape of cross section of the same teeth. Top row, Labiolingual sections of maxillary canines with cervical sections to the right. Bottom row, Mesiodistal sections of similar canines flanked by midroot sections.

Figure 13–47. Variations in size and shape of cross sections of the same teeth. Top row, Buccolingual sections of the maxillary first premolar, with cervical sections to the right. Bottom row, Mesiodistal sections of similar premolars flanked by midroot sections.

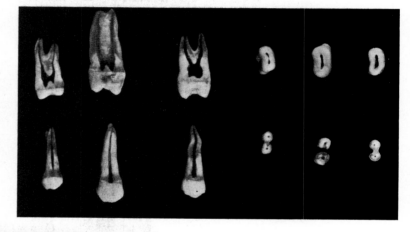

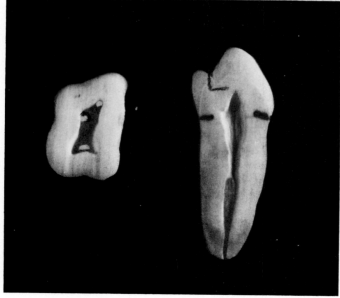

Figure 13–48. *A.* Cervical cross section of a maxillary first molar, showing the tendency of the pulp chamber to adapt itself to the cervical outline of the tooth. The white dots indicate the approximate entrances to the root canals in the pulp chamber floor. *B.* A buccolingual section of a mandibular first premolar. The cervical markings indicate the proximity of the cementoenamel junction to the pulp chamber. The occlusal marking suggests an estimated cut for cavity preparation and its proximity to the buccal pulp horn accommodation in the pulp chamber.

A   **B**

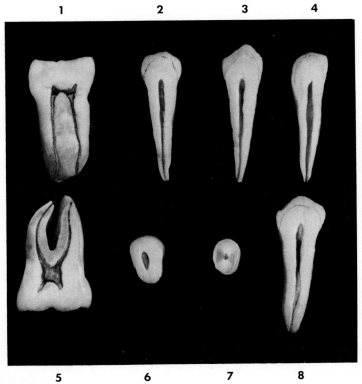

Figure 13–49.   Clear illustrations of various types of specimens which may be of interest. 1, Abraided mandibular first molar with parallel canals in the mesial root. 2, 3, 8, Mesiodistal cross sections of mandibular premolars. 4, Maxillary lateral incisor (improperly posed). 5, Maxillary first molar, mesiodistal cross section with root canals open with smooth walls. The pulp chamber shows prominent extensions for pulp horns. In fact, all molars will tend to keep some vestige of these extensions throughout life. 6, 7, Maxillary canine root. 6, Cervical section. 7, Midroot section.

MANDIBULAR THIRD MOLAR (FIG. 13–50, A, B, C, D, E)

Mandibular third molars vary greatly in development. Fig. 13–50 will display the same number and kind of cross sections as the other mandibular molars, which they resemble. These illustrations should be studied and comparisons made.

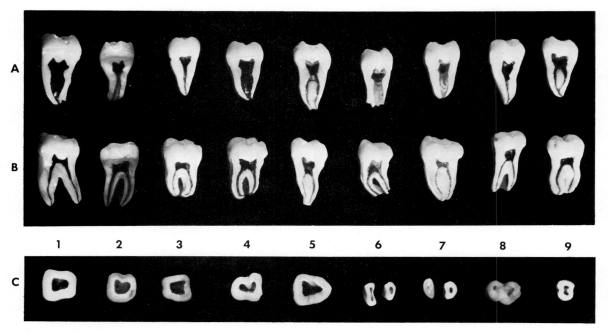

Figure 13–50. *Mandibular Third Molar.*

A. Buccolingual cross section, exposing the mesial or distal aspect of the pulp cavity. This aspect does not show on the dental radiograph.
B. Mesiodistal cross section, exposing the buccal or lingual aspect of the pulp cavity.
C. Five transverse cross sections at cervical line and four transverse sections at midroot.
D. Buccolingual cross section, exposing the mesial or distal aspect of the pulp cavity.
E. Mesiodistal cross section, exposing the buccal or lingual aspect of the pulp cavity.

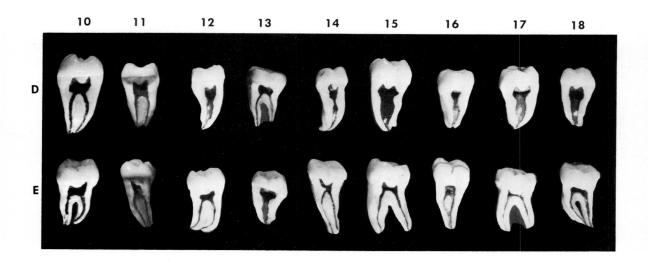

When the development and eruption of the mandibular third molar is comparable to the other mandibular molars it will resemble the second mandibular molar mostly, but will look like a tooth somewhat out of proportion at the same time. The crown may be overly large when associated with the root form; the roots may be short, curved, and inclined toward fusion (A, 2, 3, 7, etc.)

Cross sections will show all kinds of variations in pulp chambers and root canals. Nevertheless, there are instances where the retention of this tooth may be of great value to the patient. If the tooth is in good alignment, with favorable retention, it has one factor in its favor. It has the advantage shared by all third molars; it is the youngest by some years of all the individual's other teeth. Therefore, the supposition might be made that the pulp canals, although odd in formation, might well be reasonably accessible.

14

Dento-Osseous Structures

The osseous structures which support the teeth are the maxilla and the mandible. The maxilla, or upper jaw, consists of two bones: a *right maxilla* and a *left maxilla* sutured together at the median line. Both maxillae in turn are joined to other bones of the head. The *mandible,* or lower jaw, has no osseous union with the skull and is movable.

A description of the maxilla and the mandible must include the normally developed framework encompassing the teeth in complete dental arches. *This establishes the teeth as foundation tissues to be included with the bones for jaw support and as a part of the framework for the mobile portion of the face. The root forms with their size and angulation will govern the shape of the alveoli in the jaw bones, and this in turn shapes the contour of the dento-osseous portions facially.*

The loss of teeth brings about an atrophic reduction of valuable portions of the maxilla and mandible, adding disfigurement and psychological injury to the more obvious one of masticatory malfunction.

THE MAXILLAE

The maxillae make up a large part of the bony framework of the facial portion of the skull. They form the major portion of the roof of the mouth, or hard palate, and assist in the formation of the floor of the orbit and the sides and base of the nasal cavity. They bear the sixteen maxillary teeth.

Each maxilla is an irregular bone somewhat cuboidal in shape which consists of a body and four processes: the *zygomatic, nasal,* or *frontal, palatine* and *alveolar processes.* It is hollow and contains the *maxillary sinus* air space, also called the *antrum of Highmore.* From the dental viewpoint, in addition to its general shape and the processes mentioned, the following landmarks on this bone are among those most important:

1. Incisive fossa
2. Canine fossa
3. Canine eminence
4. Infra-orbital foramen
5. Posterior alveolar foramina
6. Maxillary tuberosity
7. Pterygopalatine sulcus
8. Incisive canal

The *body* of the maxilla has four surfaces:

1. Anterior or facial surface
2. Posterior infratemporal surface
3. Orbital or superior surface
4. Medial or nasal surface

The maxilla has four *processes:*

1. Zygomatic process
2. Frontal process
3. Palatine process
4. Alveolar process

ANTERIOR SURFACE

The *anterior* or *facial surface* is separated above from the orbital aspect by the *infra-orbital ridge.* Medially it is limited by the margin of the nasal notch, and posteriorly it is separated from the posterior surface by the anterior border of the zygomatic process, which has a confluent ridge directly over the roots of the first molar. The ridge corresponding to the root of the canine tooth is usually the most pronounced and is called the *canine eminence* (Figs. 14–1 and 14–2).

Mesial to the canine eminence, overlying the roots of the incisor teeth, is a shallow concavity known as the *incisive fossa.* Distal to the canine eminence on a higher level is a deeper concavity called the *canine fossa.* The floor of this canine fossa is formed in part by the projecting zygomatic process. Above this fossa and below the infra-orbital ridge is the *infra-orbital foramen,* the external opening of the infra-orbital canal. The major portion of the canine fossa is drectly above the roots of the premolars.

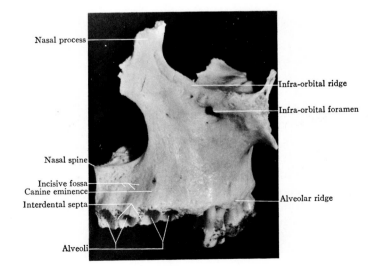

Figure 14–1. Frontal view of maxilla.

Nasal process

Infra-orbital ridge

Infra-orbital foramen

Nasal spine

Incisive fossa
Canine eminence
Interdental septa

Alveolar ridge

Alveoli

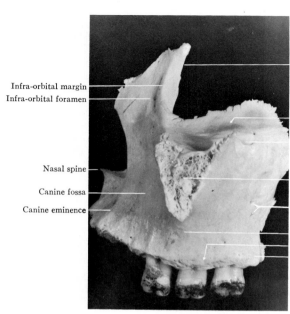

Infra-orbital margin
Infra-orbital foramen

Nasal spine

Canine fossa

Canine eminence

Frontal process

Orbital surface

Infra-orbital groove

Zygomatic (malar) process

Posterior alveolar foramina

Zygomatic ridge
Alveolar ridge
Maxillary tuberosity

Figure 14–2. Lateral view of maxilla.

POSTERIOR SURFACE

The *posterior* or *infratemporal surface* is bounded above by the posterior edge of the orbital surface. Inferiorly and anteriorly it is separated from the anterolateral surface by the zygomatic process and its lower border. This surface is more or less convex and is pierced in a downward direction by the apertures of the *posterior alveolar foramina*, which are two or more in number (Figs. 14–2 and 14–5).

These two canals are on a level with the lower border of the zygomatic process and are somewhat distal to the roots of the last molar. The lower part of this area is slightly more prominent where it overhangs the root of the third molar and is called the *maxillary tuberosity*. Medially this tuberosity is limited by a sharp, irregular margin with which the palate bone articulates (see Fig. 14–5).

ORBITAL OR SUPEROLATERAL SURFACE

This surface is smooth and forms part of the floor of the orbit. The anterior edge of this surface corresponds to the infra-orbital margin or ridge as it travels up to become part of the nasal process. Its posterior border or edge coincides with the inferior boundary of the inferior orbital fissure.

Its thin medial edge is notched in front to form the *lacrimal groove*, behind which groove it articulates with the lacrimal bone for a short distance, then for a greater length with a thin portion of the ethmoid bone, and terminates posteriorly in a surface which articulates with the orbital process of the palate bone. Its lateral area is continuous with the base of the zygomatic process.

Traversing part of this area to the distal is the *infra-orbital canal*, the anterior opening of which is located directly below the infra-orbital ridge in the anterolateral area. Distally, however, owing to a deficiency of its covering, the canal forms a groove on the orbital surface toward the uppermost boundary of the posterolateral surface.

If the covered portion of this canal were to be laid open, the orifices of the middle and anterior alveolar canal would be seen transmitting the corresponding vessels and nerves to the premolars, canines and incisor teeth.

NASAL OR MEDIAL SURFACE

This surface is directed medially toward the nasal cavity. It is bordered below by the superior surface of the palatine process; anteriorly it is limited by the sharp edge of the nasal notch. Above and anteriorly it is continuous with the medial surface of the frontal process; behind this it is deeply channeled by the *lacrimal groove,* which is of course converted into a canal by articulation with the lacrimal and inferior turbinate bones.

Behind this groove the upper edge of this area corresponds to the medial margin of the orbital surface, and the maxilla articulates in this region with the lacrimal bone, a thin portion of the ethmoid bone and the orbital process of the palate bone.

The posterior border of the maxilla, which articulates with the palate bone, is traversed obliquely from above downward and slightly medially by a groove which, by articulation with the palate bone, is converted into the *posterior palatine canal.*

Toward the posterior and upper part of this nasal surface an irregular or angular opening of the *maxillary sinus* or *antrum of Highmore* may be seen. In front of the lacrimal groove the nasal surface is ridged for the attachment of the *inferior turbinate* bone. Below this the bone forms a lateral wall of the *inferior nasal meatus.* Above the ridge for some little distance on the medial side of the nasal process, the smooth lateral wall of the *middle meatus* appears.

PROCESSES

The *zygomatic process* may be seen in the lateral views of the bone. Illustrations show it to be rough and spongelike in appearance where it has been disarticulated

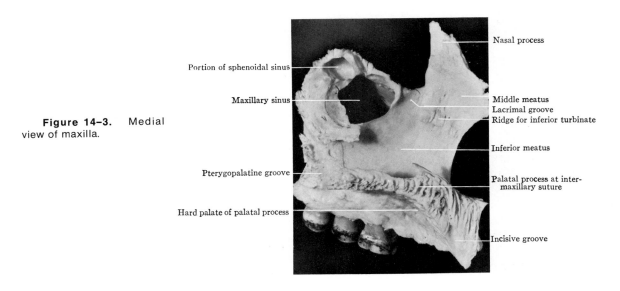

Figure 14–3. Medial view of maxilla.

Portion of sphenoidal sinus

Maxillary sinus

Pterygopalatine groove

Hard palate of palatal process

Nasal process

Middle meatus
Lacrimal groove
Ridge for inferior turbinate

Inferior meatus

Palatal process at inter-maxillary suture

Incisive groove

from the zygomatic or cheek bone (Fig. 14–2).The lower border of this process, directly over the first molar, is considered to be an important landmark.

The *frontal process* arises from the upper and anterior part of the body of the maxilla. Part of this extension is the upward continuation of the infra-orbital margin laterally. Its anterior edge articulates with the nasal bone. Superiorly the summit of the process articulates with the frontal bone. The medial surface of the frontal process is directed toward the nasal cavity.

The *palatine process* has two surfaces, the superior and the inferior. Its superior surface helps form the floor of the nasal cavity. Its inferior surface when sutured with the maxilla of the opposite side forms the anterior three-fourths of the hard palate. The posterior portion of the hard palate is formed by the horizontal part of the palate bone. The inferior surface of the palatine process is rough and pitted for the glands of the mucous membrane in the roof of the mouth and by small foramina for rich blood and nerve supply. As mentioned before, the posterior palatine canal makes its appearance where the palate bones have been disarticulated from the palatine process of the maxilla.

The posterior edge of the palatine process becomes relatively thin where it joins the palatine bone at the point of the greater palatine foramen. The palatine process becomes progressively thicker anteriorly from the posterior border. Anteriorly it becomes quite thick, its thickness being measured from the alveolar border of the anterior teeth to the nasal sinus. This portion of the palatal process is confluent with the alveolar process surrounding the roots of the anterior teeth.

Immediately posterior to the central incisor alveolus, when looking at the medial aspect of the maxilla, one sees a smooth canal which is half of the *incisive canal*, when the two bones are joined together. The *incisive fossa* into which the canals open may be seen immediately lingual to the central incisors at the median line or *intermaxillary suture*, when the maxillae are joined.

The posterior border of the palatine process, when observed from the inferior aspect, falls in line with the second molar and articulates with the horizontal part of the palatal bone (see Fig. 14–4). The intermaxillary suture and the suture joining the palate bone to the palatal process of the maxilla (transverse palatine suture) are nearly at right angles.

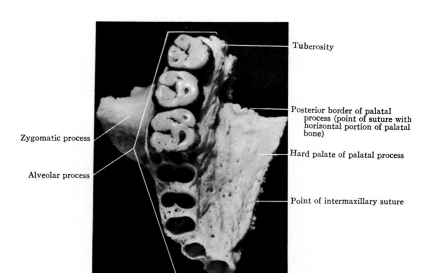

Tuberosity

Posterior border of palatal process (point of suture with horizontal portion of palatal bone)

Hard palate of palatal process

Zygomatic process

Alveolar process

Point of intermaxillary suture

Figure 14–4. Palatal view of maxilla. Note the dental foramina in the deepest portion of the canine alveolus.

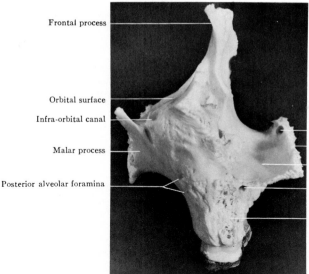

Frontal process

Orbital surface

Infra-orbital canal

Malar process

Posterior alveolar foramina

Nasal foramen of incisive cana

Palatine process

Floor of nose

Part of pterygopalatine cana

Roughened area for attachment of palatine bone

Figure 14–5. Posterior view of maxilla.

The *alveolar process* makes up the inferior portion of the maxilla; it is that portion of the bone which surrounds the roots of the maxillary teeth and which gives them their osseous support. The process extends from the base of the tuberosity posterior to the last molar to the median line anteriorly, where it articulates with the same process of the opposite maxilla (Figs. 14–4, 14–6 and 14–7). It merges with the palatine process medially and with the zygomatic process laterally (Fig. 14–7).

When one looks directly at the inferior aspect of the maxilla toward the alveoli with teeth removed, it is apparent that the alveolar process is curved to conform with the dental arch. It completes, with its fellow of the opposite side, the alveolar arch supporting the roots of the teeth of the maxilla.

The process has a facial (labial and buccal) surface and a lingual surface with ridges corresponding to the surfaces of the roots of the teeth invested in it. It is made up of labiobuccal and lingual plates of very dense but thin cortical bone separated by interdental septa of cancellous bone.

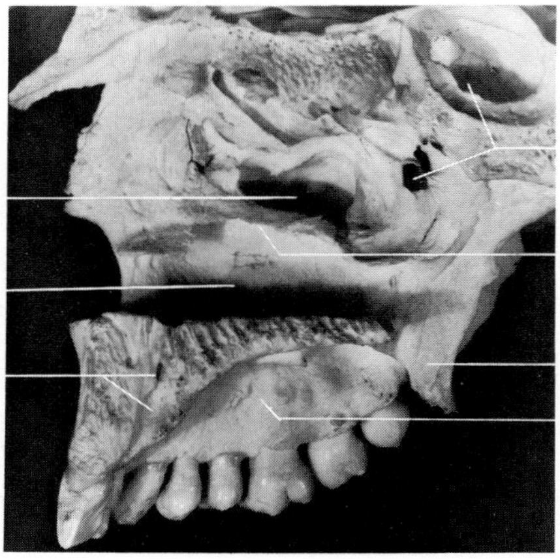

Figure 14–6. Medial view of maxilla. This specimen has not been disarticulated completely and has the maxillary teeth in situ.

Maxillary sinus

Inferior meatus

Incisive canals

Sphenoidal sinus

Inferior nasal **turbinate**

Medial lamina of pterygoid process

Hard palate

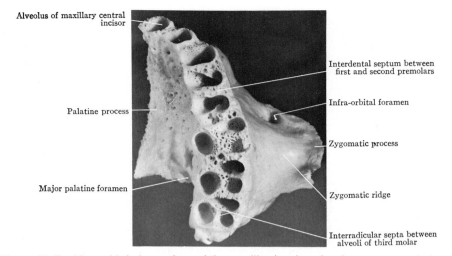

Alveolus of maxillary central incisor

Palatine process

Major palatine foramen

Interdental septum between first and second premolars

Infra-orbital foramen

Zygomatic process

Zygomatic ridge

Interradicular septa between alveoli of third molar

Figure 14–7.   View of inferior surface of the maxilla showing alveolar process and alveoli.

The facial plate is thin, and the positions of the alveoli are well marked on it by visible ridges as far posteriorly as the distobuccal root of the first molar (Fig. 14–1). The margins of these alveoli are frail and their edges sharp and thin. The buccal plate over the second and third molars, including the alveolar margins, is thicker. Generally speaking, the lingual plate of the alveolar process is heavier than the facial plate. In addition, it is longer where it surrounds the anterior teeth, and sometimes this added coverage includes the premolars. In short, it extends farther down in covering the lingual portion of the roots.

The bone is very thick lingually, over the deeper portions of the alveoli of the anterior teeth and premolars. This formation is brought about by the merging of the alveolar process with the roof of the mouth. The lingual plate is paper thin over the lingual alveolus of the first molar, however, and rather thin over the lingual alveoli of the second and third molars. This thin lingual plate over the molar roots is part of the formation of the *major palatine canal* (Fig. 14–7).

THE ALVEOLI, OR TOOTH SOCKETS

These cavities are formed by the facial and lingual plates of the alveolar process and by connecting septa of bone placed between the two plates. The form and depth of each alveolus is regulated by the form and length of the root it supports. (See table, "Measurements of the Teeth," Chapter 1.)

The *alveolus* nearest the median line is that of the *central incisor*. The periphery is regular and round, and the interior of the alveolus is evenly cone-shaped.

The second *alveolus* in line is that of the *lateral incisor*. It is generally cone-shaped. It is narrower mesiodistally than labiolingually and is smaller on cross section, although it is often deeper than the central alveolus. Sometimes it is curved at the upper extremity.

The *canine alveolus* is the third from the median line. It is much larger and deeper than those just described. The periphery is oval and regular in outline with the labial width greater than the lingual. The socket extends distally. It is flattened mesially and somewhat concave distally. The bone is so frail at the canine eminence on the facial surface of the alveolus that the root of the canine is often exposed on the labial surface near the middle third (Fig. 14–1).

The *first premolar alveolus* is kidney-shaped, with the cavity partially divided by a spine of bone which fits into the mesial developmental groove of the root of this tooth. This spine divides the cavity into a buccal and a lingual portion. If the tooth root is bifurcated for part of its length, as is often the case, the terminal portion of the cavity is separated into buccal and lingual alveoli. The socket is flattened distally and much wider buccolingually than mesiodistally. (See "Measurements of the Teeth," Chapter 1.)

The *second premolar alveolus* is also kidney-shaped, but the curvatures are in reverse to those of the first premolar alveolus. The proportions and depth are almost the same. The septal spine is located on the distal side instead of the medial, since the second premolar root is inclined to have a well-defined developmental groove distally. This tooth usually has one broad root with a blunt end, but it is occasionally bifurcated at the apical third.

Figures 14–8 to 14–10

Close-up views of three separate divisions of maxillary alveoli. The attempt was made to point the camera lens into the alveoli in such a way that the bottom of the sockets might be seen. Three views were only partially successful because, as was discussed previously, seldom does one find roots parallel, even in the same jaw.

However, some interesting and significant observations are possible. A few of these are as follows: (1) The facial cortical plate of bone is thin over the anterior teeth only. (2) The bone formation covering buccal surfaces of all posterior teeth is much thicker and is supplied rather evenly over premolar and molar roots. Cancellous as well as cortical bone seems involved. (3) Inter-radicular septa between all roots are

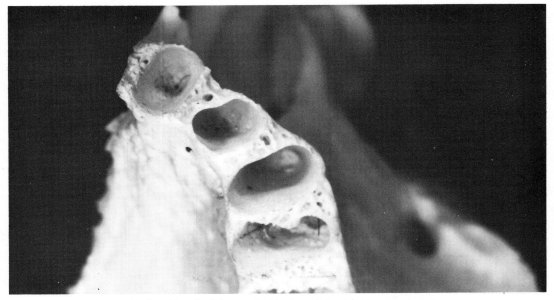

Figure 14–8. Alveoli of the central incisor, lateral incisor, and canine.

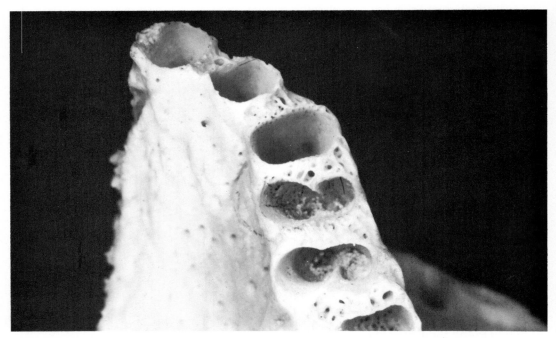

Figure 14–9. Alveoli of the premolar area.

thick, with a rich blood supply guaranteed by the visible openings in the cancellous bone. (4) Cancellous bone furnishing a good blood supply is evident in the apical portions of the tooth sockets near root ends. The anterior alveoli are lined on the sides with a hard, smooth cortical layer; the alveoli of posterior teeth, less so.

The *first molar alveolus* is made up of three distinct alveoli widely separated. The *lingual alveolus* is the largest; it is round, regular and deep. The cavity extends in the direction of the hard palate, having a lingual plate over it which is very thin. The lingual periphery of this alveolus is extremely sharp and frail. This condition may contribute to tissue recession often seen at this site.

The *mesiobuccal* and *distobuccal alveoli* of the first molar have no outstanding characteristics except that the buccal plates are thin. The bone is somewhat thicker at the peripheries than that found on the lingual alveolus. Nevertheless it is thinner farther up on the buccal plate. It is not uncommon for one to find the roots uncovered by bone in spots when examining dry specimens.

The forms of the buccal alveoli resemble the forms of the roots they support. The mesiobuccal alveolus is broad buccolingually, with the mesial and distal walls flattened. The distobuccal alveolus is rounder and more conical.

The *septa* which separate the three alveoli (interradicular septa) are broad at the area which corresponds to the root bifurcation, and they become progressively thicker as the peripheries of the alveoli are approached. The bone septa are very cancellous, denoting a rich blood supply, as is true of all the septa, those separating the various teeth as well.

A general description of the alveoli of the *second molar* would coincide with that of the first molar; these alveoli are closer together, since the roots of this tooth do not spread as much. As a consequence, the septa separating the alveoli are not so heavy.

The *third molar alveolus* is similar to that of the second molar except that it is

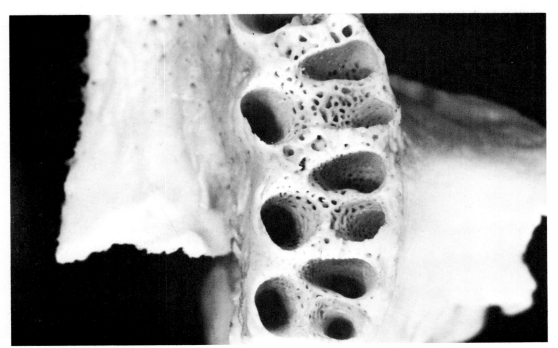

Figure 14–10. Alveoli of the molar area. Note the thinness of buccal plates over the first molar roots when compared with those of the second and third maxillary molars. The third alveoli are rarely separated as distinctly as in this specimen.

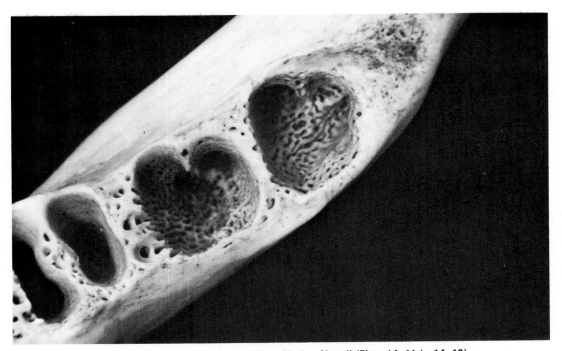

Close-Up Views of Three Separate Divisions of Mandibular Alveoli (Figs. 14–11 to 14–13).

Figure 14–11. Alveoli of the first, second and third molars. Items for special attention: the thin and perforated surface of the retromolar triangular space distal to the third molar alveolus; the cancellous formation in the alveoli proper and also in the interdental septa, which would allow a rich blood supply.

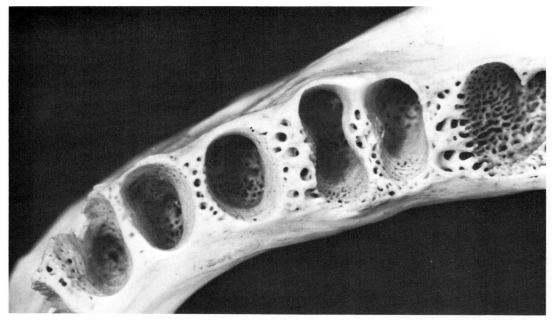

Figure 14-12. This view includes the canine, first and second premolar, and a clear view of the mandibular first molar alveoli. Note the excellent design for the anchorage of first molar roots. Apparently the blood supply for the interseptal bone lessens as anterior teeth are approached. The apical portion of the canine alveolus displays the single opening in the bone for the blood and nerve supply to the tooth pulp.

somewhat smaller in all dimensions. Figure 14–7 shows a third molar socket to accommodate a tooth with three well-defined roots, a rare occurrence. Usually the roots will be fused, the buccal roots at least, and often all three. The interradicular septum changes accordingly. If the roots of the tooth are fused, a septal spine will appear in the alveolus at the points of fusion on the roots marked by deep developmental grooves.

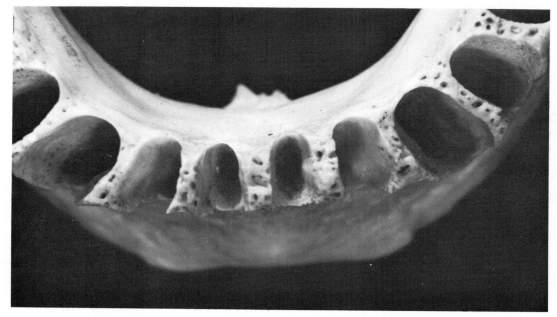

Figure 14-13. A close-up view of the mandibular anterior tooth alveoli. This picture indicates the relative sizes and shapes of the incisors for comparison with other mandibular teeth.

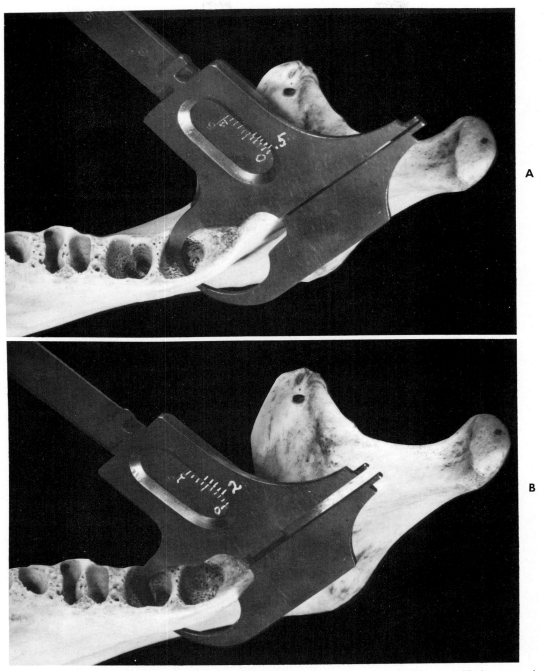

Figure 14–14. Illustration of the relative thickness of bone covering lingual mandibular second and third molar roots. *A,* Measurement of the thickness of bony cover lingual to the apex of the third mandibular molar immediately below the mylohyoid ridge. It measured only .5 millimeter. *B,* Repetition of measurement in the deepest portion lingually of the second molar alveolus. It measured fully two millimeters.

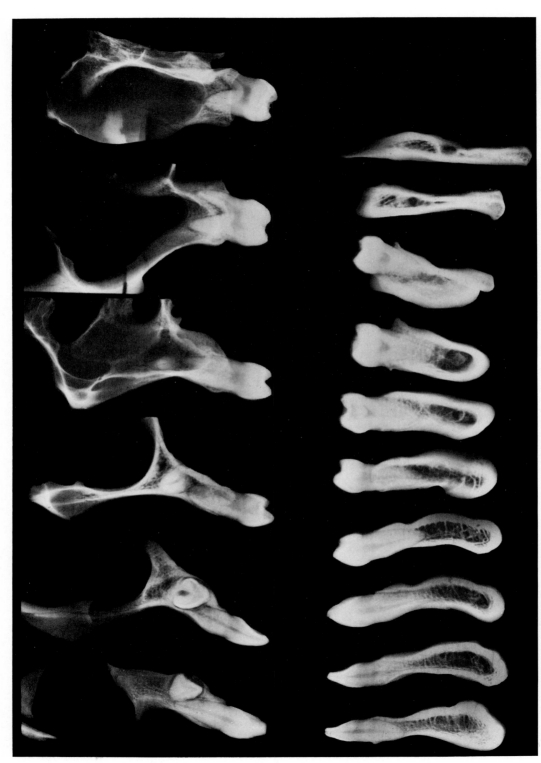

Figure 14–15. Some fine vertical sections of a skull made with radiographic problems in view. Faciolingual views of the teeth and their attachment cannot be obtained by clinical radiographic methods.

These radiographs of faciolingual sections are interesting. They show the extent of tooth attachment, how individual teeth compare with each other, and the variances between cortical and cancellous bone in anchorage. (See also Figs. 14–29 to 14–36.) The maxillary third molars were missing. Maxillary third molars were missing in this specimen. The maxillary canine was impacted in this specimen. (From "Dental Radiography and Photography," Vol. 31, No. 4, 1958. Permission granted by William J. Updegrave, D.D.S., F.A.A.O.R., Temple University School of Dentistry, Philadelphia, Pa.)

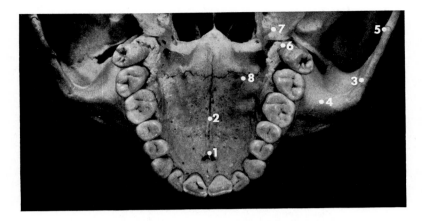

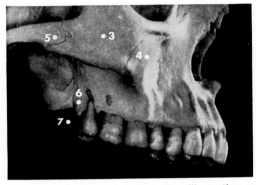

Figure 14-16. Photographs of dry specimen of maxilla, illustrating anatomic landmarks. (By H. Berton McCauley, D.D.S., in *Dental Radiography and Photography,* Eastman Kodak Co.)

1, Incisive fossa. 2, Median palatine suture. 3, Zygomatic (malar) bone. 4, Zygomatic process of maxilla. 5, Zygomaticotemporal suture. 6, Tuberosity of maxilla. 7, Hamular process of sphenoid bone. 8, Major (or greater) palatine foramen.

MAXILLARY SINUS

The maxillary sinus lies within the body of the bone and is of corresponding pyramidal form; the base is directed toward the nasal cavity. Its summit extends laterally into the root of the zygomatic process. It is closed in laterally and above by the thin walls which form the anterolateral, posterolateral and orbital surfaces of the body. The sinus overlies the alveolar process in which the molar teeth are implanted, more particularly the first and second molars, the alveoli of which are separated from the sinus by a thin layer of bone. Occasionally the maxillary sinus will extend forward far enough to overlie the premolars also. It is not uncommon to find the bone covering the alveoli of some of the posterior teeth extending above the floor of the cavity of the maxillary sinus, forming small hillocks.

Regardless of the irregularity and the extension of the alveoli into the maxillary sinus, there is always a layer of bone separating the roots of the teeth and the floor of the sinus in the absence of pathologic conditions. There is always, also, a layer of sinus mucosa between the root tips and the sinus cavity.

MAXILLARY ARTICULATION

The maxilla articulates with the nasal, frontal, lacrimal and ethmoid bones, above, and laterally with the zygomatic bone and occasionally with the sphenoid

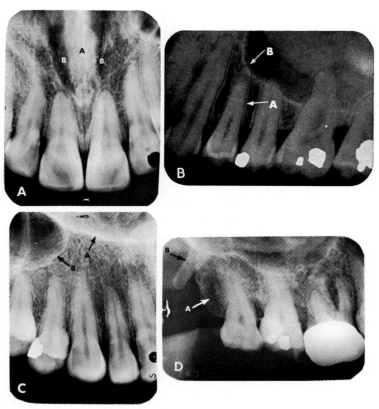

Figure 14–17, I. *A*, Radiograph of central incisor region that visualizes the nasal septum (A) and fossae (B). *B*, Radiograph that demonstrates the normal appearance of (A) the lamina dura, (B) the periodontal membrane. *C*, Radiograph that depicts the Y (inverted) formed by the junction of the lateral wall (A) of the nasal fossa and the antemedial wall (B) of the maxillary sinus. *D*, Radiograph that visualizes (A) the tuberosity of the maxilla, (B) the hamular process of the spheroid bone. (By H. Berton McCauley, D.D.S., in *Dental Radiography and Photography,* Eastman Kodak Co.)

bone. Posteriorly and medially it articulates with the palate bone besides joining the maxilla on its medial side. In addition, it supports the inferior turbinate and the vomer medially.

LANDMARKS AND BONY PROCESSES OF BOTH JAWS — A CLINICAL APPROACH (Fig. 14–18, A, B, C, D)

Before going into all of the details involved in describing bony processes of the mandible, it was thought advisable to pause at this point, and approach the subject of dento-osseous structures of *both* jaws from a clinical and diagnostic point of view.

In this the reader will be favored by being able to study some graphic illustrations borrowed from "X-rays in Dentistry," published by Eastman Kodak Company, 1972 (Fig. 14–18).

The illustrations with their explanatory legends will make further comment unnecessary. Text continued on page 370.

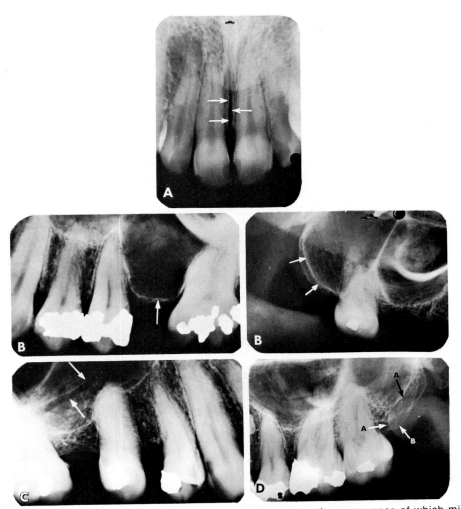

Figure 14–17, II.   *A*, Radiograph of the medial palatine suture, the appearance of which might be interpreted as a fracture. *B*, Radiographs that visualize various extensions of the maxillary sinus; left, alveolar extension; right, tuberosity extension. *C*, Radiograph in which the canal for a superior alveolar artery is seen. *D*, Radiograph showing typical superimposition of the coronoid process: (A) of the mandible on the tuberosity, (B) of the maxilla. (By H. Berton McCauley, D.D.S., in *Dental Radiography and Photography,* Eastman Kodak Co.)

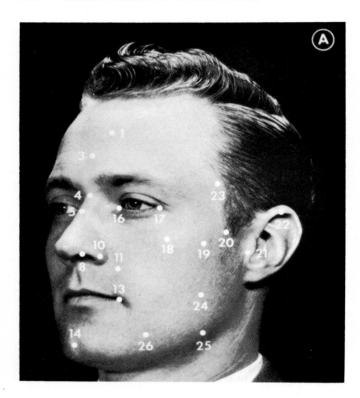

Figure 14–18.   *Surface Landmarks.**

Various dental structures in the patient's face can be quickly located by means of surface landmarks. Surface landmarks are identified in *A*. The photograph of the bony skull (*B*) was made from the same angle of view. Features of both are numbered and identified in the legend. The medial aspect of the mandible *(C)* shows anatomic details not clearly seen in the other illustrations. The bony anatomy of the hard palate and its adjoining structures are shown in *D*. Structures are identified by numbers in the legend.

Although the anatomical landmarks of the entire skull are important, most dental radiography is primarily concerned with the dentition.

*(Courtesy of Dr. Silha, *X-rays in Dentistry*, published by Radiography Markets Division, Eastman Kodak Co., 1972, pp 14–15.)

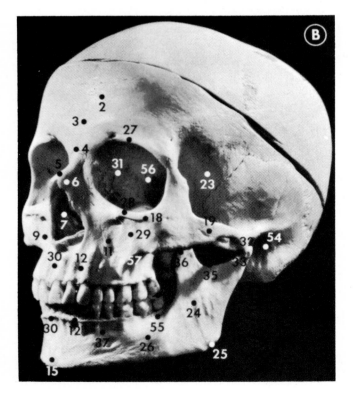

Legend
  1 Forehead
  2 Frontal bone
  3 Glabella
  4 Frontonasal suture (nasion)
  5 Bridge of nose
  6 Nasal bone
  7 Nasal cavity
  8 Nostrils
  9 Anterior nasal spine
 10 Ala of nose
 11 Canine fossa
 12 Alveolar ridges
 13 Labial commissure
 14 Chin
 15 Symphysis menti
 16 Inner canthus of eye
 17 Outer canthus of eye
 18 Cheekbone (zygomatic bone)
 19 Zygomatic arch
 20 Temporomandibular articulation

(Illustration continued on opposite page.)

Figure 14–18. *Continued.*

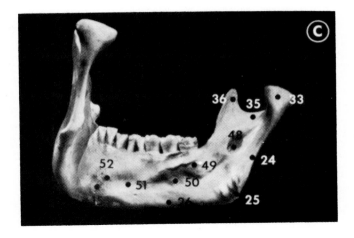

21 Tragus
22 Auricle
23 A Temple; B Temporal fossa
24 Ramus of mandible
25 Angle of mandible
26 Body of mandible
27 Supraorbital ridge
28 Infraorbital ridge
29 Zygomatic process of maxilla
30 Alveolar process
31 Orbit
32 Articular eminence
33 Mandibular condyle
34 Glenoid fossa
35 Mandibular notch
36 Coronoid process
37 Mental foramen
38 Median palatine suture
39 Palatine bone
40 Transverse palatine suture
41 Posterior palatine foramen
42 Anterior palatine foramen
43 Nasal septum
44 Posterior nasal spine
45 Vomer
46 Lateral pterygoid plate
47 Medial pterygoid plate
48 Mandibular foramen
49 Internal oblique ridge
50 Submaxillary depression
51 Sublingual depression
52 Genial tubercles
53 Styloid process
54 External auditory meatus
55 External oblique ridge
56 Optic foramen
57 Maxilla

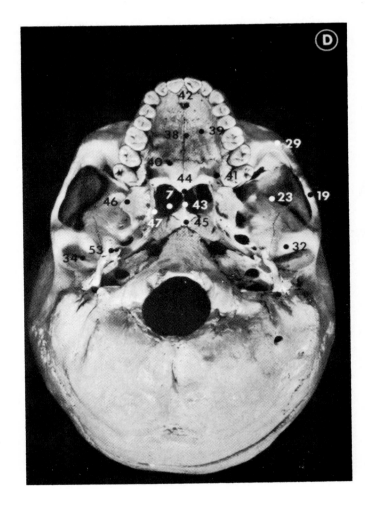

THE MANDIBLE

The mandible is horseshoe-shaped and supports the teeth of the lower dental arch. This bone is movable and therefore has no bony attachment to the skull. It is the heaviest and strongest bone of the head and serves as a framework for the floor of the mouth. It is situated immediately below the maxillary and zygomatic bone, and its *condyles* rest in the *glenoid fossa* of the temporal bone, a formation which makes possible a movable articulation (Figs. 14–19 to 14–27).

The mandible has a horizontal portion or *body* and two vertical portions or *rami*. The rami join the body at an obtuse angle.

The *body* consists of two lateral halves, which are joined at the median line shortly after birth. The line of fusion, usually marked by a slight ridge, is called the symphysis. The body of the mandible has two surfaces, an external and an internal, and two borders, a superior and an inferior.

To the right and left of the symphysis, near the lower border of the mandible, are two prominences called *mental tubercles*. A prominent triangular surface made by the symphysis and these two tubercles is called the *mental protuberance* (Fig. 14–20).

Immediately posterior to the symphysis and immediately above the mental protuberance, there is a shallow depression called the *incisive fossa*. The fossa is immediately below the alveolar border of the central and lateral incisors and anterior to the canines. The alveolar portion of the mandible overlying the root of the canine is prominent and is called the *canine eminence* of the mandible. This eminence does not extend down very far toward the lower border of the mandible, however, before it is lost in the prominence of the mental protuberance and the lower border of the mandible in this area.

The external surface of the mandible from a lateral viewpoint presents a number of important areas for examination:

The *external oblique ridge* (external oblique line) extends obliquely across the external surface of the mandible from the mental tubercle to the anterior border of the

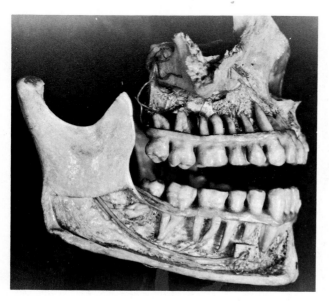

Figure 14–19. Dissected specimen of maxilla and mandible. This specimen illustrates the extent of the alveolar processes, the angulation of the long axes of the teeth, the relative lengths of the roots and the spacing of those roots, which of course governs the size, form and direction of the alveoli.

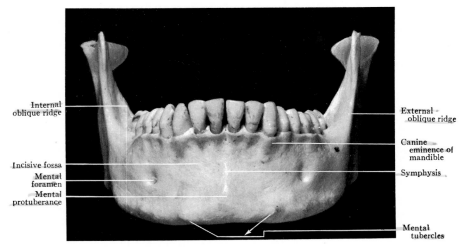

Figure 14–20.   Frontal view of mandible.

ramus, with which it is continuous. It lies below the mental foramen. It is usually not prominent except in the molar area (Figs. 14–20 and 14–21).

This ridge thins out as it progresses upward and becomes the anterior border of the ramus and ends at the tip of the *coronoid process*. The coronoid process is one of two processes making up the superior border of the ramus. It is a pointed, smooth projection flattened externally and internally, and it is roughened toward the tip to give attachment for a part of the temporal muscle.

The *condyle, or condyloid process*, on the posterior border of the ramus, is variable in form. It is divided into a superior or articular portion and an inferior portion or *neck*. Although the articular portion, the condyle, appears as a rounded knob when one sees the mandible from the side, exteriorly, from a *posterior* aspect the condyle is much wider and is oblong in outline (compare Figs. 14–21 and 14–22).

The condyle is convex above, fitting into the glenoid fossa of the temporal bone when the mandible is articulated to the skull, and forms, with the interarticular

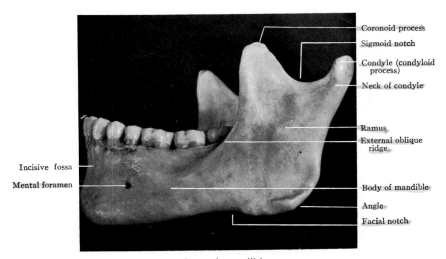

Figure 14–21.   Lateral view of outer surface of mandible.

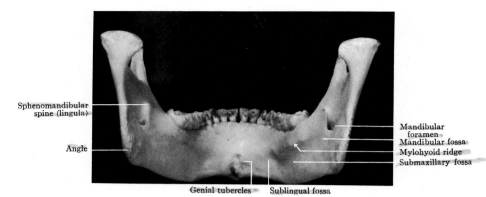

Figure 14–22.   Posterior view of mandible.

cartilage which lies between the two surfaces and with the tissue attachment, the *temporomandibular articulation.*

The neck of the condyle is a constricted portion immediately below the articular surface. It is flattened in front and presents a concave pit medially—the *pterygoid fossa.* A smooth semicircular notch, the *sigmoid notch,* forms the sharp upper border of the ramus between the condyle and coronoid process.

The distal border of the ramus is smooth and rounded and presents a concave outline from the neck of the condyle to the angle of the jaw, where the posterior border of the ramus and the inferior border of the body of the mandible join. The border of this angle is rough, being the attachment of the masseter muscle and the stylomandibular ligament.

An important landmark on the external aspect of the mandible is the *mental foramen.* It should be noted that this opening of the anterior end of the mandibular canal is directed upward and backward as well as laterally. The foramen is usually located midway between the superior and inferior border of the body of the mandible when the teeth are in position, and most often it is below the second premolar tooth, a little below the apex of the root. The position of this foramen is not constant and it may be between the first premolar and the second premolar tooth. After the teeth are lost and resorption of alveolar bone has taken place, the mental foramen may appear near the crest of the alveolar border. In childhood, before the first permanent molar has come into position, this foramen is usually immediately below the first deciduous molar and nearer the lower border.

It is interesting to note, when one observes the mandible from a point directly opposite the first molar, that most of the distal half of the third molar is hidden by the anterior border of the ramus. When looking at the mandible from in front, directly opposite the median line, the student sees the second and third molars located 5 to 7 mm. lingually to the anterior border of the ramus. (Compare Figs. 14–20 and 14–21.)

THE INTERNAL SURFACE OF THE MANDIBLE

Observation of the mandible from the rear shows that the median line is marked by a slight vertical depression, representing the line of union of the right and left halves of the mandible, and immediately below this, at the lower third, that the bone is roughened by eminences called the *genial tubercles* (Fig. 14–22).

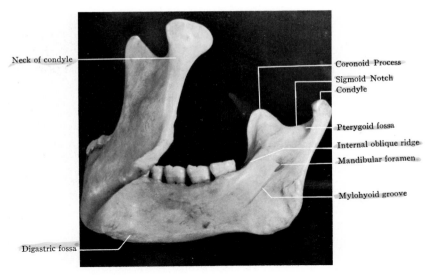

Figure 14–23. Postero-lateral view of inner surface of mandible.

Neck of condyle

Coronoid Process
Sigmoid Notch
Condyle

Pterygoid fossa
Internal oblique ridge
Mandibular foramen

Mylohyoid groove

Digastric fossa

The internal surface of the body of the mandible is divided into two portions by a well-defined ridge, the *mylohyoid or internal oblique ridge.* It occupies a position closely corresponding to the external oblique ridge on the external surface. It starts at or near the lowest part of the genial tubercles and passes backward and upward, increasing in prominence until the anterior portion of the ramus is reached; there it smooths out and gradually disappears (Fig. 14–23).

This ridge is the point of origin of the mylohyoid muscle, which forms the central portion of the floor of the mouth. Immediately posterior to the median line and above the anterior part of the mylohyoid ridge a smooth depression, the *sublingual fossa,* may be seen. The sublingual gland lies in this area.

A small oval roughened depression, the *digastric fossa,* is found on each side of the symphysis immediately below the mylohyoid line and extending onto the lower border. Toward the center of the body of the mandible, between the mylohyoid ridge and the lower border of the bone, a smooth oblong depression is located, called the *submaxillary fossa.* It continues back on the medial surface of the ramus to the attachment of the internal pterygoid muscle. The submaxillary gland lies within this fossa.

The *mandibular foramen* is located on the medial surface of the ramus midway between the sigmoid notch and the angle of the jaw and also midway between the internal oblique line and the posterior border of the ramus. The mandibular canal begins at this point, passing downward and forward horizontally.

The anterior margin of the foramen is formed by the *lingula or mandibular spine,* which gives attachment to the *sphenomandibular ligament.* Coming obliquely downward from the base of the foramen beneath the spine is a decided groove, the *mylohyoid groove.* Behind this groove toward the angle of the mandible, a roughened surface for the attachment of the internal pterygoid muscle may be seen.

THE ALVEOLAR PROCESS

The border of this process outlines the alveoli of the teeth and is very thin at its anterior portion around the roots of the incisor teeth but thicker posteriorly where it encompasses the roots of the molars. The alveolar process which composes the supe-

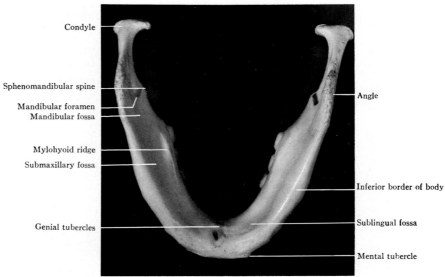

Figure 14–24.   View of mandible from below.

rior border of the body of the mandible differs from the same process in the maxillae in one very important particular: It is not so cancellous, and instead of the facial plate being thin and frail it is equally as heavy as the lingual plate. Although the bone over the anterior teeth, including the canine, is very thin and over the cervical portion of the root may be entirely missing, yet the bone which does cover the root is the compact type of bone.

The inferior border of the mandible is strong and rounded and gives to the bone the greatest portion of its strength (see Fig. 14–24).

When looking down on the mandible from a point above the alveoli of the first molars (Fig. 14–25), one may notice that, although the alveolar border may be thinner anteriorly than posteriorly, the body of the bone is uniform throughout. The lines of direction of the posterior alveoli are inclined lingually to conform to the lingual inclination of the teeth when they are in position. The anterior teeth, of course, have their alveoli tipped labially; therefore when one looks down upon the mandible from above the alveolar process, more of the bone may be seen lingual to the anterior teeth than lingual to the posterior teeth. In contrast posteriorly, more of the bone may be seen buccal to the teeth than lingual. *Therefore, the outline of the arch of the teeth does not correspond to the outline of the arch of the bone.* The dental arch is narrower posteriorly than the mandibular arch.

The lingual walls of the alveoli of the second and third molars are relatively thin near the bottoms of the sockets, although the bone near the periphery is somewhat thicker and very compact. If a specimen of the mandible from which the third molar has been removed is held up to the light, the bone at the bottom of the socket is so thin that light will penetrate it. This is caused by the mandible being undercut at this point for the submaxillary fossa below the mylohyoid ridge (Figs. 14–14, A, B and 14–24).

The bone buccal to the last two molars is very heavy and thick, being reinforced by the external oblique ridge. Posterior to the third molar a triangular shallow fossa is outlined; it is called the *retromolar triangle.* The cortical plate over this fossa is not so heavy as the bone surrounding it, and it is more cancellous under the thin cortical plate covering it.

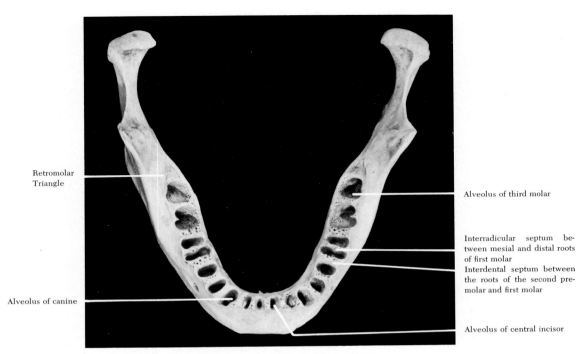

Retromolar
Triangle

Alveolus of third molar

Interradicular septum be-
tween mesial and distal roots
of first molar
Interdental septum between
the roots of the second premolar and first molar

Alveolus of canine

Alveolus of central incisor

Figure 14–25.   The alveolar process of the mandible showing alveoli.

THE ALVEOLI

The first alveolus right or left of the median line is that of the *first* or *central incisor*. The periphery of the alveolus often dips down lingually and labially and exposes the root for part of its length. This arrangement makes an interdental spine out of the interdental septum separating the alveoli of the mandibular central incisors. The central incisor alveolus is flattened on its mesial surface and is usually somewhat concave distally to accommodate the developmental groove on the root (Fig. 14–25).

The alveolus of the mandibular *second* or *lateral incisor* is similar to that of the central incisor. It usually has the following variations: The socket is larger and deeper to accommodate a larger and longer root; the periphery does not dip down so far on the lingual but may dip more on the labial, exposing more of the root of the lateral incisor. The interdental septum extends up just as high between the teeth as that between the central incisors.

The *canine alveolus* is quite large and oval and of course deep to accommodate the root of the mandibular canine. The lingual plate is stronger and much heavier than over the alveoli just described, although the thin labial plate may thin out at its edges and expose just as much of the canine root on the labial side. The labial outline of the alveolus is wider than the lingual outline, and the mesial and distal walls of the sockets will be irregular to accommodate developmental grooves, both mesially and distally, on the canine root.

The alveoli of the *first* and *second premolars* are similar in outline. The outline is smooth and rounded, although the dimensions are greater buccolingually than mesiodistally. The alveolus of the second premolar is usually somewhat larger than that of the first premolar. The buccal plate of the alveoli is relatively thin, but the lingual plate is heavy; the interdental septum has become heavier at this point when

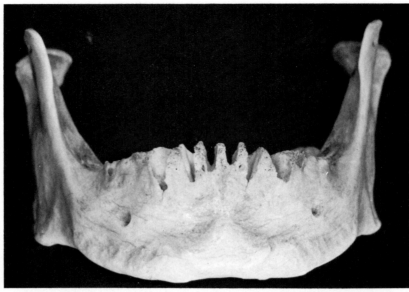

Figure 14–26. Anterior view of empty anterior tooth sockets. There was no evidence present to indicate pathological involvement. The cortical layer of bone labially and lingually over the roots of mandibular incisors and canines is very thin and often fails to cover, as indicated in this specimen. (See also Fig. 16–58.)

one compares it with the interdental septa found between the anterior teeth. The interdental septum between the canine and first premolar is relatively thin although uniform in outline. The septum between the first premolar and second premolar is nearly twice as thick.

Progressing posteriorly, one finds that the interdental septum between the second premolar socket and the alveolus of the mesial root of the *first molar* is twice as thick as that found between the first and second premolars. The socket of the first molar is divided by an interroot septum which is strong and regular. The alveolus of the mesial root is kidney-shaped, much wider buccolingually than mesiodistally and

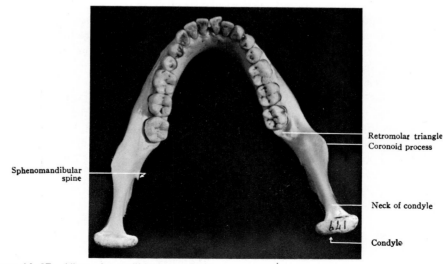

Sphenomandibular spine

Retromolar triangle
Coronoid process

Neck of condyle

Condyle

Figure 14–27. View of mandible from above.

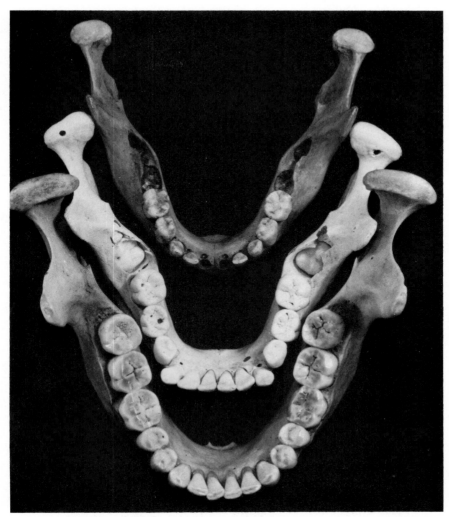

Figure 14–28. Comparison of size and shape of mandibles at various ages. *Top*, mandible of five-year-old. Notice the rounded bowlike form. Notice also the amount of space between the second deciduous molar and the ramus. *Middle*, mandible of nine-year-old. Notice the angular outline with constriction at the point of second permanent molar development. *Lower*, well-developed mandible of an individual approximately fifty years of age. The bone is regular in outline. The lingual constriction has lessened and has retreated to the third molar area.

constricted in the center to accommodate developmental grooves found mesial and distal to the mesial root of the first molar. The alveolus of the distal root of the first molar is evenly oval with no constriction, conforming to the rounded shape of this root. The interdental septum between the alveoli of the mandibular first molar and the socket of the second molar is thick mesiodistally although cancellous in character.

The mandibular *second molar alveolus* may be divided into *two* alveoli, as was the case in the first molar. However, often it is found to be one compartment near the periphery of the alveolus, but divides into two compartments in the deeper portions. A septal spine occurs where the developmental grooves on the root are deep enough, or an interradicular septum will appear where the roots are entirely divided. The interdental septum between the second molar sockets and the third molar sockets is not so thick mesiodistally as the two interdental septa immediately anterior.

The mandibular *third molar alveolus* is usually irregular in outline. Usually it is much narrower toward the distal than toward the mesial. It may have interradicular septa or septal spines to accommodate itself to the irregularity of the root.

Classical illustrations by Dr. Hugh W. MacMillan are shown in Figs. 14–29 to 14–36. The sections demonstrate the directional lines of the axes of the teeth and their alveoli. In addition, the radiographs of the sections graphically illustrate the relative densities of the teeth and supporting structures and show the outline and relative thickness of the bone over the various teeth at the site of each section.

ARTERIAL SUPPLY TO THE TEETH

The arteries and nerve branches to the teeth are mere terminals of the central systems. This book must confine itself to dental anatomy and the parts immediately associated, and references will therefore be made only to those terminals which supply the teeth and the supporting structures.

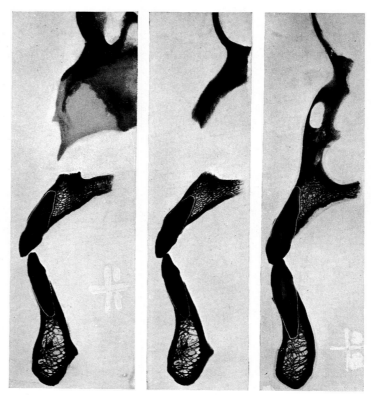

Fig. 14–29.   Fig. 14–30.   Fig. 14–31.

Figure 14–29 to 14–31.   Note the axial relations of the superior and inferior teeth, the relative thickness of labial and lingual alveolar plates, the characteristics of the cancellous tissue, the relative densities and the relation of the teeth to important structures. Compare the changes in the external contour and internal architecture of the adjacent sections. The sections in this series, with the exception of Fig. 14–32, were taken from the same cadaver and are from the left side. A plaster cast was made before sectioning. The sections were reassembled in the cast and held in exact relation while being X-rayed.

Figure 14–29.   The central incisor regions, showing relation of superior central incisor to inferior lateral incisor.

Figure 14–30.   The lateral incisor regions. Note position of apex of superior lateral incisor.

Figure 14–31.   The canine regions. Note anterior extremity of maxillary antrum.

Copyright 1924 by Hugh W. MacMillan.

Figure 14–32. The first premolar regions.

Figure 14–33. The second premolar regions.

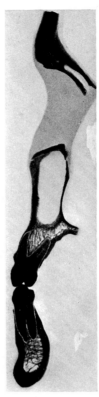 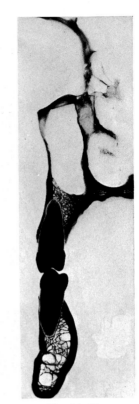

Fig. 14–32.   **Fig. 14–33.**

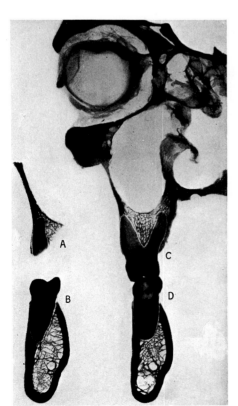

Figure 14–34. The first molar regions, showing relations of (C) mesiobuccal and lingual root with (D) mesial half of lower molar, (A) distobuccal root, (B) distal half.
Copyright 1924 by Hugh W. MacMillan.

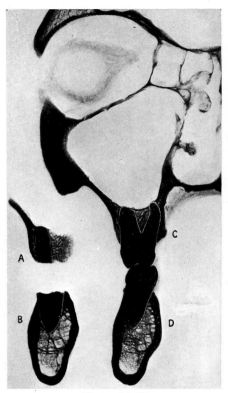
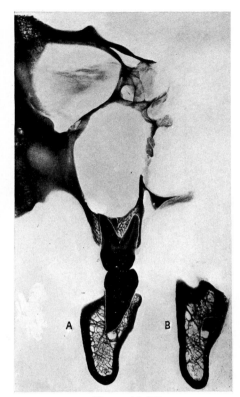

Figure 14–35.   **Figure 14–36.**

Figure 14–35. The second molar regions, showing relations of (C) mesiobuccal and lingual roots with (D) mesial half, (A) distobuccal root, (B) distal root.

Figure 14–36. The third molar regions, (A) mesial root, (B) apex of distal root. Note deep groove for descending palatine artery.

INTERNAL MAXILLARY ARTERY (FIG. 14–37)

The arterial supply to the jaw bones and the teeth comes from the *internal maxillary artery,* which is a branch of the *external carotid artery.* The *branches* of the internal maxillary artery which feed the teeth directly are: (1) the *inferior alveolar artery* and (2) the *superior alveolar arteries.*

Inferior Alveolar Artery

The *inferior alveolar artery* branches from the internal maxillary artery medial to the ramus of the mandible. Protected by the sphenomandibular ligament, it gives off the *mylohyoid branch,* which rests in the mylohyoid groove of the mandible and continues along on the medial side under the mylohyoid ridge. After giving off the mylohyoid branch, it immediately enters the mandibular foramen and continues downward and forward through the mandibular canal, giving off branches to the premolar and molar teeth. In the vicinity of the mental foramen it divides into a *mental* and an *incisive branch.* The mental branch passes through the mental foramen to supply the tissues of the chin and to anastomose with the *inferior labial* and *submental arteries.*

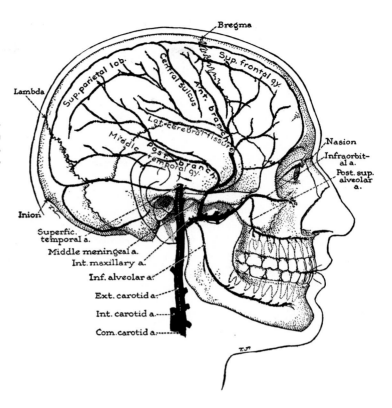

Figure 14–37. Projection of internal maxillary artery and its branches in relation to brain, skull, and mandible, including the teeth. (Jones and Shepard, *A Manual of Surgical Anatomy.*)

The incisive branch continues forward in the bone to supply the anterior teeth and bone and to form anastomoses with its fellows of the opposite side.

The anastomoses of the mental and incisive branches furnish a good collateral blood supply for the mandible and teeth.

In their canals, the inferior alveolar and incisive arteries give off *dental* branches to the individual tooth roots for the supply of the pulp and of the periodontal membrane at the root apex. Other branches enter the interdental septa supplying bone and adjacent periodontal membrane and terminating in the gingivae. Numerous small anastomoses connect these vessels with those supplying the neighboring alveolar mucosa.

Superior Alveolar Arteries

The *posterior superior alveolar artery* branches from the internal maxillary at the posterior of the maxillary tuberosity along with the alveolar nerves and supplies the maxillary teeth, alveolar bone and membrane of the sinus. A branch of variable size runs forward on the periosteum at the junction of the alveolar process and maxillary body supplying the gingiva, alveolar mucosa and cheek. When it is large, it may supplant in part the buccal artery.

A *middle superior alveolar branch* is usually given off by the infra-orbital branch of the internal maxillary artery somewhere along the infra-orbital groove or canal. It runs downward between the sinus mucosa and bone or in canals in the bone and joins the *posterior* and *anterior alveolar vessels*. Its main distribution is to the maxillary teeth.

Anterior superior alveolar branches arise from the infra-orbital artery just before this vessel leaves its foramen. They course down the anterior aspect of the maxilla in bony canals to supply the maxillary anterior teeth and their supporting tissues and to join the *middle* and *posterior superior alveolar branches* in completing an anastomotic plexus.

Branches to the teeth, periodontal membrane and bone are derived from the superior alveolar in the same manner as described for the inferior alveolar artery.

Descending Palatine and Sphenopalatine Arteries

The palatal blood supply comes from two sources but chiefly from the *descending palatine* artery, which descends from its origin from the internal maxillary through the pterygomandibular canal. Its *major* (greater) *palatine* branch enters the palate through the greater palatine foramen and runs forward with its accompanying vein and nerve in a groove at the junction of the palatine and alveolar processes. It is distributed to the bone, glands and mucosa of the hard palate and to the bone and mucosa of the alveolar process, in which it forms anastomoses with fine branches of the superior alveolars. Minor branches of the descending palatine pass to the soft palate through minor palatine canals in the palatine bone.

Terminal branches of the *nasopalatine* branch of the *sphenopalatine artery:* The *nasopalatine* courses obliquely forward and downward on the septum and enters the palate through the incisive canal. It has a limited distribution to the incisive papilla and adjacent palate and forms an anastomosis with the major palatine.

NERVE SUPPLY

The sensory nerve supply to the jaws and teeth is derived from the *maxillary* and *mandibular* branches of the *fifth cranial,* or *trigeminal,* nerve, whose ganglion, the *gasserian,* is located at the tip of the petrous portion of the temporal bone.

MAXILLARY NERVE

The *maxillary* nerve courses forward through the wall of the cavernous sinus and leaves the skull through the foramen rotundum. It crosses the pterygopalatine fossa, where it gives branches to the *sphenopalatine* ganglion, a parasympathetic ganglion. This ganglion gives off several branches, now containing visceral motor as well as sensory fibers, to the mucous membrane of the mouth, nose and pharynx.

Its branches of practical significance in the mouth are the *descending palatine* branches. Of these the *anterior palatine* enters the hard palate through the major palatine foramen, to be distributed to the hard palate and palatal gingivae as far forward as the canine tooth. *Middle* and *posterior* palatine branches from the ganglion enter the soft palate through minor palatine foramina. A *nasopalatine* branch of the *sphenopalatine* branch of the ganglion runs downward and forward on the nasal septum. Entering the palate through the incisive canal, it is distributed to the incisive papilla and to the palate anterior to the anterior palatine nerve.

The maxillary nerve also has a *posterior superior alveolar* branch from its pterygopalatine portion. This nerve divides, enters foramina on the posterior surface of the maxilla and, forming a plexus, is distributed to the molar teeth and the supporting tissues.

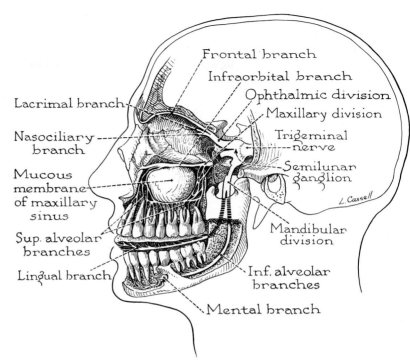

Figure 14–38. Diagram showing distribution of the trigeminal nerve. (King and Showers, *Human Anatomy and Physiology*, 5th Edition.)

The maxillary nerve enters the orbit and, as the *infra-orbital nerve,* runs forward in its floor first in the infra-orbital groove and then in the infra-orbital canal. It terminates at the infra-orbital foramen in branches distributed to the upper face. At a variable distance after it enters the orbit, a *middle superior alveolar* branch arises from the infra-orbital nerve and runs through the lateral wall of the maxillary sinus. It is distributed to the premolar teeth and surrounding tissues and joins the alveolar plexus. The middle alveolar nerve may be associated closely with the posterior alveolar nerve as its origin but frequently branches near the infra-orbital foramen.

An anterior alveolar branch leaves the infra-orbital nerve just inside the infra-orbital foramen and is distributed through bony canals to the incisor and canine teeth. All three superior alveolar nerves join in a plexus above the process. From the plexus *dental branches* are given off to each tooth root and *interdental branches* to the bone, periodontal membrane and gingivae; the distribution being similar to that described for the arteries.

MANDIBULAR NERVE

The *mandibular nerve* leaves the skull through the foramen ovale and almost immediately breaks up into its several branches. The chief branch to the lower jaw is the *inferior alveolar* nerve, which at first runs directly downward across the medial surface of the external pterygoid, at the lower border of which it is directed laterally and downward across the outer surface of the internal pterygoid muscle to reach the mandibular foramen. Just before entering the foramen it releases the mylohyoid branch, which is primarily a motor branch to the mylohyoid muscle and anterior belly of the digastric muscle.

The inferior alveolar nerve continues forward through the mandibular canal beneath the roots of the molar teeth to the level of the mental foramen. During this part of its course it gives off branches to the molar and premolar teeth and their supporting bone and soft tissues. The nerve to the teeth does not arise as individual branches but as two or three larger branches which form a plexus from which *inferior dental* branches enter individual tooth roots and *interdental* branches supply alveolar bone, periodontal membrane and gingivae.

At the mental foramen the nerve divides, and a smaller incisive branch continues forward to supply the anterior teeth and bone and a larger mental branch emerges through the foramen to supply the skin of the lower lip and chin.

Other branches of the mandibular nerve contribute in some degree to the innervation of the mandible and its investing membranes. The *buccinator (long buccal) nerve,* while chiefly distributed to the mucosa of the cheek, has a branch which is usually distributed to a small area of the buccal gingiva in the first molar area, but in some cases its distribution may extend from the canine to the third molar. The *lingual nerve* as it enters the floor of the mouth lies against the body of the mandible and has mucosal branches to a variable area of lingual mucosa and gingiva. The *mylohyoid nerve* may sometimes continue its course forward on the lower surface of the mylohyoid muscle and enter the mandible through small foramina on either side of the midline. It has been implicated in the innervation of central incisor teeth and their periodontal membranes.

15

Temporomandibular Articulation — Muscles of Mastication and Facial Expression — Oral Pharynx — Analysis of Mandibular Movements

THE TEMPOROMANDIBULAR ARTICULATION

The temporomandibular articulation is closely associated with the functioning of the teeth. It receives its name from the two bones which enter into its formation, namely, the temporal bone and the mandible. The temporomandibular joint allows a wide range of motion to the mandible. Entering into its construction are bone, ligaments, cartilage and synovial membrane; these tissues are all essential to any movable articulation.

The temporomandibular joint is an example of diarthrosis, and its movements are a combination of gliding movements and a loose hinge movement. The osseous portions of the joint are the anterior portion of the *glenoid fossa* and *articular eminence* of the temporal bone and the *condyloid process* of the mandible. Both the condyle and the glenoid fossa are covered with a layer of fibrous tissue over the usual articular cartilage. There is a cushion of interarticular fibrocartilage called the *meniscus* between the condyle and the glenoid fossa (Figs. 15–6, 15–7 and 15–8).

THE GLENOID FOSSA

The glenoid fossa is an oval or oblong depression in the temporal bone just anterior to the auditory canal (Fig. 15–2). It is bounded anteriorly by the *eminentia ar-*

385

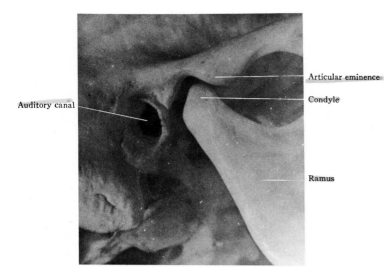

Auditory canal

Articular eminence

Condyle

Ramus

Figure 15–1. The relation of the condyle of the mandible to the glenoid fossa and the articular eminence of the temporal bone when the teeth are in *centric occlusal relation.*

ticularis (articular eminence), externally by the middle root of the zygoma and the auditory process, and posteriorly by the tympanic plate of the petrous portion of this bone. The shape of the glenoid fossa conforms to some extent, though not exactly, to the posterior and superior surfaces of the condyloid process of the mandible (Fig. 15–1).

THE CONDYLOID PROCESS

The condyloid process of the mandible is convex on all bearing surfaces, although somewhat flattened posteriorly, and its knoblike form is wider lateromedially

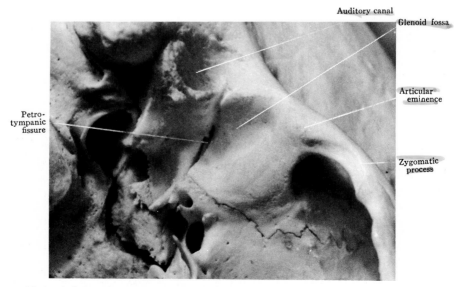

Auditory canal

Glenoid fossa

Articular eminence

Petro-tympanic fissure

Zygomatic process

Figure 15–2. Inferior view of the glenoid fossa of the temporal bone.

than anteroposteriorly (see Figs. 14–19 to 14–27, Chapter 14). It is perhaps two and one-half times as wide in one direction as in the other. Although the development of this condyle differs in individuals, the functional design remains the same. The long axes of the condyles are in a lateral plane, and at first sight they seem to be out of alignment, since the long axes, if the lines were prolonged, would meet at a point posterior to the condyles of the mandible (Fig. 16–94). However, on closer observation it is noted that the plane of the posterior surface of each condyle or a line through the long axis of the condyle is almost perpendicular to the axis of the main portion of the body of the mandible (Figs. 14–24, 14–27 and 14–28).

LIGAMENTS

The temporomandibular articulation is maintained by ligaments and by the powerful muscles of mastication. The ligamentous attachments are: the *capsular* ligament, the *sphenomandibular* ligament, the *stylomandibular* ligament and accessory fibers of the stylomandibular called the *stylohyoid* ligament.

The *capsular ligament* is a synovial capsule which completely surrounds the condyle. It has fibers divided into four portions: anterior and posterior portions, and internal and external portions. The anterior portion is attached below to the anterior margin of the condyle and above to the front of the glenoid ridge. The posterior portion is attached above just in front of the glenoid fissure and is inserted into the posterior margin of the ramus of the mandible just below the neck of the condyle (Fig. 15–3).

The internal portion of the capsular ligament is composed of well-defined fibers and has a broad attachment above to the inner edge of the glenoid fossa and is inserted below into the inner side of the neck of the condyle.

The *temporomandibular ligament,* which is the external portion of the capsular ligament and continuous with it, is the strongest portion of the capsular ligament. It has a broad attachment above the zygomatic process of the temporal bone, the anterior fibers attaching forward well beyond the articular eminence (Fig. 15–3). These fibers, slanting downward and backward, converge with more vertical fibers and are inserted into the outer side and posterior margin of the neck of the condyle. The temporomandibular ligament acts as the main suspensory ligament of the mandible during moderate opening movements, commonly referred to as the "hinge movements," when the forward movement of the condyle is very slight. With wider opening of the jaw, the condyles move forward rapidly, relaxing the external lateral ligament as the *sphenomandibular ligament* becomes taut.

The *sphenomandibular ligament* is situated some distance from the temporomandibular joint, and, as its name implies, it has its attachment above to the sphenoid bone and below to the mandible. Actually its main origin is from the spinous process of the sphenoid bone with lateral fibers from the temporal bone in the immediate vicinity. The ligament passes downward and forward and is inserted into the lingula of the mandible, with some fibers attached below the mandibular foramen and some posterior to it. The attachment of the sphenomandibular ligament is round and cordlike at its origin; it takes on more of a ribbonlike form at its insertion from the lingula backward on the inner surface of the ramus (Fig. 15–4).

The *stylomandibular ligament* extends from the styloid process of the temporal bone downward and forward to be inserted into the posterior border of the ramus of the mandible just above the angle. Just before the stylomandibular ligament makes its insertion, it gives off accessory fibers which continue downward to the posterior border of the hyoid bone. This accessory ligament is called the *stylohyoid* ligament.

Temporomandibular ligament   Capsular ligament

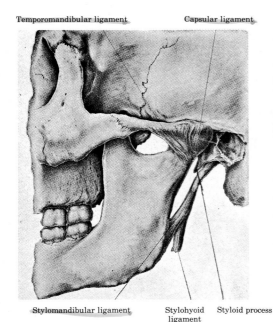

Figure 15–3. Temporomandibular articulation–external view of the ligamentous attachment of the condyle of the mandible to the zygomatic process. Note the strong attachment of the temporomandibular ligament laterally and posteriorly to the neck of the condyle. (Deaver.)

Stylomandibular ligament   Stylohyoid   Styloid process
                                  ligament

The temporomandibular ligament and the sphenomandibular ligament (the latter to a much smaller degree) apparently act as suspensory ligaments, whereas the stylomandibular ligament with its accessory stylohyoid ligament acts as a checkrein on the mandible and helps to prevent excessive anterior drift at the angle during the more extreme opening movements.

The *interarticular fibrocartilage* or *meniscus* is a tough fibrous disk placed between the condyle and its temporal bearing areas, the glenoid fossa and the articular eminence of the zygomatic process, adapting itself exactly to the two bony surfaces, making up for any discrepancy in these two surfaces and promoting smooth articula-

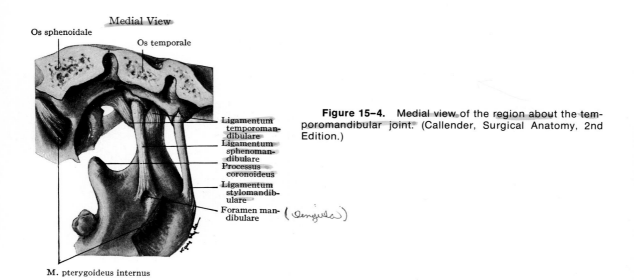

Medial View

Os sphenoidale   Os temporale

Ligamentum
temporoman-
dibulare
Ligamentum
sphenoman-
dibulare
Processus
coronoideus
Ligamentum
stylomandib-
ulare
Foramen man-
dibulare   (lingula)

M. pterygoideus internus

Figure 15–4. Medial view of the region about the temporomandibular joint. (Callender, Surgical Anatomy, 2nd Edition.)

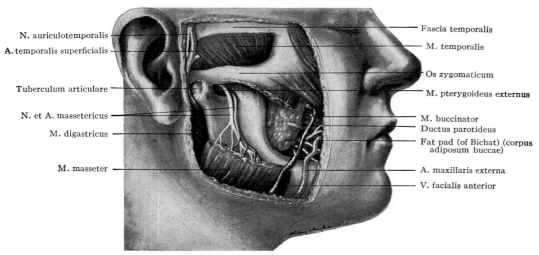

N. auriculotemporalis

A. temporalis superficialis

Tuberculum articulare

N. et A. massetericus

M. digastricus

M. masseter

Fascia temporalis

M. temporalis

Os zygomaticum

M. pterygoideus externus

M. buccinator

Ductus parotideus

Fat pad (of Bichat) (corpus adiposum buccae)

A. maxillaris externa

V. facialis anterior

Figure 15–5.   Deep structures of the masseter region. (Callender, Surgical Anatomy, 2nd Edition.)

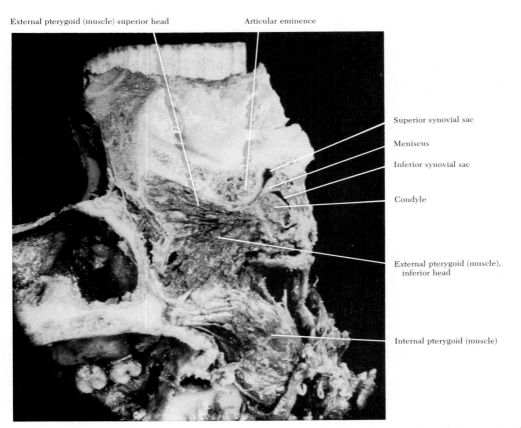

External pterygoid (muscle) superior head

Articular eminence

Superior synovial sac

Meniscus

Inferior synovial sac

Condyle

External pterygoid (muscle), inferior head

Internal pterygoid (muscle)

Figure 15–6.   A sagittal section of a prepared anatomic specimen, sectioned through the center of the right mandibular condyle.

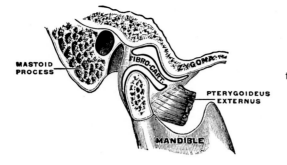

Figure 15–7. Temporomandibular articulation in sagittal sections. (Testut.)

tion and movement. It is attached at its periphery to the capsule, and a section of these tissues shows a superior joint compartment above the meniscus and an inferior joint compartment below (Figs. 15–6, 15–7 and 15–8). These are synovial cavities lined with synovial membrane and lubricated by synovial fluid. The upper compartment is the larger. However, neither compartment exhibits an actual space during life when there is normal articulation of the parts.

The foregoing is the usual description of the joint.

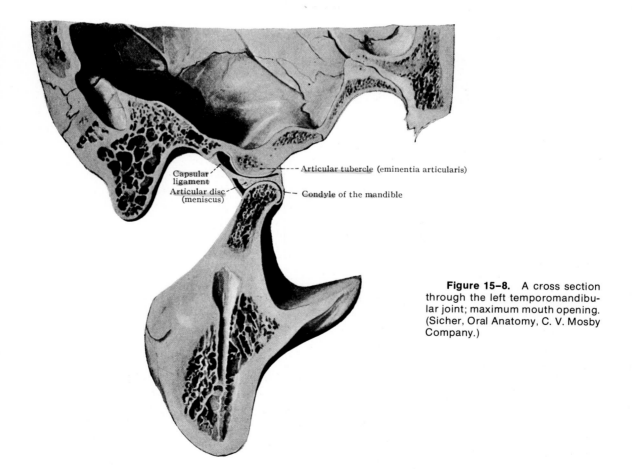

Figure 15–8. A cross section through the left temporomandibular joint; maximum mouth opening. (Sicher, Oral Anatomy, C. V. Mosby Company.)

Robinson states it thus: "The inferior synovial cavity is the smaller of the two joint cavities, and it is here that the ginglymoid, or hinge, action takes place. In the larger upper synovial cavity, the arthrodial, or gliding action occurs. There are no true 'spaces' or 'cavities,' only potential cavities existing. All surfaces are in contact. These are lubricated by a small amount of synovial fluid.

"The disk (meniscus) is not composed of fibrocartilage, which is known not to be repairable. It is composed of a specialized connective tissue. Fibrocartilage is characterized by oval cells with homogenous capsules arranged in groups extending lengthwise in rows. Typical fibrocartilage was not found in any of the disks examined. There are no homogenous capsules.

"A transition type between fibrocartilage and fibrous connective tissue is increasingly evident in disks of persons over twenty years of age."

THE MUSCLES OF MASTICATION AND FACIAL EXPRESSION

The muscles of mastication are those muscles which, through their contraction, bring about the opening and closure of the jaws. It is these muscles that apply the forces which act through the teeth of the mandibular dental arch against the teeth of the maxillary dental arch during the various movements of mastication.

The muscles of mastication comprise the following:

1. Masseter
2. Temporal
3. External pterygoid
4. Internal pterygoid

The external pterygoids aid in depressing the mandible by drawing the condyles forward so that the ramus is freed from pressures of tissues behind it and so that the hinge action in the lower joint compartment is permitted.

The suprahyoid and infrahyoid muscles, including the platysma muscle, function by asserting some control over the act of mastication through their activity in applying counter forces against those greater forces which are brought to bear by the more powerful muscles of mastication. These muscles come into play during extreme depression of the mandible when the mouth is opened its widest during lateral movements of the mandible beyond the functional movements of mastication, when the mandible is attempting to close against unusual resistance, and during the act of swallowing.

Nevertheless, in the final analysis, the functional form of the teeth and their alignment in the jaws are designed to co-operate during mastication with the functional forces brought upon them by the four muscles of mastication only, in a relatively limited range of jaw movement.

For reference purposes, therefore, and to complete this text, the muscles of mastication are the only ones which will be considered, since it is not the purpose of this book to be a complete anatomic treatise on the head and neck.

The *buccinator muscle*, mentioned occasionally as a muscle of mastication, belongs to the muscles of facial expression. This muscle is located in the cheek and functions with the tongue in the placement of food between the teeth during mastication. Nevertheless, it is neither a levator nor a depressor of the mandible.

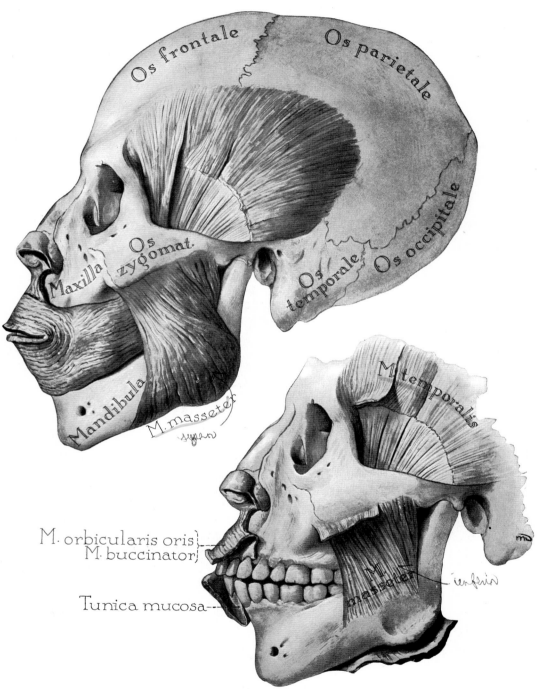

Figure 15–9. Muscles of mastication; lateral views. (Anson, An Atlas of Human Anatomy, 2nd Edition.)

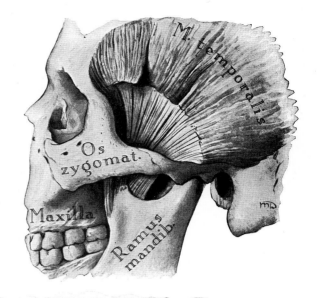

Figure 15–10. Muscles of mastication; lateral view. (Anson, An Atlas of Human Anatomy, 2nd Edition.)

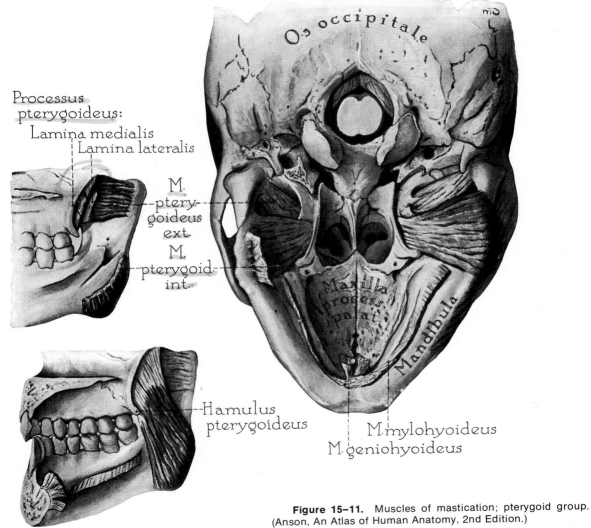

Figure 15–11. Muscles of mastication; pterygoid group. (Anson, An Atlas of Human Anatomy, 2nd Edition.)

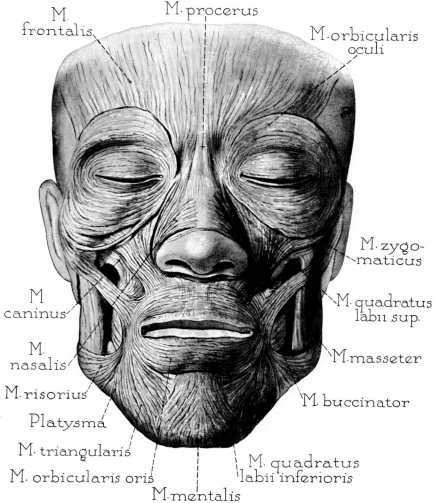

Figure 15–12.   Muscles of facial expression; anterior view. (Anson, An Atlas of Human Anatomy, 2nd Edition.)

AN ANALYSIS OF MANDIBULAR MOVEMENTS

Anatomically or architecturally considered, the human dental mechanism consists of a fixed base, the maxillae, which bear the maxillary teeth, and a movable arm, the mandible, which bears the mandibular teeth.

The *fixed base* of the masticating mechanism, the maxillae, is supported through articulations with other bones of the skull. The maxillae are united at the median line.

The *movable arm*, or mandible, is a single bone. The teeth in the mandible are so placed that they oppose those of the fixed base when they are brought into contact during the various mandibular movements of mastication.

The teeth serve as the armament of the masticating apparatus, affording hard surfaces between which food material is reduced for assimilation by the organism. The relation of the mandibular portion of the dental apparatus to the maxillary or fixed portion is maintained by ligamentous attachments and the powerful muscles of mastication.

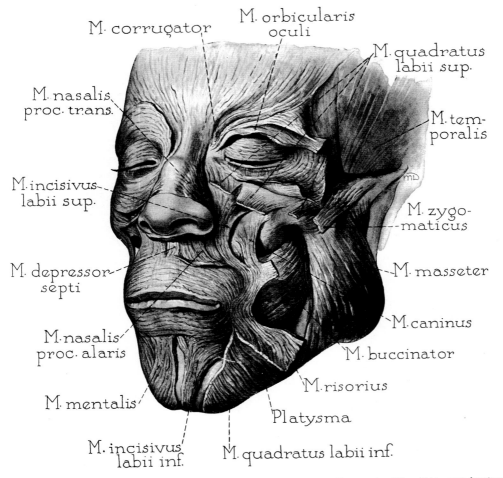

Figure 15-13. Muscles of facial expression; anterolateral view. (Anson, An Atlas of Human Anatomy, 2nd Edition.)

As mentioned heretofore, the mandible is freely movable, the temporomandibular joint being the most flexible joint in the body. Because of its mobility, the various movements are difficult to describe. The attempt will be made to classify and explain the most obvious movements which are most important in the study of the function of the teeth and jaws.

The mandibular movements may be classified under two headings: (1) those which are *bilaterally symmetrical* and (2) those which are *bilaterally asymmetrical*.

Those movements which are bilaterally *symmetrical* are:

Depression	Protrusion
Elevation	Retraction

The movements which are bilaterally *asymmetrical* are:

Lateral movements $\begin{cases} \text{right} \\ \text{left} \end{cases}$

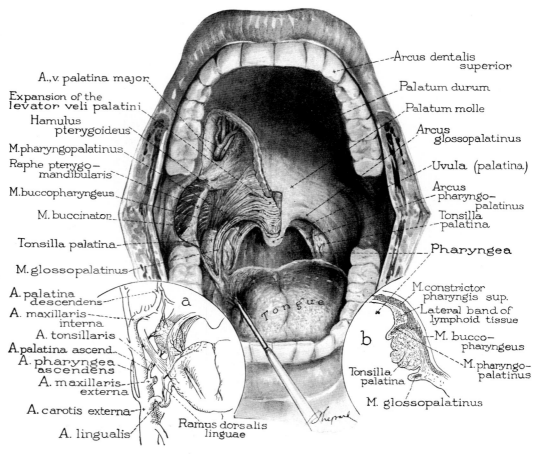

A.,v. palatina major
Expansion of the levator veli palatini
Hamulus pterygoideus
M. pharyngopalatinus
Raphe pterygo-mandibularis
M. buccopharyngeus
M. buccinator
Tonsilla palatina
M. glossopalatinus
A. palatina descendens
A. maxillaris interna
A. tonsillaris
A. palatina ascend.
A. pharyngea ascendens
A. maxillaris externa
A. carotis externa
A. lingualis

Arcus dentalis superior
Palatum durum
Palatum molle
Arcus glossopalatinus
Uvula (palatina)
Arcus pharyngo-palatinus
Tonsilla palatina
Pharyngea
M. constrictor pharyngis sup.
Lateral band of lymphoid tissue
M. bucco-pharyngeus
M. pharyngo-palatinus
M. glossopalatinus

Tongue
Ramus dorsalis linguae
Tonsilla palatina

Figure 15–14. Oral pharynx, with special reference to the palatine tonsil and the musculature of the palate. (Anson, An Atlas of Human Anatomy, 2nd Edition.)

It is the purpose in this section of the book to make an analysis of the dynamics of occlusion and occlusal relations with mandibular movements which have a bearing on the physiologic form of the teeth, their alignment and their occlusion. The mandible is capable of movements which are not related to tooth function: wide opening, excessive protrusion, etc. Repeating some lines of the functional anatomy of the teeth in Chapter 4: The anatomy is such that teeth are enabled to perform two major functions during life: they incise and reduce food material during mastication, and they help sustain themselves in the dental arches by assisting in the development and protection of the tissues which support them. Protection of the investing tissues and stabilization of the alignment of the teeth are provided by the normal form of the individual teeth in proper alignment with the others in the same jaw, by *normal development* of the jaws, and by the proper *relation of one jaw to the other during functional movements.*

When the mandibular teeth come into contact with the maxillary teeth, they are said to be in *occlusion.* One definition of occlusion could be "the relation of the mandibular teeth to the maxillary teeth when in functional contact during the activity of the mandible."

The dental arches have several *functional relations* which are brought about by mandibular movements. They are as follows:

> Centric occlusal relation (centric or central occlusion)
> Right lateral occlusal relation
> Left lateral occlusal relation
> Protrusive occlusal relation
> Retrusive occlusal relation

Centric occlusal relation of the dental arches (centric occlusion, central occlusion), is the concluding terminal relation of the teeth. It is the culmination of all of the other occlusal relations. The entire dental mechanism is designed to co-operate with the design of, and to achieve finally, centric occlusion as the ultimate goal in function.

In normal centric occlusion there is an intercusping contact relation between all of the posterior teeth of both dental arches on both right and left sides. At the same time all of the anterior teeth of one arch are in contact with those of the other arch. In centric occlusion, lines of force brought to bear upon the fixed base or maxillary arch by the movable or mandibular arch are equalized and absorbed by the mutual aid of all of the teeth.

Protrusive occlusal relation is achieved by means of protrusion of the mandible. Such movement places the mandibular teeth in an anterior relation to centric occlusion. *Retrusive occlusal relation* is brought about by retrusion of the mandible. The mandibular teeth are placed by retrusion in a posterior relation to centric occlusion. Retrusion is limited by the compressibility of the tissues posterior to the condyle heads; therefore the movement is so limited it can be said to be nonfunctional.

Right lateral and left lateral occlusal relations are achieved by right lateral and left lateral movements of the mandible. The mandibular dental arch, through these movements, is placed in a right or a left lateral relation to centric occlusion.

Centric, protrusive and retrusive relations of the dental arches may be achieved by mandibular movements which are *symmetrical*—in short, those movements in which both condyles of the mandible make equidistant excursions in sagittal planes of the body. The symphysis of the mandible also moves in a sagittal plane. Right lateral and left lateral relations are achieved by a circular movement to right or left by one condyle of the mandible while the other condyle pivots. These movements are *asymmetrical.*

As was mentioned before, the temporomandibular articulation allows a great range of movement. The mandible is made capable of the central opening movement (so called "hinge" movement, which is an inaccurate term); the joint allows extension of the mandible forward, which movement is called "protrusion"; the mandible may be retracted to some extent in the retrusive movement and it may be rotated from side to side in the right and left lateral movements.

All of the mandibular movements have individual limitations, depending upon the ligamentous attachments and upon the functional range of the muscles of mastication, the origin and insertion of the muscles, their length, directional pull, tonus (counter tension), etc.

Quoting from Thompson and Brodie:* "It was thoroughly established by Sherrington that the same motor impulse that caused one set of muscles to contract caused

---

*Thompson, J. R., and Brodie, A. G.: Factors in the Position of the Mandible. J. Am. Dent. A. 29:925, 1942.

an inhibition of tonus in their antagonists. Thus, the rest position of any movable part may be taken as an equilibrium between all of the forces operating upon it. If these forces happen to be entirely muscular, there is an equal pull on both sides of the part through a state of tonus. Thus, even a rest position must be viewed as a dynamic condition. Steindler points out that for every movement of the body there is a definite amount of inertia to be overcome, a definite amount of balance to be disturbed. Let us now imagine the head being held normally and motionless in the position of erect posture. Such a position is maintained by the antagonistic pull of the muscles of the back of the neck on the one hand, and the force of gravity plus the three enumerated sets working together on the other hand (muscles of mastication, suprahyoids and infrahyoids). Suppose we disturb this balance by swallowing. In deglutition, it is necessary to elevate the hyoid bone, which means the contracting of the suprahyoid muscles. If this group is contracted, it would have just as strong a tendency to depress the mandible as to elevate the hyoid. It seems obvious, therefore, that additional tension must be generated in the masticatory group to prevent the downward displacement of the mandible. The fact that this is true can be easily demonstrated by placing the fingers lightly on the temples and swallowing. At the instant of elevation of the hyoid, a pulse of contraction will be felt in the temporalis.

"A similar phenomenon may be demonstrated in mastication. In spite of the rather extensive and violent movements of the mandible, the hyoid bone is relatively stable. Indeed, it is only in wide opening movements that the hyoid bone shifts to any extent, and even this shift is unexpected. An excellent fluoroscopic moving picture, 'Physiology of Mastication,' by Klatsky, shows these points.

"Thus it is seen that the muscles lying anteriorly from the vertebral column, *i.e.*, the masticatory, suprahyoid and infrahyoid groups, have, as their roles, not only their own specific functions, but also a team play behind these which helps to maintain the posture of the head. This coordination permits of mastication, deglutition and speech without any accompanying nodding of the head.

"We have been thinking of the mandible too much as a bone concerned with a single function, rather than as a connecting link in the anterior muscle chain. The muscle tension acting on the mandible is balanced; that is, there is just as much downward pull as there is upward pull on this bone."

FUNCTIONAL MANDIBULAR MOVEMENTS

(A Description of the Association of the Activity of the Temporomandibular Articulation with the Functional Activity of the Muscles of Mastication and the Ligamentous Attachments)

When the mandible is at rest with its musculature relaxed the mandibular teeth are not in contact with the maxillary teeth. Thompson estimates an opening of 2 mm. on the average. This relation is borne out by Higley, Kurth and other investigators. The relation is called the *physiologic rest position* of the mandible.

When the teeth are together in centric relation, that relation is called the *physical rest position* of the mandible.

All mandibular movements start with the physiologic rest position with the teeth disengaged. When the mandible is depressed, each condyle moves forward on the disk, the disk or meniscus moving with it. Since the condyles move during all manipulations, the points of rotation on the mandible are not within the condyle heads, which arrangement might be expected from the study of some other joints. The mandible is a single bone with bilateral joints which have to be independent of one an-

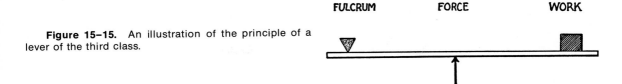

Figure 15–15. An illustration of the principle of a lever of the third class.

other at times in order to allow the flexibility that is necessary for proper functional movements.

The mandible is still regarded by some as a lever of the third class (Fig. 15–15). The *fulcrum* of the mandible shifts its location, however, during functional activity because of the flexibility of the bilateral joints and the independent action of all the muscles involved. The position of the fulcrum is dependent entirely on the location of the *work*, anteriorly, posteriorly or laterally.

If the mandible were regarded as a simple lever of the third class, the condyles in the glenoid fossa would have to be regarded as a fixed fulcrum, with the muscles providing the power for force at a point between the fulcrum and the work. The work is placed at some point on the teeth over the body of the mandible.

In a lever of the third class the fulcrum absorbs a large portion of the force, depending upon (1) the location of the force between the fulcrum and the work, (2) the amount of force generated and (3) the weight or resistance of the work.

Examination of the parts of the temporomandibular joint shows that the area of the glenoid fossa of the temporal bone, which is situated just above the condyle of the mandible, is quite thin. This area is not designed to support the condyle as a fulcrum of a lever of the third class. In fact, any attempt to describe the activity of the mandible as a lever of any one class is oversimplification of jaw movements.

It must be remembered that the mandible is suspended by soft tissues (ligaments and muscles). The ligamentous attachments are not fixed points mechanically; in other words, the individual muscles may contract or relax independently of one another, changing the points of rotation of the mandible within certain limitations.

The mandible has a "bow" form, one bone with two condyloid joints, which permits the "points of rotation," "power arms," "fulcra" or "location of the work" to be shifted from one position to another in a most flexible manner. The two temporomandibular joints may have similar movements simultaneously, as in the central opening movements, or they may work independently of each other, as in lateral movements; and each masticatory muscle of either right or left side may contract or relax independently. In addition, the point or points of rotation of the mandible change their locations according to the extent of opening and position of the jaw during depression, protrusion or right and left lateral relations. Because of the flexibility, it may be more correct to speak of rotation "areas" of the mandible rather than rotation "points," since it is impossible to locate definite points of rotation as final as in a strictly mechanical problem.

In the instances just described, the mandible approaches the second class lever in function. The components of the lever are as follows: the *fulcrum*—muscles of the left side, near the left molars; the *work*—molars and premolars of the right side; the *force*—muscles of the right side buccal to the right posterior teeth. The work is not precisely located between the fulcrum and the force, as is true in a second class lever, but the example of activity as outlined more nearly approaches a second class lever in function than it does the third class lever.

The point or points of rotation of the mandible also change their locations—a fact dependent upon the relation of the mandibular dental arch to the maxillary dental arch during depression, protrusion or right and left lateral relations, and upon the extent of depression of the symphysis of the mandible (point of chin).

Depression of the Mandible

During simple depression of the mandible (central opening movement) from its rest position, both condyles move forward, the menisci moving with them. It is generally agreed by many authorities (Prentiss, Lord, Chissin, Brodie, Higley, Stimson, Sicher and others) that both condyle heads are pulled forward in this initial opening movement by the external pterygoid muscles.

While the condyle is being pulled forward in opening the jaw by the inferior head of the external pterygoid, the meniscus is being pulled forward by the superior head of the external pterygoid muscle. When the condyle approaches the articular eminence it rides forward on the thinner portion of the meniscus—an arrangement which makes allowances for the downward protuberance of the eminence.

When in "rest position," each condyle rests upon a thick posterior portion of the meniscus which fills the space between the condyle and the deeper portion of the glenoid fossa. Anteriorly, the meniscus is much thinner at the portion which approximates the dorsal area of the articular eminence and the frontal area of the condyle (Figs. 15–6 and 15–8).

The relative thickness of the meniscus anteroposteriorly, plus the compensating

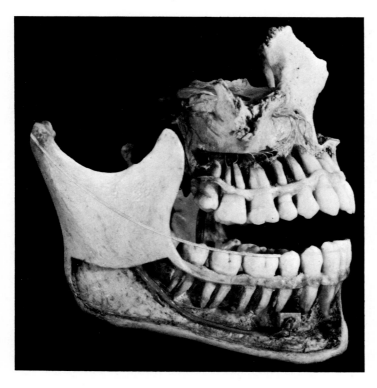

Figure 15–16. A specimen showing normal development; dissected to show crown and root development and long axis angulations. An extension of a curved line touching occlusal levels of the mandibular posterior teeth seems to bisect the neck of the condyle below the condyle head. The supposition is that if the curved occlusal surface acts as one arm of a hinge, the axis of opening would be somewhere along the extension of the arm.

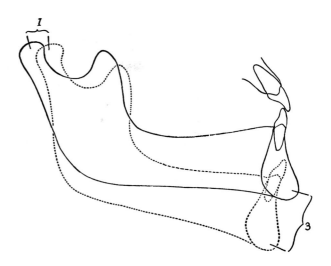

Figure 15–17. Outline tracings of mandible and central incisors in centric occlusal relation. The broken outline represents the relative position of the mandible and central incisor after the central opening movement. Note the relative position of the condyle and the central incisor. The condyle moves forward and downward approximately one-third the distance the symphysis of the mandible (point of chin) moves downward and backward. The position of the depressed mandible shows the approximate relation when the mandible has reached the lowest point during ordinary masticatory movement. The mandible is capable of depression much greater when the occasion makes it necessary. (See Figure 15–8.)

activity of the two heads of the external pterygoid muscle, allows the condyles of the mandible to move forward with a gliding movement on a "single plane" regardless of the irregularity of the surface of the glenoid fossa and of that of the articular eminence. The "plane" has an inclination downward when the head is held erect. It is interesting to note that the inclined plane of the condylar glide when the mandible is depressed is seemingly parallel to the occlusal plane of the molars and the lower border of the body of the mandible when the jaws are closed.

During the central opening movement of the mandible, the axis of movement is not in the condyle heads, since these move forward immediately, even though the initial movement forward is slight. Apparently the area of rotation approaches the attachment of the temporomandibular ligament laterally and distally to the neck of the condyle. This is a logical conclusion because of the suspensory character of this strong ligament and the general direction of its fibers (Fig. 15–3).

The central opening movement of the mandible (depression) in conjunction with the central closing movement (elevation) provides the action commonly termed "simple hinge movement." As far as the relation of the dental arches is concerned in this opening and closing movement, the action is comparable to the action of a simple hinge. The occlusal surfaces of the maxillary teeth may be considered as the upper extension of the hinge, and the occlusal surfaces of the mandibular teeth as the lower extension in the central opening movement. Owing to the involved design of the articulation and the need for jaw support, the rotation point or axis of the hinge cannot be centered in the condyles as many believe. The uneven shape of the condyle, added to its forward movement immediately upon jaw opening, would defeat this argument. The jaw has body and weight and must be suspended by ligamentous attachment in some area. The design and location of the temporomandibular ligament makes it the logical choice among condyle attachments to accomplish ligamentous suspension of the jaw in the initial opening movements. (See *Temporomandibular ligament*, page 388). The attachment superiorly is forward, wrapped around the zygomatic "bar" of the temporal bone; inferiorly, it is down and back, and is strongly attached posteriorly in a limited area to the neck of the condyle, below the condyle itself (Figs. 15–7 and 15–18).

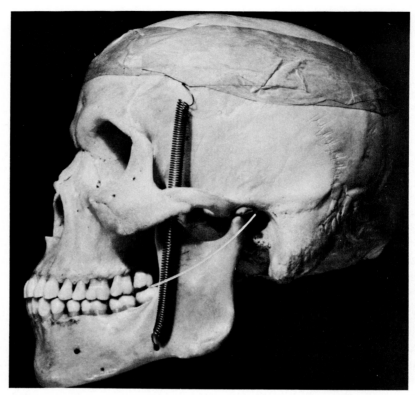

Figure 15–18.   A curved line representing an extension of the curvature of the occlusal plane will pass laterally and slightly below the neck of the condyle. See Fig. 15–7, 8. This is the area of the attachment of the temporomandibular ligament. The "point" of rotation, or "hinge axis," will be located somewhere in this area in the initial central opening movement of the mandible. See also Fig. 15–16.

When the jaw is opened no more than necessary for ordinary use in mastication (10 to 12 mm. maximum), the action of placing the teeth of one arch in and out of contact with the teeth of the opposing arch in a sagittal plane may be called a hinge movement, regardless of our inability to pinpoint the "hinge axis."

In the study of the individual masticatory movements to follow, make continuous reference to the illustrations of the muscles of mastication in Figures 15–9 and 15–11.

Elevation of the Mandible

The mandible is elevated by the temporal muscles, the masseter muscles and the internal pterygoid muscles.

The *temporal muscle* has anterior and posterior fibers. The anterior fibers exert an upward pull; the posterior fibers pull upward and backward.

The *masseter muscle* has two sets of fibers: superficial and deep fibers. The superficial fibers exert a pull upward and forward on the mandible. The deep fibers exert a pull vertically upward.

The *internal pterygoid muscle* has two heads, each of which pulls in the same general direction. Together they exert a pull on the mandible which is upward, forward and inward.

When the temporal, masseter and internal pterygoid muscles of the two sides contract simultaneously, the mandible is elevated and returns the teeth to occlusion.

When the teeth are brought into centric occlusion, both condyles of the mandible are moved a short distance posteriorly to their rest position.

Protrusion of the Mandible

The mandible cannot be protruded unless the cusps of the teeth are disengaged. Therefore, the mandible must be depressed slightly, the condyles moving forward before the protrusive movement is begun.

The muscles which promulgate the protrusive movement which brings about the protrusive occlusal relation of the teeth are the *external pterygoid* muscles, which are assisted by the *anterior fibers* of the *temporal muscles*. The pterygoids pull forward on the condyles and the temporals pull upward with a counter action on the coronoid processes; this prevents further depression of the mandible during the protrusive movement. The tonus and counterbalancing action of other fibers of the temporals as well as some other muscles may come into play during the protrusive movement.

During this movement the condyles are pulled forward with their menisci, but their forward movement is quite limited (Fig. 16–114, Chapter 16).

Retraction of the Mandible

In retraction, the mandible returns along the same path it traveled in the protrusive movement. The retractive movement is, therefore, just the reverse of the protrusive movement.

The jaw is pulled back by the action of the *temporal* muscle, the posterior fibers principally. The condyles with their menisci are returned to rest position.

If it is the purpose of this movement to bring the teeth back into centric occlusion, the *masseter* and *internal pterygoid* muscles join the activity of the temporals in the culmination of the act.

The mandible may be retracted a very small degree posteriorly to centric occlusal relation of the teeth. This movement is nonfunctional and consequently very limited. Movement of the condyles distally is resisted by the posterior wall of the glenoid cavity; the movement is limited to the compressibility of the soft tissues intervening between the bony parts.

Lateral Movements of the Mandible

The lateral movements (right and left) of the mandible are *asymmetrical* movements; the right and left condyles do not follow similar paths. These movements are made possible by the ability of one temporomandibular joint to move independently of the other.

Each *internal pterygoid* muscle exerts a medial pull on the mandible, since it does not operate on a line with the forward or protrusive movement of the jaw. Its action pulls the condyle inward as well as forward.

The right lateral movement of the mandible is affected, therefore, by a slight depressive movement of the mandible, both external pterygoids operating, which action depresses the mandible and moves both condyles forward. At this point the left *internal* pterygoid contracts independently, the right internal pterygoid and other muscles relaxing. The activity of the left internal pterygoid pulls the left condyle forward and inward in a circular path which rotates about a point in the right condyle, the right condyle turning on the pivotal point. This action results in the rotation of the mandible about the pivotal point in the right condyle, moving the mandible to the right.

In the return movement, the condyles retrace their path. The mandible is returned to rest position, or the teeth into centric occlusion, through the activity of the left temporal muscle (mainly posterior fibers), other muscles of mastication of both sides joining forces as the teeth approach central occlusion with a final masticatory thrust.

The left lateral movement of the mandible is affected in the same manner. In this instance the right condyle is pulled forward and inward while the left condyle pivots. The right internal pterygoid muscle contracts and causes the movement of the mandible to the left. The right temporal is the muscle mainly operative which affects the return of the mandible to centric relation with the assistance of the other muscles in balance with it.

16

The Arrangement of the Teeth and Occlusion

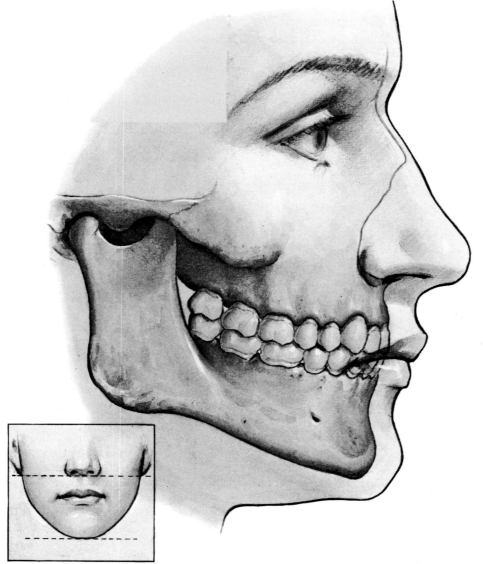

The face is man's most individual characteristic. The jaws and teeth comprise two-thirds of its structure.

Normal occlusion of the teeth and jaws is essential to a pleasing appearance of the entire face and to efficiency in mastication.

Abnormal occlusion may result from the abnormal positioning of the teeth alone or from abnormality in the growth of the jaws.

From Massler and Schour, *Atlas of the Mouth.* 2nd Ed. American Dental Assoc., 1958.

A simple definition of *biology* is that it is the "science which deals with the phenomena of life and living organisms." Man, who must be included in the study, exhibits many phenomena within himself, and there are many problems that concern him that are not understood. One of the most frustrating of these problems and at the same time one of the most fascinating, is the phenomenon called the *human dental mechanism.*

The objective of any properly designed mechanism is that it not only function as intended but also that its design assist in prolonging its own life and usefulness. Man's dental equipment should qualify in the same manner.

In order to analyze properly anything made to function, one must list specific questions for analysis. Concerning the human dental mechanism, the following questions are applicable:
1. What is its function?
2. Which part is basic in design?
3. Which portions (accessories) of the mechanism are necessary to safeguard the basic part?
4. Which collateral parts or attachments can be listed that seem important during use?

It has always been this writer's opinion that when *question one* is answered when relating to the dental mechanism, the basic part asked for in *question two* is *"the tooth and its multiples."*

The *third question* would involve the *periodontium,* the foundation which provides security for the basic part. This includes bone and soft tissue in which blood and nerve supply are incorporated.

Question four is the least important in the study of the design which affects function. Neither the ligamentous attachments of the mandible nor the muscles of mastication are part of the "useful tool" at all. They are important tissues but their sole function is to hold and manipulate the mandible in any manner which seems to be indicated in order to properly occlude the teeth of the dynamic lower jaw with the teeth in the static upper jaw. The temporomandibular attachment tissues are very flexible and adaptable in use (and necessarily so) but their very mobile make-up defeats attempts to make accurate clinical surveys which would indicate their importance as gauges of the physiologic form of the occlusal design of tooth crowns. These surfaces are hard and unyielding, and to complicate matters further they are measured in *millimeters* and *fractions of millimeters.* Whether or not at any one moment an analysis of movable tissues involving the face and jaws can be used, as a rule, to indicate normalcy or abnormalcy in occlusal relations is questionable. An analysis of the minutiae of occlusal form and function of the teeth has to be more consistent and more definite.

Because the teeth, once formed, do not change *macroscopically,* except from destructive causes outside themselves, it follows that in each individual they must have been intended to last a lifetime with a minimum of change and that the static form was supposed to be functional. Each permanent tooth takes approximately ten years to mature, and since its design for occlusal form is established years before it has to be put into service, part of the "plan" of occlusion is incorporated and "frozen" in the unyielding surface of each tooth crown. *Therefore the part the tooth crowns are to play in occlusion is foreordained before eruption.*

The overall plan for the cooperation of all of the teeth in occlusal relations is finally consummated by *normal* jaw and facial development.

There has been much time spent on the study of occlusion and many points of view have been offered, by prosthetists, orthodontists, periodontists, dental technicians, tooth manufacturers, and so on. Strangely, few have been interested enough in the specialized study of individual tooth form to discover whether or not its design needs to be that unique in order to be part of one of the two units making up that wondrous creation known as the human dental mechanism.

We have some of the answers to queries concerning occlusion, but many more need answering. First, it must be understood that the principles of occlusion of the teeth cannot be understood until each tooth *in its entirety* is studied in order to determine its share in the unit effort. Too many studies of occlusion have been confined to the occlusal third of the teeth, an area which represents only a portion of the whole story. Also, the tendency has been to stress the importance of picturing the dental arch as a whole, sometimes ignoring the unique design of each tooth.

Here are just a few questions that are of interest, and which, if answered, might solve some problems in occlusion:

1. Why is each tooth in the maxillary dental arch (the whole tooth, root and all), different from each antagonist in the opposite dental arch?

2. Why is each tooth in the same arch shaped differently from its neighbor in that arch?

3. Since in each arch the teeth have "offset" relations with the opposing teeth, why are they not of standard dimensions with simpler forms, and "offset" evenly one-to-two, similar to standard bricks in a wall? Since they are not arranged this way, what would an analysis indicate?

4. Since escapement to lessen pressures is incorporated in the tooth form, why are the facial embrasures, especially posteriorly, narrower than the lingual embrasures everywhere?

5. What is the value of the *occlusal escapement* that is incorporated in crown design; the occlusal escapement aided moreover by the alignment of the crowns in arch formations?

All of these questions have been presented in order to arouse thoughtful interest in the fascinating subject called *occlusion*.

Definition: Occlusion may be defined as that situation which is created when the teeth in the mandibular dental arch come into contact with the teeth in the maxillary dental arch in a functional relationship.

It has not been sufficiently realized that normal occlusion of the teeth is the result of many of the same factors that influence and control the growth and development of the whole body: nutrition, internal secretions, environment, and so on. Various considerations must be borne in mind in seeking to determine "ideal" occlusion. There are changes taking place with the transition from the deciduous to the permanent dentition (Fig. 3–37), and in addition to this major alteration there are changes in the occlusion of the *deciduous teeth* with the growth of the jaws and the wear of the separate teeth in use; furthermore, there is change in occlusion of the *permanent teeth* as a result of wear or accident.

It is essential therefore to list some stages in the development of occlusion. Here are five important phases:

1. The occlusion of the deciduous teeth after their complete eruption

2. Changes that occur in the occlusion previous to the eruption of the permanent incisors and first permanent molars

3. Changes that occur in the occlusion following the loss of deciduous canines and the first and second deciduous molars

4. The occlusion of the permanent teeth in a young adult

5. The changes which occur in the occlusion as the result of aging, wear, or accident.

There are many changes in occlusion at various periods in life, ranging from the very young to the older stages. There are no changes macroscopically in tooth form (except through wear or accident), but all soft tissues and bones which support them are subject to changes in form and function any time they are affected by circulatory and metabolic problems.

At two and a half years of age, all the deciduous teeth should have erupted and should have made proximal contact with one another in each arch (Figs. 3–34 and 3–35). Among the stages of occlusion just mentioned for normal development, numbers two and three might be regarded as being the most important. To repeat: number two marks the changes that occur in the occlusion previous to the eruption of permanent central incisors and first molars. Number three marks the changes that occur following the loss of deciduous canines and the first and second deciduous molars. (The latter are replaced mainly by permanent premolars).

It is at this time that the occlusion and development of the teeth and jaws are undergoing elaborate change in a tremendous state of flux. It is the period in life from six or seven years until 12 years that is often spoken of as the comic or ugly period in facial appearance. It is at this time that vacant spaces appear; the teeth seem too large for the face, with little occlusal or incisal level to be seen anywhere. This stage in development must be looked upon as normal and as nothing to be alarmed about unless development later seems deficient. It is necessary that the diagnostician, general practitioner or specialist, take into consideration the normal expectations to come in development, so that unqualified observations shall not be made. Time must be allowed for all of the adjustments that are necessary for development of the jaws and for the proper placement of the teeth. Therefore, the stages and possible changes in individual cases must be carefully weighed in diagnosis and prognosis until an "ideal" or normal situation is created by maturation.

Good occlusion contributes to the welfare of the individual in other ways besides its usefulness in mastication: it helps to bring about symmetry and good appearance in facial development, and promotes good enunciation in speech, two important aspects which come about as the result of normal development and stabilization of tissues. *Stability of jaw relations* is another condition which cannot be secured without normal tooth form, proper alignment, and of course, good occlusion.

Although we may postulate a hypothetical ideal occlusion, observation of tooth relations in individuals points to something which must be recognized and treated seriously and that is that occlusion is ever changing; slowly and imperceptibly, even though dental arches are intact and pathology plays no part, but much more rapidly if conditions for stability are unfavorable. It must be kept in mind continually that occlusion must obey the general biologic principle of physiologic change and adjustment.

Physiological Mesial Drift

One of the most interesting of the functional responses of the alveolar bone, *physiological mesial drift*, occurs during a period of relative stability and inactivity. The teeth normally tend to drift toward the median line. In this way they help maintain their proximal contact. In the case of missing teeth, the distal teeth tend to drift mesially and fill in the space formerly occupied by the missing tooth. (This is true particularly in molar areas).

While such a drift cannot be noted macroscopically, histological examination gives proof of its existence in almost all normal dentures. When physiological movement occurs the mesial periodontal membrane fibers are slackened and resorption of the alveolar bone along the mesial periodontal surface takes place. On the distal aspect, however, tension of the periodontal membrane occurs and is translated into a stimulating effect on the alveolar bone with a consequent appositional response and bundle bone is formed. Thus normally, the alveolar bone on the mesial surface of teeth shows resorption, the distal, apposition of bundle bone.

This constant adjustment reveals the dynamic quality of bone. The alveolar process is not a static support of the teeth and its structure, and position is determined by the functional demand of the moving dentition.*

---

*From "Dental Histology and Embryology" by Noyes, Schour, and Noyes, 5th Edition (page 223). Lea & Febiger, Philadelphia, Pa.

The "ideal" arrangement of teeth as hypothesized by a general consensus of opinion may be used as a basis for the planning of dental treatment. Unless some agreement is accepted as being properly descriptive of the norm, comparisons leading to problem evaluation cannot be made successfully in diagnosis.

It is common knowledge that there are many adults whose dental apparatus is far from ideal, but who are happy with their teeth and jaws as they are. The teeth and jaws seem to function well and the host enjoys healthy periodontal tissues at the same time. Usually a fortunate, though variable, situation such as this may be explained by pointing to some fundamentals of good functional occlusion which are operating, even though the case departs from the "ideal" plan.

An understanding of dental anatomy and physiology stands one in good stead when variables are to be contended with in problems dealing with alignment and occlusion. This holds true, whether the dental treatment is preventive or restorative.

The teeth are arranged in two opposing series; one is fixed (maxillary series), and the other is movable (mandibular series). Each series is made up of sixteen teeth arranged so that they form a dental arch. Generally speaking, each dental arch conforms to a parabolic curve (Figs. 16–1, 16–2, 16–3, 16–4 and Fig. 1.1).

The mandibular arch, which is movable, operates against the maxillary arch, which is fixed. This obvious fact is sometimes overlooked. The main reason for the oversight is this: dental articulators used in dental prosthesis have the maxillary member movable, with the mandibular member fixed, which is just the opposite arrangement from that found in the human jaws. Mechanically, the dental articulator design simplifies the instrument for use in the laboratory. Nevertheless, this can affect the user's thinking, unless he is careful to keep the true state of affairs in mind. It is important in the study of occlusion that one realize that the primary forces of occlusion are brought to bear against the *static* maxillary dental arch by the *dynamic* mandibular arch. (Consult "An Analysis of Mandibular Movements," page 394.)

Normal tooth form (plus proper alignment) assures efficiency in the comminution of food. The form of each tooth in each dental arch must be recognized as an important integral part in the total design of the arches. The form of each of the sixteen teeth, in

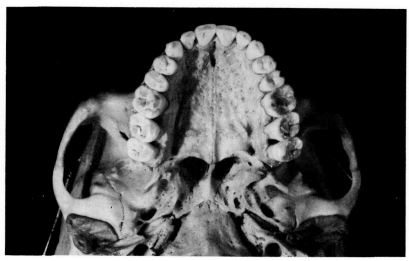

Figure 16–1. An occlusal view of maxillary teeth (same specimen as Figs. 16–2, 16–3, and 16–4). This specimen shows considerable wear of the occlusal surfaces. It demonstrates the surfaces of the maxillary teeth which are in contact during occlusal relations by the areas showing abraded facets.

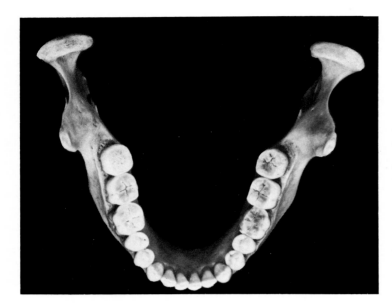

Figure 16-2. An occlusal view of the mandibular teeth. The facets of occlusal wear appear on the labioincisal portions of anterior teeth and the occlusal and bucco-occlusal surfaces of posterior teeth.

addition to the proper positioning and angulation of each tooth, creates overall functional form. If the dental arch is properly designed, through normal development and positioning of all its parts, the dental arch *in toto* becomes an efficient unit for service. *Stability and efficiency will be assured only as long as the normal arrangement is maintained.*

The stability of the dental arch is dependent to a great extent on good form and development. However, these assets would be ineffective without the periodontal support that is furnished by healthy tissue with good blood and nerve supply.

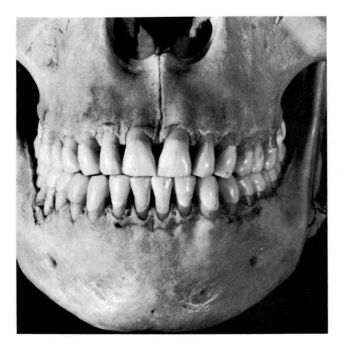

Figure 16-3. A view of the teeth at the median line, or maxillary suture. Note the acute angulations of the anterior teeth to the suture. This specimen shows considerable occlusal wear, balanced occlusion and a minimum of overbite or overjet of the maxillary anterior teeth.

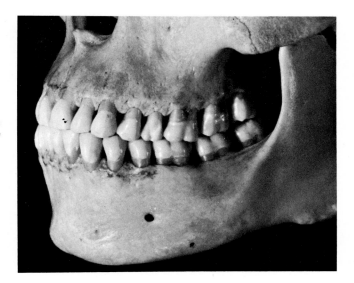

Figure 16–4. Lateral view of the specimen shown in Figs. 16–1, 16–2, and 16–3. Note the curve of Spee.

Figure 16–5. An illustration of normal occlusion—anterior and lateral views. This specimen demonstrates a different type of tooth and a different type of occlusion from the specimen shown in Fig. 16–3. These teeth show little occlusal wear and considerable overjet* and overbite† to anterior and posterior teeth. Note the extreme angulation of anterior teeth from the lateral view; this angulation is characteristic when overbite and overjet are greater than usual.

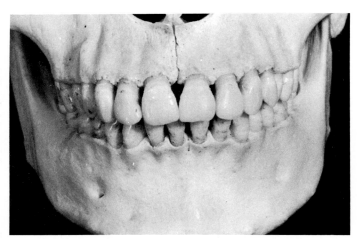

Overjet is that characteristic of the teeth in which the incisal ridges or buccal cusp ridges of the maxillary teeth extend labially or buccally to the incisal ridges or buccal cusp ridges of the mandibular teeth, when the teeth are in centric occlusal relation.

†*Overbite* is that characteristic of the teeth in which the incisal ridges of the maxillary anterior teeth extend below the incisal ridges of the mandibular anterior teeth when the teeth are placed in centric occlusal relation.

We speak of the relative degree of overbite or overjet.

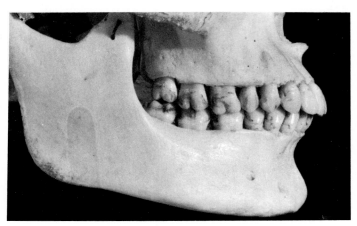

If the development of teeth and jaws is *abnormal*, the final result is a poorly formed dental apparatus capable only of *malocclusion*. However, a diagnosis of malocclusion cannot be made unless the diagnostician is cognizant of the normal development in occlusion. Most of this chapter will be concerned with an analysis of dental anatomy and physiological form which creates the values accepted generally under the term *normal occlusion*.

Functional relations during jaw movements affect the directional forces brought to bear upon the teeth, and normal jaw relationships apply the forces equally in directions which the teeth, being in proper alignment, are prepared to withstand. If each tooth is able to retain its established place, the stability and permanence of the entire dental arch as a functioning unit remains assured.

EIGHT ITEMS WHICH MUST BE INCLUDED IN THE STUDY OF OCCLUSION (Fig. 16–6)

1. *Dental arch formation (alignment of the teeth)*
2. *Compensating curvatures of the dental arches (curved occlusal planes)*
3. *Compensating curvatures of the individual teeth (curved axes)*
4. *Angulation of individual teeth in relation to various planes (including root form)*
5. *Functional form of the teeth at their incisal and occlusal thirds*
6. *Facial relations of each tooth in one arch to its antagonist or antagonists in the opposing arch in centric occlusion*
7. *Occlusal contact and intercusp relations of all the teeth of one arch with those in the opposing arch in centric occlusion*
8. *Occlusal contact and intercusp relations of all the teeth during the various functional mandibular movements*

1. DENTAL ARCH FORMATION (ALIGNMENT OF THE TEETH) (Fig. 16–6, 1, P. 413)

In general, the alignment of the teeth in both dental arches follows a parabolic curve. This is especially true of the alignment of facial surfaces (Figs. 16–1 and 16–2). The figure describing the maxillary arch facially is somewhat larger than that of the mandibular dental arch facially. When the teeth are in centric occlusal relation, the maxillary arch "overhangs" labially and buccally; this arrangement is called the *overjet* of the maxillary teeth. The difference in outside size allows extensions in the direction of mandibular movements (Fig. 16–7).

This arch relation has another useful feature: during opening and closing movements of the jaws, the cheeks, lips and tongue are less likely to be clipped. Since the occlusal margins facially of the maxillary teeth extend beyond the facial occlusal margins of the mandibular teeth, and since the linguo-occlusal margins of the mandibular teeth extend lingually in relation to the linguo-occlusal margins of the maxillary teeth, the soft tissues are displaced during the act of closure until the teeth have had an opportunity to come together in occlusal contact. The overjet relation facially and lingually of one dental arch to the other might be compared roughly to the relation of the teeth of gear wheels opposing each other. The design avoids the clashing of points and edges during contact (Figs. 16–10, 16–59, and 16–61), as long as the relationship exists.

The teeth of each arch are arranged in an unbroken series of occlusal surfaces, each tooth being in close contact with neighboring teeth. The last molar in either arch

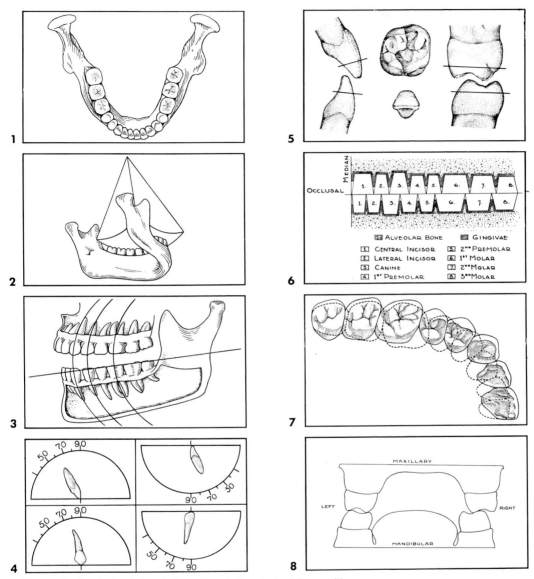

Figure 16–6.   1. Dental arch formation (alignment of the teeth).
2. Compensating curvatures of the dental arches (curved occlusal planes).
3. Compensating curvatures of the individual teeth (curved axes).
4. Angulation of individual teeth in relation to various planes. Root form.
5. Functional form of the teeth at their incisal and occlusal thirds.
6. Facial relations of each tooth in one arch to its antagonist or antagonists in the opposing arch in centric occlusion. (Schematic drawing.)
7. Occlusal contact and intercusp relations of all the teeth of one arch with those in the opposing arch in centric occlusion.
8. Occlusal contact and intercusp relations of all the teeth during the various functional mandibular movements. "Balance" in lateral occlusal relations.

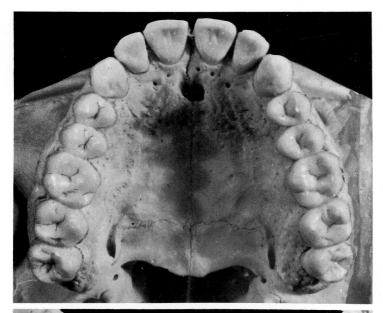

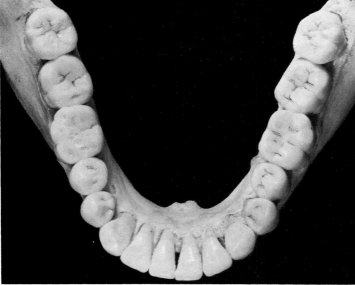

Figure 16–7. A very fine anatomic specimen showing normal alignment for good occlusion (see also Figs. 16–8 and 16–9). Although the mandibular arch gives the impression that it is longer from the median line to the distal of the third molars, this is an optical illusion. Because the teeth adapt themselves to compensating occlusal curvature, the mandibular arch is spoken of as being "concave." This comes close to putting the axis of each posterior tooth in the line of vision; this also puts each occlusal surface of a posterior mandibular tooth in "perfect profile," which registers mesiodistal measurements completely. Because the maxillary curvature is the reverse of the mandibular and "convex" rather than "concave," the mesiodistal measurement of maxillary posterior teeth is foreshortened in the camera lens, creating the misconception.

is in contact only with the tooth mesial to it. Each of the other teeth has adjoining members in contact both mesially and distally.

The contact relation between teeth in the same dental arch serves two purposes: (1) it protects the gingival papillae in interproximal spaces, thereby avoiding periodontal involvement which could be destructive; and (2) the collective activity of all the teeth in contact "shoulder to shoulder," stabilizes each tooth in the dental arch. The firmness of this arrangement prevents tooth migration and supplies the necessary jaw support for security. (Proximal Contact Areas, Chapter 5.)

The teeth are divided into four classifications anatomically, and they function in accordance with those classifications. The four classifications are: (1) incisors, (2) canines, (3) premolars and (4) molars.

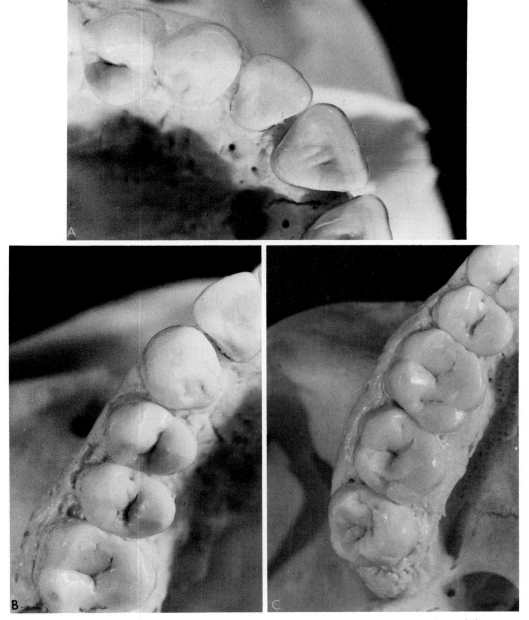

Figure 16–8.   Close-up views of sections of a dental arch. These pictures were taken of the same specimens shown in Fig. 16–7. They show the variations in the design of individual units in the arch, contact form, occlusal form, group alignment, and so forth. The photographs of the teeth of one half of the arch were taken by means of three different angulations of camera focus. Even by this means, it is impossible to get more than one or possibly two teeth in direct profile. A more perfect approach would require a view of each of the teeth in direct alignment with individual axes. Later in the chapter the variance in axial alignment will be discussed.

   A. This section includes maxillary central incisor, lateral incisor, canine and first premolar. The focus was made in line with the long axis of the canine.

   B. A view of the maxillary lateral incisor, canine, first and second premolars. The angle was in line generally with the first premolar.

   C. This section includes the maxillary second premolar and all three of the molars. The camera was focused on the first molar, putting it in profile.

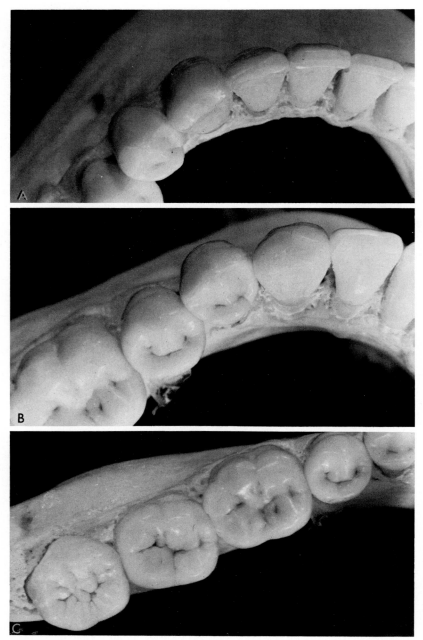

Figure 16–9. Sectional views of the mandibular teeth of the specimen as described in Fig. 16–8.
A. This section includes the mandibular dental incisors, the lateral incisor, canine and first premolar. The camera was aligned axially with the lateral incisor.
B. A view of the mandibular lateral incisor, canine, first and second premolars. The view is directly in line with the long axis of the first premolar.
C. Primarily a molar "setup." The angle is in line with the long axis of the mandibular first molar. The second and third molars enjoy a more acute angulation.

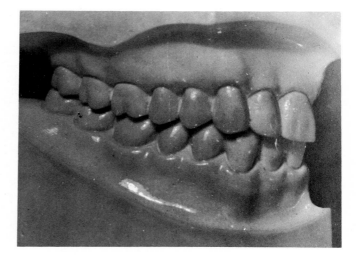

Figure 16–10. A cast of the teeth showing normal overjet of the maxillary arch. The lighting for the photograph was arranged for emphasis. (This is a duplicate of the cast shown in Fig. 16–110.)

The *incisors* are designed to function as shears or blades when they come in contact with opposing incisors. (See Chapters 6, 7.)

The *canines* have single cusps, more or less pointed, with sloping cusp ridges. These teeth serve by piercing and holding food material, in addition to using an incising action similar to that of the incisors. The canines, by means of their structure and their excellent root anchorage, support the incisors during the stresses of incision or prehension of food which might be resistant in character (Chapter 8).

The *premolars* have from one to three functioning cusps, and they are intermediate between canines and molars. The first premolars particularly, both maxillary and mandibular, have cusps which are long and sharp. They assist the canines in their function. The second premolars have cusps which in general correspond in form with those of the molars; therefore they may be considered as complementary in function to the molars. The premolars, by their intercusping relation and because of advantages inherent in their location posteriorly, are of more assistance in the comminution of food than the incisors or canines (Chapters 9 and 10).

The *molars* are multicusped teeth, with broad occlusal surfaces. They are the most efficient of all the teeth in chopping and reducing food material to proper consistency for assimilation. Each molar has several points or areas of occlusal contact dur-

Figure 16–11. Note how the curved teeth of one gear wheel fit into the curved embrasures of the other without clashing the edges. Compare this design with Figs. 16–10 and 16–35.

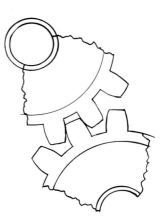

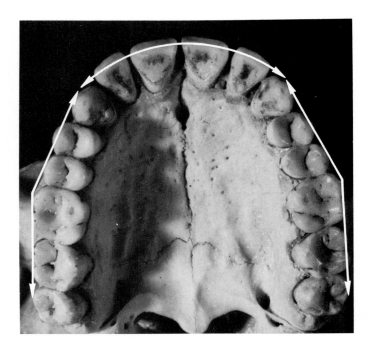

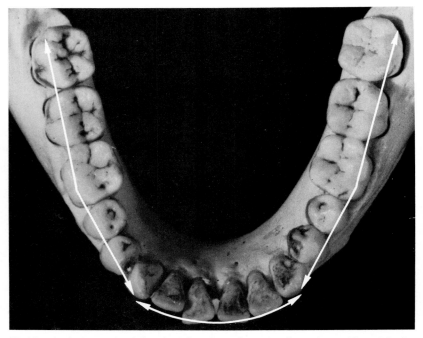

Figure 16–12. A photograph of the dental arches of a natural specimen. The white lines show the approximate alignment in segments of the labial and buccal surfaces of the dental arches. See text for details.

ing mastication. *The molars collectively show more points of occlusal contact in centric occlusion than all of the other teeth combined* (Fig. 16–29). Premature loss of molars is a severe handicap (Fig. 16–47).

The tooth alignment in the arches is divided into *three segments: anterior segments, middle segments* and *posterior segments.* Actually, since the teeth are in close contact relation, the lines, curved and straight, which are used to describe and divide the segments, will overlap slightly, portraying canines and first molars as cooperating in more than one division. This arrangement serves to indicate a supposition held by most, that the first molars and canines serve as anchor supports for both dental arches. Their roles during development bear out the contention (Fig. 16–12).

A curved line describing the *anterior segments* includes the anterior teeth ending at the labial ridge of canines. A straight line describing the *middle segments* will include the distal portion of the canines, the premolars, and the buccal ridge of the mesiobuccal cusps of first molars. The *posterior segments* can be illustrated by a straight line from the buccal cusps of first molars, the line remaining in contact with buccal surfaces of second and third molars.

At first sight the overall picture in Figure 16–12 gives one the impression that the alignment of the two arches is dissimilar. This is an optical illusion caused by the arrangement of dissimilar teeth in each arch. No one tooth in the maxillary arch looks like any one tooth in the mandibular dental arch, and they differ axially as well. Yet the teeth are arranged in such a way that they function and "fit" together. This wondrous plan of design requires further study in research before some of its secrets are known.

In a study of the arch segments the two dental arches are comparable. The mandibular arch segments differ from the maxillary in two small details only. The variation is mainly one of relative measurement labially and buccally because the mandibular arch is smaller. The *anterior segment* covers the same area but is quite a bit smaller than the comparable maxillary segment. The *middle segment* extends distally to the *distobuccal* cusp of the *mandibular* first molar, the *posterior segment* starting at that point, whereas the *maxillary middle segment* ends at the *mesiobuccal* cusp of the *maxillary* first molar, the posterior segment extending posteriorly from that point.

The form of the individual teeth, the arrangement into segments of arch form, and the angulation of tooth axes, make for efficiency in mastication. At the same time, the teeth seem to be arranged for other biologic needs. As an example, the shape and alignment of molars in each jaw provide for freedom of movement of the tongue and also for the expansion and contraction of masticatory muscles. The taper of maxillary molar crowns, narrowing from mesial to distal, allows for increased expansion of the back of the tongue; in addition, buccal space is created for the accommodation of muscles.

PHASES IN THE DEVELOPMENT OF DENTAL ARCHES

There are five phases of development which establish the alignment of the permanent teeth into dental arch formation.

First Phase

The first permanent molars (sometimes termed "cornerstones") take their places immediately posterior to the second deciduous molars. This happens at about six years of age and adds considerably to chewing efficiency and jaw development during a period of rapid growth. They serve to back up the deciduous molars; together they support the jaws while anterior deciduous teeth are being exfoliated and new permanent anteriors substituted.

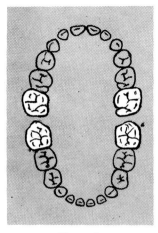

Phase 1

Second Phase

The placing of anterior permanent teeth begins near the median line. Central incisors, and then lateral incisors, develop lingually to deciduous anterior roots; but exfoliation and jaw growth finally place them labially to those places formerly held by the deciduous anterior teeth. However, the permanent location of anterior teeth is not established until the development of the dental arch form is complete.

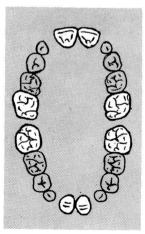

Phase 2

Third Phase

The premolars come in anterior to the first permanent molars, taking the places of deciduous molars. The host is able by this means to acquire more efficiency in his dental apparatus, with added jaw support. This is another period of rapid development occurring during the elementary school years. Developmentally, the premolar area is of special significance because of the sizes and shapes of the premolars when compared to the larger teeth they replace. The contours of bone covering the narrower roots of the premolars, plus the state of flux in bone formation in this area that furnishes adjustment for dental arch measurements, makes these sections of the dental arches of both jaws very important architecturally. The value of premolars and the premolar areas should be thoughtfully analyzed before removal of any of these teeth for "aesthetic" reasons.

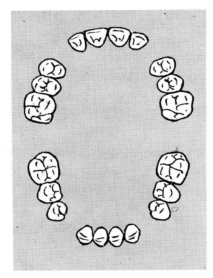

Phase 3

Fourth Phase

The smooth wedge-shaped canines (sometimes called *keystones*) force themselves between the lateral incisors and first premolars in both dental arches as they take their places. If they operate according to plan, contact relations between neighboring teeth are established and the dental arches are completed from first molars forward. Simultaneously, the second molars are due to emerge distally to first molars, backing them up during the wedging activity of the canines.

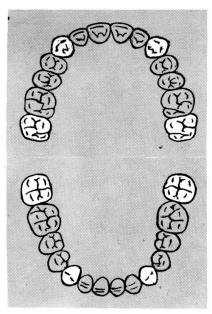

Phase 4

Fifth Phase

As the individual approaches maturity, the jaws should develop sufficiently to accommodate third molars distal to second molars. The late formation of third molars delays their schedule in the eruptive process. They are not due to show until several years after second molars are in place.

Many anatomists are of the opinion that third molars are vestigial and that our dental arches are physiologically complete without them.

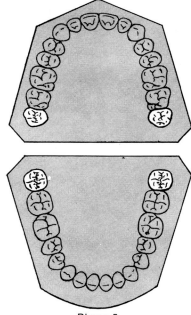

Phase 5

2. COMPENSATING CURVATURES OF THE DENTAL ARCHES (CURVED OCCLUSAL PLANES) (Fig. 16–6, 2, P. 413)

The occlusal surfaces of the dental arches do not conform to a flat plane. The mandibular arch conforms generally to one or more curved planes which appear concave, and the opposing maxillary arch, to curvature which appears convex. When the two arches are brought together in centric occlusion, these curved planes become identical.

Because the mandible is a single bow-formed bone with two joints moving independently of one another, and because the shifting of points of rotation is quite complicated during jaw movement, the adaptation of flat planes in opposing dental arches is out of the question (Fig. 16–19). In order to achieve balance by simultaneous contact in more than one area of dental arches during mastication, only curved planes can make this possible.

The movement of the mandible to the right or left during mastication is called the Bennett movement. Although Bennett of England was not the first to describe the movement, his work on the activity of the condyles established the term.

Bonwill was the first to describe the mandible and mandibular arch as adapting itself in part to an equilateral triangle (Fig. 16–13). The angles of the triangle are placed at the centers of each condyle and at the mesial contact areas of mandibular central incisors. Bonwill was of the impression that most mandibles would conform to a 4-inch equilateral triangle. Today, anatomists realize that such measurements cannot be established arbitrarily because of variables which are always likely to be present. Nevertheless, Bonwill's theory did emphasize bilateral symmetry, and although 4 inches exactly may not be accepted as the measurement, apparently more mandibles and mandibular arches conform to an approximation of a 4-inch equilateral triangle than to any other one approximation.

Later, Von Spee noted that the cusps and incisal ridges of the teeth tended to display a curved alignment when the arches were observed from a point opposite the first molars. This alignment is spoken of still as the "curve of Spee" (Fig. 4–10, Chapter 4). This curvature is within the sagittal planes only.

Monson, at a later date, connected the curve of Spee, or curvature in sagittal planes, with related compensating curvatures in vertical planes. Following up Bonwill's theorem, Monson originally described the normally developed mandibular

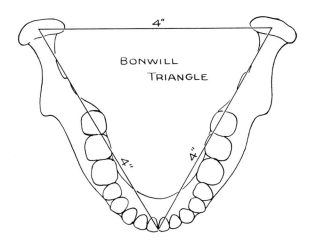

Figure 16–13. The Bonwill equilateral triangle.

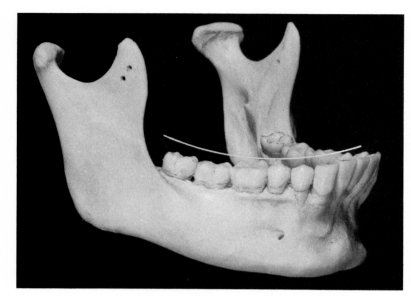

Figure 16–14. A good illustration of the arrangement of mandibular teeth which may be recognized as physically capable of establishing the compensating occlusal curvatures assumed by both dental arches (See also Fig. 4–10).

arch as adapting its occlusal surfaces to the curved surface of a segment of a sphere of a 4-inch radius. Although later developments have refuted the arbitrary 4-inch measurement, the fact remains that the occlusal surfaces of mandibular teeth do conform in a general way to a curved plane which may be represented by the curved outer surface of a segment of a sphere. The radius of the segment varies considerably in different individuals. It may be less than 3 inches or more than 4 inches. Nevertheless, it is true that there is a compensating curvature of the occlusal surfaces of the teeth—a curvature which involves more than one plane (Fig. 4–11, Chapter 4, and Figs. 16–15 and 16–16). The occlusal surfaces of the teeth do not conform to any one

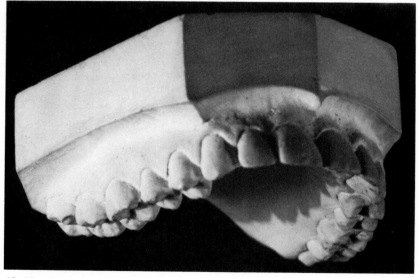

Figure 16–15.   An accurate cast of maxillary teeth demonstrating compensating occlusal curvature.

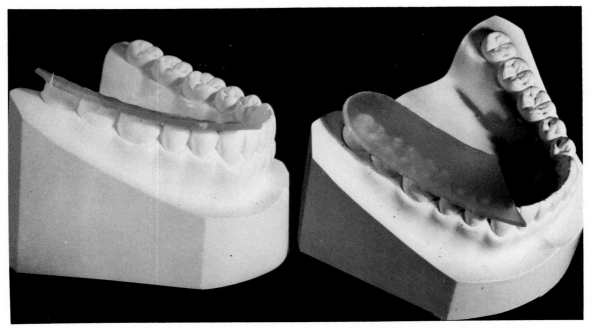

Figure 16–16.   Two views of a curved sheet of wax adapted to cusps of a cast of mandibular teeth. The right side only is covered, leaving the left side open for comparison. The curved wax, following curvatures of combined occlusal contacts, covers the canine and all of the posterior teeth, including premolars and molars.

curved plane exactly. *Nothing anatomic may be reduced to the mathematical exactitude of geometrical terms.*

The mandibular teeth are the ones which establish compensating curvature. The maxillary teeth have to adapt themselves to the mandibular teeth and to any arrangement they care to impose (Fig. 16–14).

The mandibular teeth are scheduled to appear in advance of the maxillary teeth. Therefore since they have jaw force behind them during the process of eruption and with bone development in a state of flux, the mandibular teeth provide the physical force which helps to decide the ultimate placement and angulation of their adversaries in the upper jaw.

The process will be activated by the crown forms of mandibular teeth coming into contact with the crown forms of maxillary teeth during functional jaw movement.

Finally, the establishment of compensating occlusal design is assisted by all the biologic forces at work that lead up to the terminus of maturation of parts.

AN ANALYSIS OF COMPENSATING OCCLUSAL CURVATURES

Occluding surfaces of the teeth of either jaw which are identified as functional are called *morsal surfaces* or "working surfaces."

A simplified description, which will suffice for the present, will locate the occluding surfaces as follows: the buccal cusp portion of mandibular posterior teeth contacts at some point, the central sulci of maxillary posterior teeth. These sulci lie directly between the buccal and lingual cusps.

Anteriorly, the incisal ridges of the mandibular canines and incisors contact the

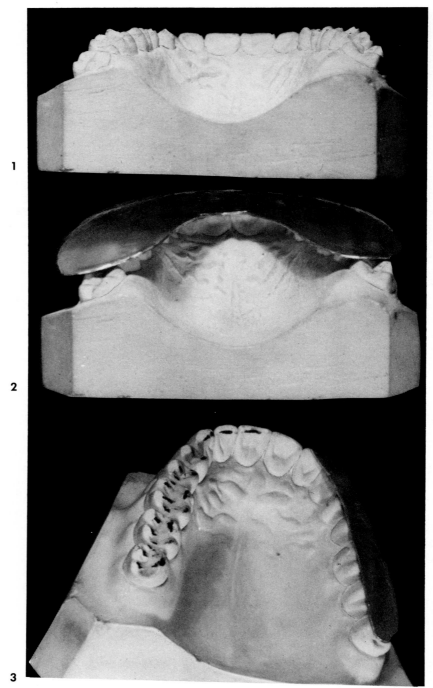

Figure 16–17.   Additional illustrations defining compensating occlusal curvature.

1. An extreme posterior view of the cast shown in Fig. 16–15. This picture affords further perspective on the occlusal curvature in this case.

2. The broad template (used in dental prosthetics) was placed over the occlusal surfaces of the cast in order to emphasize its extension in every direction beyond the confines of occlusal surfaces.

3. A narrow metal section of the template on the left side is all that is necessary to more than cover the occlusal contact surfaces of the *maxillary* teeth. The occlusal markings on the teeth on the right side, uncovered by the metal, will bear this out. Note the narrowness of the occlusal contact range from buccal to lingual. In millimeters the contact area will measure less than the measurement of the largest maxillary molar from cusp tip to cusp tip buccolingually (see also Fig. 16–101). The cast shown here is the same as that in Fig. 16–18.

maxillary canines and incisors, above their incisal and cusp ridges on lingual surfaces (Fig. 16–18,1).

As mentioned heretofore, Count Von Spee was the first to notice occlusal curvature. His attention was attracted to the molars of the maxillary dental arch, where the curvature is most noticeable (Fig. 16–15). Also, until rather recently, students of occlusion pursued the concept of cusps riding up and down over each other, in line with "planes" of occlusion. Therefore when the attempt was made to adapt a curved surface to occlusal surfaces of the teeth, the adaptation was made by contacting the tips of cusps of maxillary posterior teeth, and hoping that the incisal edges of maxillary anterior teeth would conform to the curvature also. Since "nothing is perfect in Nature," if some approximations were happily attained in any one case, it was accepted as a working hypothesis.

Some fundamental biologic rules were forgotten; mainly, that the mandibular teeth are scheduled to develop ahead of maxillary teeth, and as a consequence they are the first to erupt into the mouth. Also, the mandibular teeth are part of a movable arm capable of applying force. As the maxillary teeth (molars and premolars particularly) come in to take positions in a bone (maxilla) exhibiting no movement, the mandibular teeth with jaw force behind them proceed to manipulate the maxillary teeth into positions that correspond to the tooth form and jaw movement at work.

The description of this process has been repeated here in order to emphasize the futility of expecting the cusps of maxillary teeth to establish occlusal balance.

As a rule, the closest adaptation possible of a curved gauge (called a "template," which represents a segment of a sphere) that may be made is one which contacts buccal cusps of *mandibular posterior teeth*, hopefully with the incisal edges of anteriors, including the canines. The tips of lingual cusps of mandibular teeth usually do not touch the curved plane, because normally they are little involved in occlusal contact, especially in lateral jaw movements.

It seems as if one curved plane for all the teeth is unlikely. Many mouths are seen with complete arches and good functioning occlusion in which various segments of the arches may be cooperating with as many curved planes. Nevertheless, one thing is certain: the biologic laws involved that dictate tooth and jaw movement in man demand that occlusal relations follow curved paths. "Nature abhors straight lines"; therefore, in no place in the dental mechanism will straight lines be operative. That truism would guarantee also that if a plane involving tooth and jaw movement were to be found necessary, it without doubt would show curvature.

The curved planes traversed by the cusps of mandibular teeth over the maxillary teeth during mastication will not be dependent upon the height of cusps or upon the angulation of the inclines of cusp slopes (the so-called "inclined planes"). Occlusally, the mandibular teeth will follow a curved path through centric, in centric, and out of centric, and during this activity the buccal cusps of mandibular posteriors will be following the level of a curved plane as they contact and move across the occlusal surfaces of the maxillary teeth.

The plane might be traced by observing the occlusal contacts of *maxillary posterior* teeth, because there are more contacts to be observed over a broader level than are to be found on mandibular posteriors. Actually, however, a simpler approach would be to analyze a curved three-dimensional surface touching the *mandibular posterior* teeth, because their contacting surfaces during occlusal movements are mainly the buccal formations. Also, there are fewer contact markings to check, and these are arranged in a linear fashion (Fig. 16–78,LLOR).

It is possible to adapt a template representing a segment of the outer surface of a sphere to the main "working" occlusal surfaces of the *mandibular teeth* for an approx-

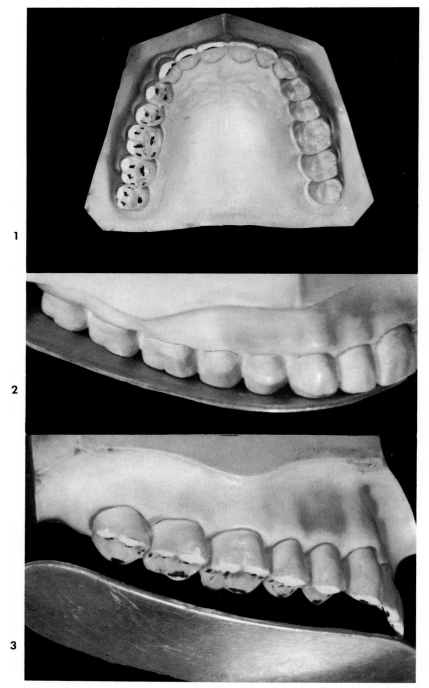

Figure 16–18. A visualization of an established curved plane adapting itself to occlusal contacts registered during mastication.

1. Two casts with "balanced" occlusion were articulated in order to register occlusal contact markings on one side—right lateral and centric relations. The left side remained free. The marked maxillary cast alone was used for this demonstration.

2. The buccal cusps of the posterior teeth and the incisal ridges of the anterior teeth on the right side were sanded off until the teeth adapted themselves to the curved template, putting the occlusal markings in contact with it.

3. The illustration here clarifies the relationship of teeth and template as shown in 2. The cast and template are posed parallel but separately. Thus, the occlusal markings as shown in 1 indicate parallelism with the curved template in 3, the instrument which represents the curved compensating occlusal plane.

imation of contact. This is one proof that the occlusal surfaces do not adapt themselves to a flat plane (Fig. 16–16). Nevertheless, our inability to earmark any one curvature that seems indicated in any single dental arch is frustrating. Also, more than one curved plane seems involved in surveys of this kind.

A template representing a curved plane that is adaptable to the markings of occlusal contacts on the teeth of the mandibular arch cannot be made to parallel similar occlusal markings on the teeth of the opposing arch because the tips of the cusps and the incisal ridges of the maxillary teeth are not a part of the compensating curved plane established by the mandibular contacts, thus they would prevent the seating of the template at proper level. The level of occlusal contacts on the maxillary teeth would be somewhere on the lingual surfaces of anterior teeth above the incisal ridges, and between the cusps of the posterior teeth (bearing lingually), within the sulci at marginal ridge levels approximately. The occlusal markings would show where the contacting surfaces of the mandibular teeth rest or glide while following the paths of occlusal relations (Figs. 16–17, 3 and 16–18).

Nevertheless, the points of occlusal contact on the maxillary teeth and the points of occlusal contact on the mandibular teeth must conform to an approximation of curved planes which are identical during the occlusal relations of both arches during mastication. Several curved planes at different angulations seem to be represented.

3. COMPENSATING CURVATURES OF THE INDIVIDUAL TEETH (CURVED AXES) (Fig. 16–6, 3, P. 413)

Vertical sections of the jaws with the teeth in centric occlusion point to the fact that the axes of the posterior teeth, maxillary and mandibular, approach alignment with each other, but that these axes are not perpendicular to a horizontal plane (Fig. 4–2, Figs. 14–29 to 14–36 and Fig. 16–23). It can be demonstrated also that any line which bisects the crown and root base of a tooth from any aspect exhibits some curvature. Therefore, the design or functional activities of the dental mechanism may never be reduced to equations in plane geometry.

A survey of the human dental mechanism, either whole or in part, will show that *curvature* is the rule in its basic design. Maxwell termed this basic phenomenon "spherical congruency." *Man-made structures* usually follow straight lines and angles to be studied in relation to straight lines, but Nature abhors such planning—which abhorrence is clearly demonstrated in anatomic structures. The human *dental mechanism* is no exception to the rule.

It is true, of course, that in the study of anatomy variations from the usual form may be expected. Nevertheless, duplications and tendencies should be considered important; and if they are repeated often it may be taken for granted that conclusions reached in this manner are of some consequence. Although it may not be advisable to accept an apparent truth as proving a rule, it should be seriously considered as knowledge which could play an important part in subsequent conclusions. The conclusions might possibly indicate a practical application.

The human dental mechanism is so complicated that it holds many secrets that go unanswered at the present time. Some conclusions which are fundamental, however, must be accepted because they can be demonstrated.

In the study of occlusion, and its association with the subject of dental anatomy and physiology, curvature is ever noticeable and obviously so, whether it be two dimensional or three dimensional in quality. The use of plane geometry as a medium for research into the intricacies of occlusion must be considered irrelevant. Supposi-

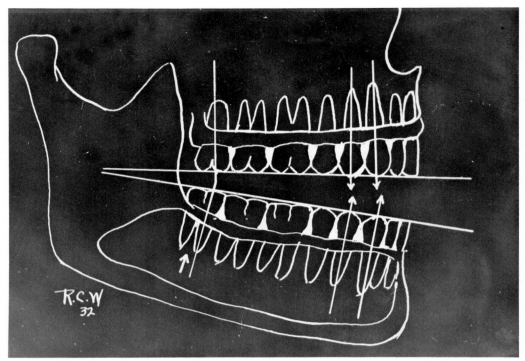

Figure 16–19. Schematic drawing of an imaginary occlusal relation. The occlusal surfaces have no compensating curvature, and the teeth have their axes at right angles to their occlusal surfaces. It will be noticed that as soon as the jaw is opened the axes of teeth in the upper jaw no longer coincide in direction with those of the lower jaw. A resistant bolus of food placed between the teeth at this opening will exert pressures unfavorable to stabilization of the various units.

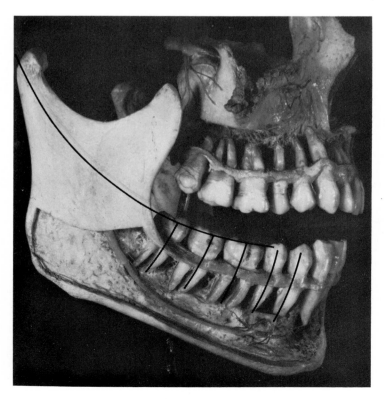

Figure 16–20. A different aspect of the specimen shown in Fig. 16–23. Here, a curved line contacts mandibular molar buccal cusps; a line representing the "Curve of Spee" for this individual is continued through the neck of the condyle. Curved lines representing axial lines are indicated on all the mandibular posterior teeth. Interestingly enough, the axial lines seem to make a ninety-degree approach toward the occlusal line; this line could indicate the level of a curved occlusal plane also. See Fig. 16–21.

tions based on flat planes and box-like forms must be accepted only as schematic demonstrations simplifying the communication of ideas. Plane geometry has been used in the past in an attempt to illustrate the design of occlusion (planes of occlusion, vertical dimension, long axes, etc.). In the main, the result has been a confusion of important issues.

The following truisms must be kept in mind:

1. Every segment of a tooth presents *curved* surfaces, except when the tooth is fractured or worn (Fig. 16–37)

2. Lines bisecting the teeth from any aspect exhibit some *curvature*

3. The teeth are aligned to form *arches*

4. The maxilla and mandible present *curved* outlines only

5. The mandible operates in paths which are *curved*

6. The occlusal and incisal surfaces of the teeth as units in the dental arch adapt themselves to *curved* planes (*compensating occlusal curvature*)

A common mistake is to assume that the forces of occlusion act upon the teeth in straight lines and also that the axes of the teeth are at right angles to their occlusal surfaces (Fig. 16–19). If the assumption were true, the arches would not be stable very long, because the forces brought to bear upon the tooth units would be tangent to their axes at any time the teeth of the two jaws were separated. Another difficulty which would be encountered is the impossibility of adapting teeth with straight axes to curved occlusal planes. Some of the roots would compete with others for the same space; and the human jaws would have to be designed differently to accommodate them. This remarkable arrangement allows proper spacing between roots for blood and nerve supply and for secure anchorage of the tooth roots in the jaw bone.

Actually, the compensating occlusal curvature of the dental arches which establishes occlusal balance could not be created unless the teeth themselves reflected those curvatures, thereby enabling them to take their places in the scheme of occlusion, a scheme built on essential curvatures. Arbitrary placement of teeth of indiscriminate form could not achieve the same result. An interesting comment might be made at this point: Practicing dentists, and dental students also, are too likely to be guided in their study of occlusion by their experiences in prosthetic technical procedure in which they "set up" manufactured artificial teeth into dental arch forms. It must be realized that in such procedures the operator is dealing with tooth crowns only, with no roots or foundation tissues to interfere. In addition, the artificial crowns usually do not conform to known anatomic values. Observations made on dissected human jaws showing the teeth *in situ* with their roots exposed prove without doubt the presence of

Figure 16–21. A schematic representation of a curved occlusal plane with curved planes above and below representing the axial curvatures of maxillary and mandibular teeth. See Fig. 16–20.

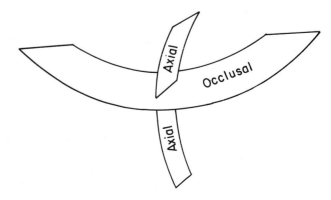

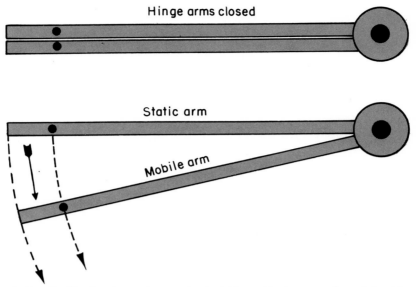

Figure 16–22.   Profile drawings of a mechanical hinge. Each arm or jaw of the hinge has been marked with dots in identical locations.

In the lower drawing, when the upper arm is held motionless and the lower arm is moved open to imitate the opening of the lower jaw, it will be seen that the dot marking, as well as the arm end of the lower member, follow curved paths.

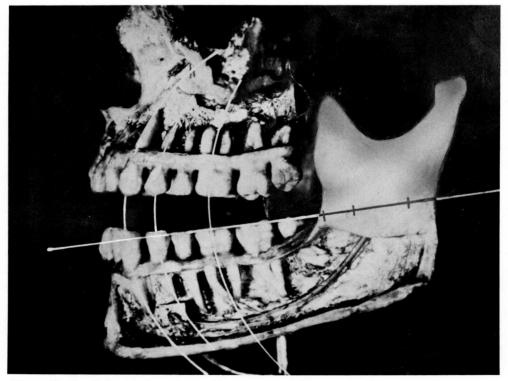

Figure 16–23.   A dissected specimen with the roots of the teeth exposed. The axes of the teeth show curvature. The axes of the arcs of the teeth for this specimen are on a line with the occlusal plane of the mandibular first molars. The marks on the ramus of the mandible represent the axes of the arcs shown.

axial curvatures and the apparent co-ordination of these curvatures with the occlusal curvatures of the arches.

A dissected specimen is shown in Figure 16–23. The line of vision is at right angles to the buccal surface of the mandibular first molar. The anterior teeth are seen from a distal aspect and the posterior teeth from a buccal aspect. Without doubt there is an accommodation in balance between the curvatures identified as occlusal levels and those identified as tooth axes. The occlusal surface of the crown portion of the tooth would tend to adapt itself to a curved plane on one level, while the curved axis of the whole tooth is representative of a different curved plane in direct apposition to the one which would be described as the occlusal plane. All this is a further demonstration of the avoidance of flat planes and straight lines (Figs. 16–20 and 16–21).

It is readily apparent that the long axes of the teeth are all curved; consequently a line bisecting any one of them describes an arc. Arcs passing through the teeth of one dental arch seem to be parallel to those passing through the teeth of the opposing arch. It just happens that in the specimen in Figure 16–23 the extent of jaw opening places the axes of the teeth in one jaw in the same curved plane with their namesakes in the opposite jaw. We know that this is not true when the teeth are in centric occlusion, because the teeth then have an offset relationship with each other. Nevertheless, *the axial arcs would have a tendency toward parallelism or concentricity with each other regardless of the extent of jaw opening.*

Evidently the axial curvature is necessary in order to stabilize each tooth in its location in the arches. In this specimen curved lines passing through the first molars (if viewed from the buccal aspect), and any of the teeth anterior to them, describe arcs that are related (the central and lateral incisors are viewed from distal aspects). The axes of these circles happen to be a line parallel with the occlusal surface of the mandibular first molar.

The second and third molar axes are arc segments of smaller circles. *It is interesting to note in this connection that the position and design of the second and third molars are such that they can act as braces for the other teeth in the arch, forbidding any tendency of the posterior teeth to drift in a distal direction.* The mandibular second and third molars have an extra inclination mesially. During mandibular activity, they strike the maxillary second and third molars with a mesial inclination of force. This may explain the tendency of molars to drift mesially as age advances, especially when space is created anteriorly to them. This is recognized as a physiologic change. Under certain conditions, mainly pathologic, cases may be observed in which *buccal* and *distal* drift of maxillary molars has taken place.

It is known that any one point in the mandibular dental arch follows curved paths during normal masticating movements of the mandible; the masticatory forces travel in curved paths. Therefore the axial curvatures of the individual teeth in the jaw seem to conform to the physical laws governing such an activity (Fig. 16–23).

Photographs of teeth placed within a protractor prove their axial relation to compensating occlusal curvature (Figs. 16–24, 16–25 and 16–26). In these illustrations the anterior teeth were posed in the approximate positions they assume in the jaws. The posterior teeth were posed with their marginal ridges (mesial and distal) parallel with the horizontal plane, or 0 degrees. The horizontal plane (marginal ridge levels) is taken as an approximation of the occlusal plane for each tooth.

The illustrations, as shown, must be accepted as arbitrary hypotheses only, made in order to show the adaptability of the axes of the teeth to angulation as an integral part of the compensating dental mechanism. The examples do not prove a rule of measurement in any instance.

Chances are, the angulations would vary in direct ratio to the size of teeth and jaws, genetic background, etc. This subject provides an open field for research.

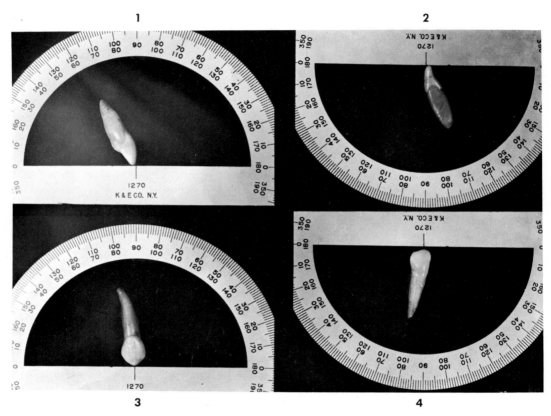

Figure 16–24. Individual teeth placed within a protractor to show their axial inclinations. The placement of the roots in relation to occlusal levels of the crowns governs the association of occlusal levels in the dental arch. The combination of occlusal levels exhibits curvature, which in turn assists in arriving at occlusal compensation during jaw movements. 1, Maxillary central incisor. 2, Mandibular central incisor. 3, Maxillary canine. 4, Mandibular canine.

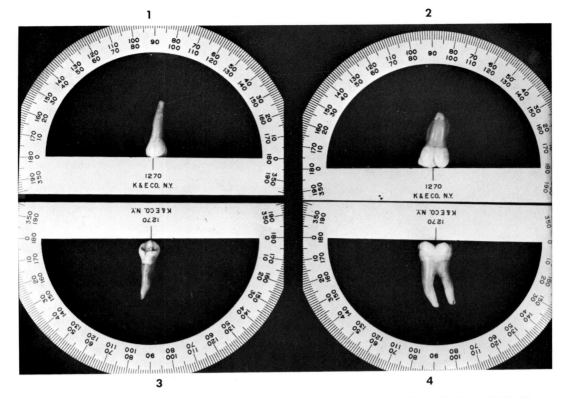

Figure 16–25. Individual teeth placed within a protractor to show their axial inclinations. 1, Maxillary first premolar. 2, Maxillary first molar. 3, Mandibular first premolar. 4, Mandibular first molar.

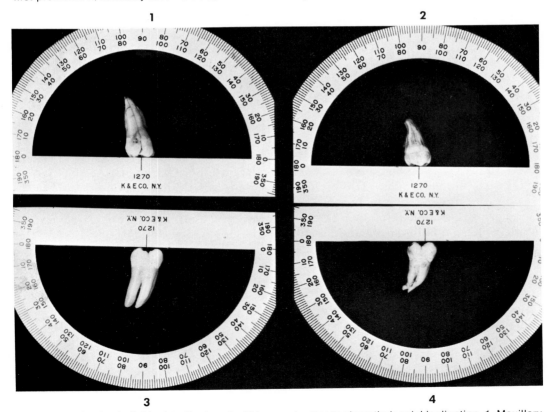

Figure 16–26. Individual teeth placed within a protractor to show their axial inclination. 1, Maxillary second molar. 2, Maxillary third molar. 3, Mandibular second molar. 4, Mandibular third molar.

4. ANGULATION OF THE INDIVIDUAL TEETH IN RELATION TO VARIOUS PLANES; ROOT FORM

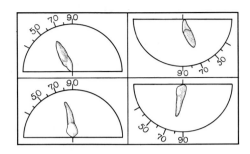

The relationship of axes of maxillary and mandibular teeth to each other varies and depends upon which tooth group or anatomic classification is to be considered.

Sections through the jaws with the teeth in centric occlusion, made to show the mesial aspect of each tooth in either arch, are shown in MacMillan's illustrations in Figs. 14–29 to 14–36, Chapter 14. The technical difficulties involved in the production of the illustrations, *Cross sections of maxillary and mandibular teeth and bone to show relationship in centric occlusion,* must have presented many problems. There is little doubt that some error could be involved. Nevertheless, the results are remarkable, and it would seem to be indicated that the occlusal relations should be accepted as approximate at least for this specimen. The acceptance of the cross sections of a rare anatomic specimen by a person of MacMillan's stature serves as a valuable aid in the study of occlusal relations, as well as tooth and bone relationships. In this specimen it may be noted that the incisors are placed with their axes at about 60 degrees to the horizontal plane at the occlusal contact, the axis of the maxillary tooth being placed at an acute angle to the axis of the mandibular tooth. The canines are placed so that the axes form angles less acute, followed by the first premolars, which resemble the canines in their placement.

The second premolars and the first molars differ from the teeth anterior to them in their axial relations to each other and in their angulations to a horizontal plane. The axes of these maxillary and mandibular teeth are nearly parallel. In studying Figure 14–34, it may be seen that there is a possibility of error here. More than likely, the second premolar mandibular and first molar maxillary should have been related as pictured in Figure 14–35, which depicts the second molar region correctly.

The second and third mandibular molars have their axes at angles somewhat more acute in relation to the horizontal than the first molar axis. Prolongations of the lines bisecting the mandibular second and third molars tend to bisect the lingual roots of the maxillary second and third molars. The axis line of the mandibular first molar, when prolonged, would tend to pass between the buccal and lingual roots of the maxillary first molar.

No absolute rules may be assumed when describing the axial relations of maxillary and mandibular teeth in centric occlusion. Nevertheless, even though skulls and specimens show some variations in the degree of angulations, normally developed specimens show angulations of crowns and roots similar to the generalizations just described.

Each tooth must be placed at the angle that best withstands the lines of forces brought against it during function. The angle at which it is placed depends upon the function the tooth has to perform. If the tooth is placed at a disadvantage, its func-

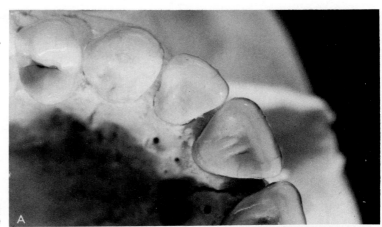

Figure 16–27. *Maxillary Teeth.*

Specimen skull photographed from three points at the same time the occlusal aspects are viewed.

The compensating occlusal curvature (Curve of Spee) makes it necessary to focus the camera parallel with tooth axes from at least three points in order to obtain some accuracy in making comparisons. The close-up is of value in noting crown form, alignment, contact area relationships and so on. A more scientific observation would require as many aspects as there are teeth in view because of individual variations in axial angulations (See also Fig. 16–7).

A. This is looking at an anterior section of the arch in line with the long axis of the canine.

B. Here the lens was centered directly opposite the contact of first and second premolars.

C. This photo is in line with the long axis of the maxillary first molar.

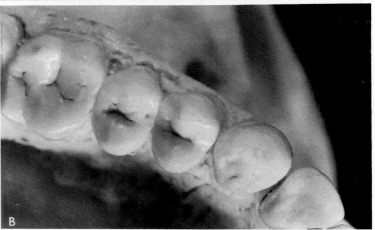

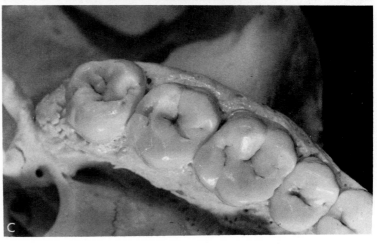

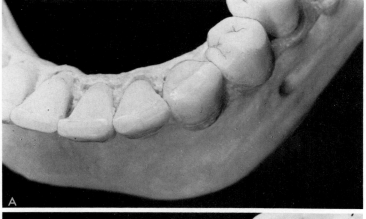

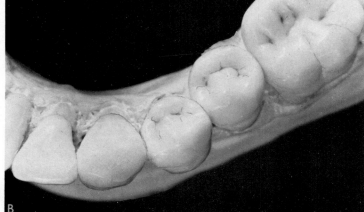

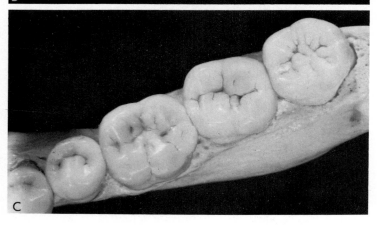

Figure 16–28.   *Mandibular Teeth.*

Close-up view of occlusal surfaces using the technique in photography mentioned in Fig. 16–27.

A. An anterior section of the mandibular dental arch. The camera is pointed in line with the long axis of the canines.

B. Here the aim was centered on the line of contact between the canine and the first premolar.

C. The posterior section, featuring the molars, was made by focusing the lens in line with the long axis of the first molar.

tional efficiency is limited to that extent, and the permanency of its position is endangered. The dental arch can be only as efficient and as permanent as its component parts.

The anterior teeth, as shown in the illustrations (Figs. 14–29, 14–30 and 14–31), seem to be placed at a disadvantage when one views them from mesial or distal aspects. The lines of force during mastication, or when the jaws are merely opened or closed, are tangent generally to the long axes of these teeth (Fig. 14–29). It must be remembered that they are designed for momentary *biting* and *shearing* only, and not

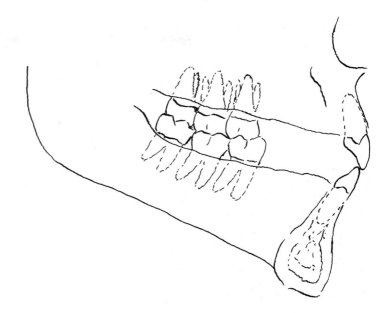

Figure 16–29. This illustration, which emphasizes the contrast in placement and angulation between molars and incisors, also emphasizes the "power ratio" of the two segments of the dental arch. It is obvious that the molars are designed to be the principal jaw support and that anterior teeth, both in design and in placement, are not capable substitutes when the molars are lost.

for the assumption of the full force of the jaws; in other words, they cannot assume jaw support under all situations.

During the act of occlusion, the approaching mandibular anterior teeth are brought against the fixed maxillary anteriors in a forward position of the mandible (protrusion). The shearing action as the mandible is closed and retruded softens the force of occlusion somewhat, and the movement is in the direction of the angulation of maxillary anterior tooth roots.

The axes of the mandibular anterior teeth, with the lines running through crown and root, are in line with the resultants of force brought against them by the reverberation of their own force against the incisal or lingual surfaces of the static maxillary anterior teeth. This analysis may give one answer to the clinical picture often observed: the smaller, weaker mandibular central and lateral incisors often prevail over the maxillaries in the presence of occlusal trauma. *Nevertheless, these smaller teeth, angled as they are, along with the maxillary anteriors, are all at a disadvantage without posterior tooth support.* If the arrangement of the teeth is proper, *the full force of the jaws is not brought to bear on anterior teeth until the posterior teeth, mainly molars, have had an opportunity to assume the jaw force.*

The greatest amount of force which the jaws are capable of applying against the teeth does not culminate until centric relation in occlusion is approached. As the teeth come into centric occlusion, the posterior teeth, and the molars especially, assume the full force of the load, supported by the arch form arrangement and the compensating curvature involved. The molars are able to withstand the maximum forces during masticatory function by virtue of their form, structure, anchorage and placement (Figs. 16–29, 16–49 and 16–66).

Loss of support, through damage or loss of molars, seriously handicaps the entire dental mechanism. The teeth anterior to the molars are not designed or placed in a manner conducive to total dental arch support.

The anterior teeth, when observed from directly in front of the median line, also demonstrate axial inclinations in relation to vertical or horizontal lines. From this point of view the degree of their inclinations is not great, but it may be readily seen that there is some inclination of the axes. The long axes of the teeth are never at right angles to the horizontal plane.

The teeth are placed so that their axes on either right or left side are at acute angles to the median line or median plane (sagittal plane) (Fig. 16–3). This arrangement makes the anterior teeth of each side of the mouth point, with their crowns, in the direction of the median line. The arrangement therefore favors the stabilization of the contact relationship of these teeth.

The teeth are inclined at angles of from 5 to 10 degrees to the median plane—which is, in effect, angulation of 85 to 80 degrees to the horizontal plane.

(*Text continued on page 444.*)

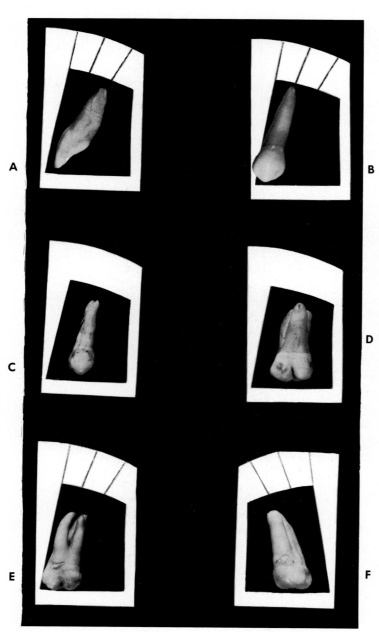

Figure 16–30. *Maxillary Teeth.*

The teeth are posed arbitrarily in the approximate angle they assume in the jaws. The straight line of the border of the white frame is made parallel with marginal ridges and contact areas and is thereby parallel to occlusal surfaces generally. This approach is experimental, and there is no assumption that it proves any certain degree of angulation of tooth axes, but these illustrations of maxillary teeth leave no doubt in mind that angulation exists, and further studies must be made in order to understand its significance in the plan of occlusion. *A.* Central incisor. *B.* Canine. *C.* First premolar. *D.* First molar. *E.* Second molar. *F.* Third molar.

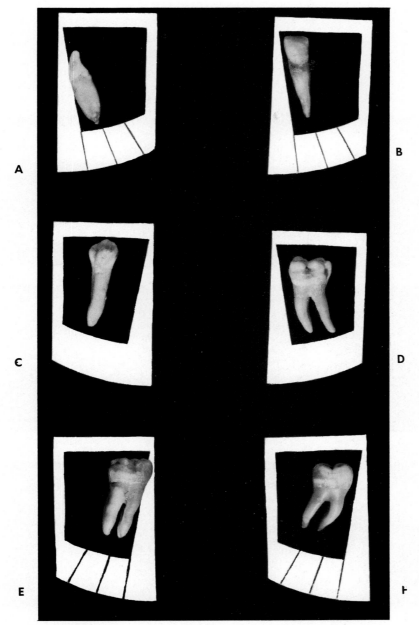

Figure 16–31. *Mandibular Teeth.*

Arrangement explained in Figure 16–30. *A.* Central incisor. *B.* Canine. *C.* First premolar. *D.* First molar. *E.* Second molar. *F.* Third molar.

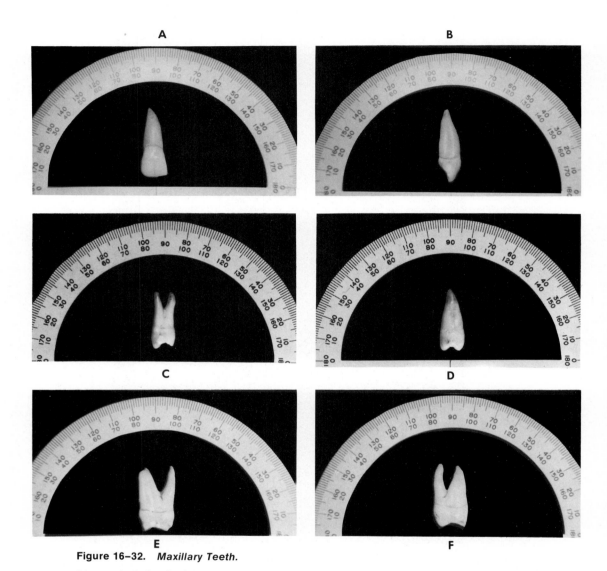

Figure 16–32. *Maxillary Teeth.*

Photos depicting further experimentation in the study of the angulation of axes, which, it is realized, could have an effect upon lines of force in occlusion. Here the approach was from different aspects (mesial and distal), placing the teeth in their approximate alignment with occlusal levels. The crown portions of the teeth, along with the cervical third of the roots, seem to be straight with the horizontal line (See Figs. 14–35 and 14–36). However, close scrutiny of the roots will suggest varied curvatures. *A.* Central incisor. *B.* Canine. *C.* First premolar. *D.* Second premolar. *E.* First molar. *F.* Another maxillary first molar showing some differentiation in form when compared with *E.*

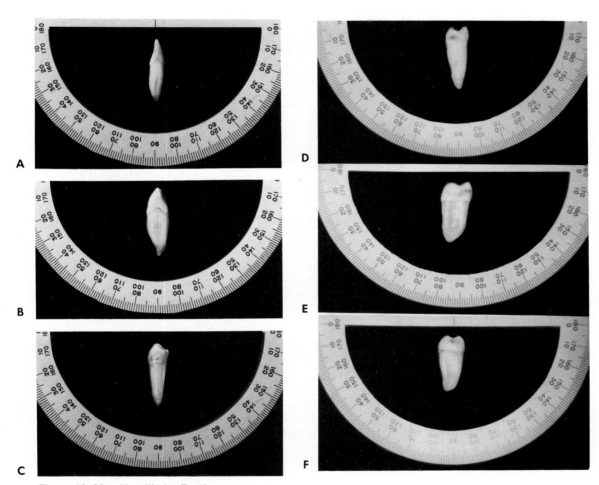

Figure 16–33. *Mandibular Teeth.*

Generally speaking, the mandibular teeth will show angulation similar to the maxillary when viewed from mesial or distal aspects. However, the root forms must conform to the manner in which the teeth are anchored, so the teeth in the two jaws differ; the mandibular has no spreading roots from mesial or distal aspects. The developmental grooves and depressions in many roots on mandibular teeth furnish anchorage akin to fused roots; the somewhat kidney-shaped roots (on cross section) resist movement when imbedded in bone. Also, close scrutiny here will demonstrate some curvature from the cervical third of the root to the apex (*E*) when the crest of contour is followed on each side of the developmental depression, as if following the direction of fused roots. *A.* Central incisor. *B.* Canine. *C.* First premolar. *D.* Second premolar. *E.* First molar. *F.* Another first molar, smaller and differing somewhat from *E*.

5. THE FUNCTIONAL FORM OF THE TEETH AT THEIR INCISAL AND OCCLUSAL THIRDS

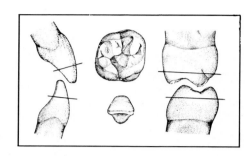

Items 5, 6, 7 and 8 in the study of tooth form, arrangement and occlusion have to do with the crown forms of the teeth and their alignment for function, the practical aspects of occlusion to be observed in the mouth. (See also page 412.)

However some of the basic concepts of design, which have just been described under items 1, 2, 3, and 4, must be realized and respected, in order for one to understand certain fundamentals of form which contribute to stability. These stabilizing principles are reflected in the crown forms also.

The incisal and occlusal thirds of the tooth crowns present convex or concave surfaces at all contacting occlusal areas (Fig. 16–34). When the teeth of one jaw come into occlusal contact with their antagonists in the opposite jaw during various mandibular movements, curved surfaces come into contact with curved surfaces. These curved surfaces may be convex or concave. A convex surface, representing a segment of the occlusal third of one tooth, may come into contact with a convex or a concave segment of another tooth; always, however, curved segments contact curved segments, large or small (Fig. 16–35).

There are no flat planes on the incisal or occlusal surfaces of any of the teeth unless there are some created by wear or accident. When such planes are created, the efficiency of the occlusal form is lessened in direct proportion to the extent of the deterioration.

Every segment of a cusp, marginal ridge or incisal ridge is a segment of a spheroid regardless of the size of the segment (Fig. 16–37).

Lingual surfaces of maxillary incisors present some concave surfaces where convex portions of the incisal ridges of mandibular incisors come into occlusal contact.

The posterior teeth show depressions in the depths of sulci and developmental grooves; nevertheless, the enamel sides of the sulci are formed by convexities which point into the developmental grooves. Cusps that are rather pointed will contact the rolls of hard enamel which make up marginal ridges on posterior teeth. Until the cusps are worn flat, the deeper portions of the sulci and grooves act as escapements for food, since the convex surfaces of opposing teeth are prevented from fitting into them perfectly by the curved sides of the sulci (Figs. 16–38 and 16–43).

The crown of a human tooth, with its occlusal form, is at its most efficient period immediately following its eruption and its occlusion with its antagonists. *The curved hard surfaces, coming into contact with like surfaces, permit the teeth to be used as cutters; when convexities come into contact with other convexities or with concavi-*

(Text continued on page 448.)

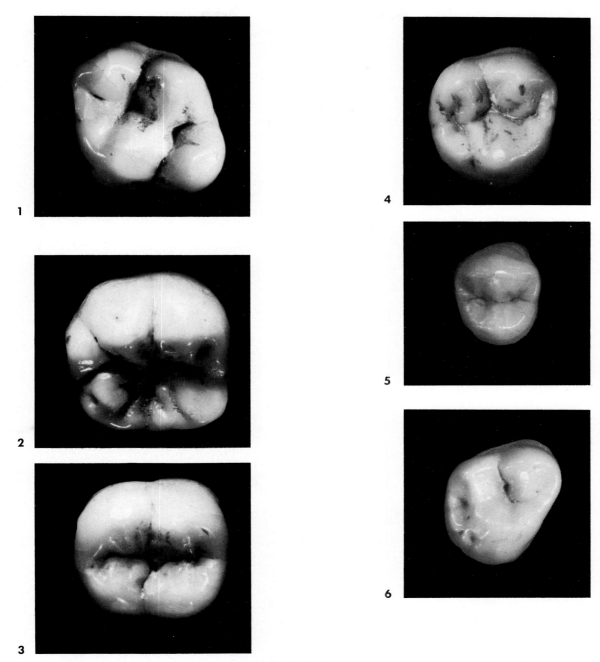

Figure 16–34.   Occlusal views of some posterior teeth showing convex and concave surfaces and no vestige of flat planes or sharp angles. 1. Maxillary first molar. 2. Mandibular first molar. 3. Mandibular second molar. 4. Maxillary second molar. 5. Maxillary first premolar. 6. Maxillary third molar.

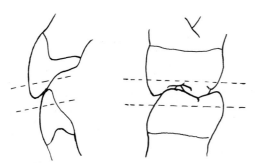

Figure 16–35. The incisal or occlusal thirds of the tooth crowns present convex or concave surfaces at all contacting occlusal areas.

Figure 16–36. Natural tooth specimens set up as they approach each other in occlusion. The relatively sharp lingual cusps of maxillary premolars usually contact the hard rounded marginal ridges of mandibular premolars. In an ideal situation, the tips of lingual cusps would approach or rest in the disto-occlusal fossae of mandibular premolars.

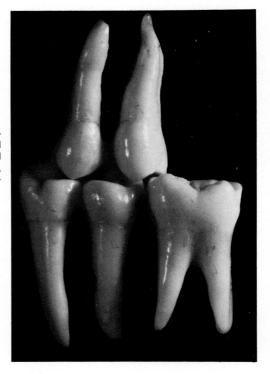

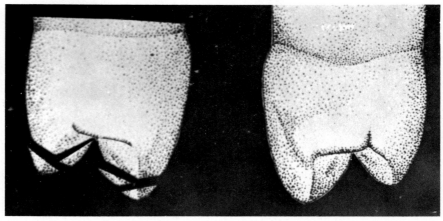

Figure 16–37. A diagrammatic representation of spheroidal segments sectioned from the occlusal portion of a maxillary premolar.

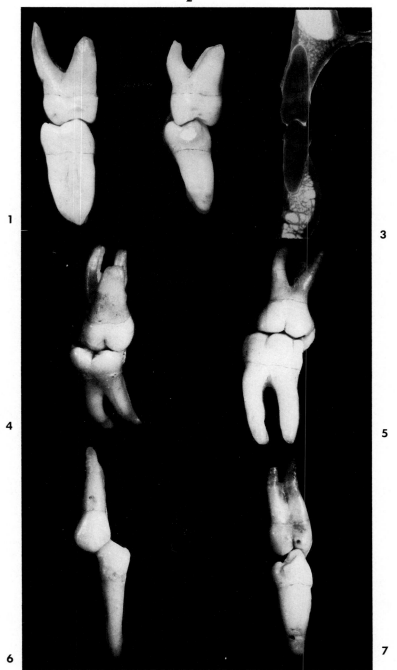

Figure 16–38. Maxillary and mandibular first molars and maxillary and mandibular premolars placed in centric occlusal relation.

1. Mesial aspect of first molars in centric occlusion. Compare this picture with 4.

2. Distal aspect of first molars in centric occlusion. Compare 2 with 5.

3. A radiograph of a section of a specimen showing the approximate relation of second premolars in centric viewed from the mesial aspect. (After MacMillan.)

4. Lingual aspect of first molars in centric occlusion, taken at an unusual angle to emphasize occlusal contacts and escapement spacing. Compare with 1.

5. Unusual angle of first molars in centric occlusion showing that the cusps do not fit together closely, but that limited spots of enamel come into contact with space around them. Study the four aspects of first molars in occlusion by comparing 1, 2, 4, and 5.

6. Buccal aspect of first premolars in centric occlusal relation. Compare 6 with 7.

7. Mesial aspect of first premolars in centric occlusal relation. Note the approximation of the buccal cusp of the mandibular premolar to the mesial marginal ridge of the maxillary first premolar.

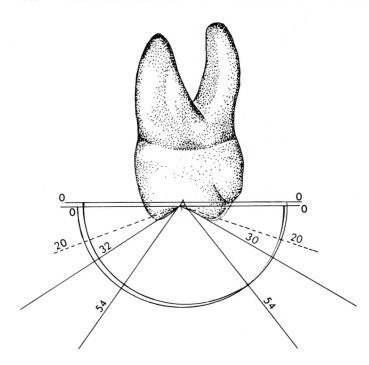

Figure 16–39. An idealized drawing of a maxillary first molar with markings depicting the approximate angulation of occlusal slopes.

The steepest angulation would be attributed, first, to the walls of developmental grooves, 50° to 55° to the horizontal; next, to the slopes represented by the triangular ridges of cusps, 30° to 32°; and last, to the angulation of marginal ridges, which seem to average about 20°. The horizontal line represents the base line of cusps.

Although we no longer think of the cusps in one jaw as sliding up and down the sides or "planes" of the cusps in the opposite jaw, an illustration such as this, necessarily approximate, will help to establish a sense of proportion in the study of dental anatomy and occlusion.

ties, *they touch in points or in small circumscribed areas only. When the contacting areas are hard and unyielding, they cut or shred any penetrable material when, in addition to their contact, they are moved over each other with considerable shearing force.*

The cusps, marginal ridges and sulci on multicusped posterior teeth may be compared favorably with the eminences and spillways of the schematic drawings in Figs. 16–42, 16–43 and 16–44.

The cusps of the schematic tooth are made to resemble spheres which approximate each other. The opposing tooth is similarly drawn and placed in occlusal contact. One may see that the cusps touch in circumscribed areas or points, with spillways appearing where the spheres of one tooth fail to penetrate the deeper portions of the sulci of the other.

Although the cusps and rounded eminences of the occlusal surfaces of natural teeth may not be comparable to sections of spheres, the various segments of the rounded eminences are comparable to sections of spheroids of greater or lesser dimensions; their comparison with the schematic cusps is therefore a logical one. The curvatures formed at the occlusal portions of the teeth conform to the physiologic entity of the entire dental mechanism, which, as has been mentioned before, is based on curvature.

Another aspect of importance: *Curved contacting surfaces of opposing teeth allow greater facility of adjustment to changing conditions involving the dental mechanism with less sacrifice of efficiency than any design which might include flat planes.* Any mechanism, to be practicable in use, allows ease of adjustment of parts during its assembly, and the completed mechanism allows proper facilities for adjustment to changing conditions which are brought about by wear or accident. The design of the human tooth forms and the design of the temporomandibular articulation make these allowances in a most complete manner. The articulation allows the maximum

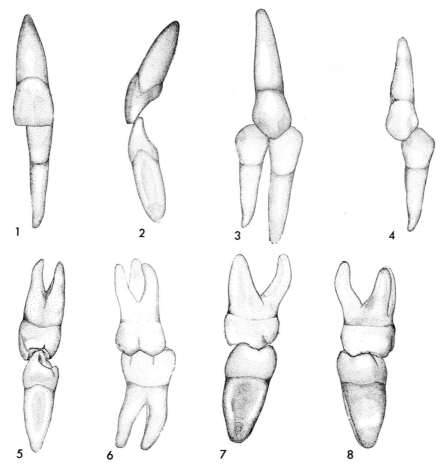

Figure 16–40. *Drawings Showing Normal Intercuspation of Maxillary and Mandibular Teeth.*

1. Central incisors, labial aspect.
2. Central incisors, mesial aspect.
3. Maxillary canine, in contact with mandibular canine and first premolar, facial aspect.
4. Maxillary first premolar and mandibular first premolar, buccal aspect.
5. Maxillary first premolar and mandibular first premolar, mesial aspect.
6. First molars, buccal aspect.
7. First molars, mesial aspect.
8. First molars, distal aspect.

adjustment; it adjusts itself with limitations to movement in various planes, flat or curved. The curved occlusal surfaces allow the individual teeth to be adjusted to various angulations of their long axes with the minimum of variance in their placement; simultaneously, with a minimum lack of occlusal efficiency.

The occlusal design of the crowns of the permanent teeth is established several years before the teeth have an opportunity to complete occlusal relations with their antagonists. In the meantime, the bones of the jaws and the temporomandibular articulation are developing and are subject to changes which must take place during the years when the teeth are erupting and establishing their relations to each other.

Pointing to the chronology of the development of the parts and the fact that the occlusal design of the teeth is permanently fixed in unchangeable form years before

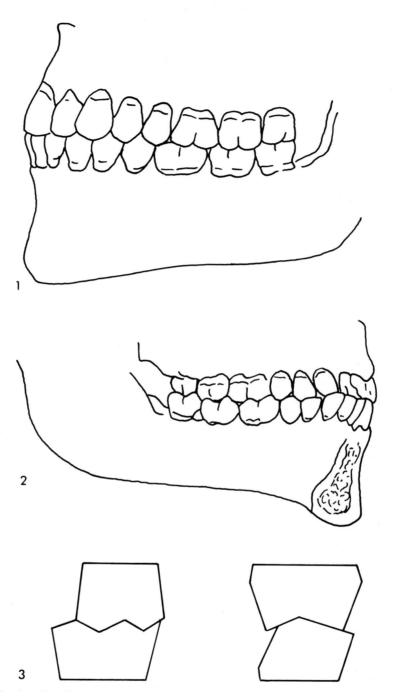

Figure 16–41. *Drawing Purporting to Show Teeth in Functional Contact as They Might Appear When in Centric Occlusal Relation.*

1. A drawing of the teeth in occlusion observed from the buccal aspect. The first impression by an observer would be favorable, for he might believe that here was a good illustration. In fact it is a fair example of the type of illustration of occlusion used most often. Because the teeth and jaws, showing one half the dental arches, have considerable breadth and thickness, a flat two-dimensional drawing such as this gives an erroneous impression. The study of occlusion demands that three-dimensional images be created in the mind. Good photographs with proper lighting will be an improvement over the two-dimensional drawing (Fig. 16–48).

(*Legend continued on opposite page.*)

Figure 16–42. Schematic drawing of the mesial aspect of first molars in occlusion, illustrating the cusp forms as perfect circles. With this arrangement, escapement spaces would be larger, but the centric occlusal relation would be too unstable and the cusps would be too flat. Also, "mortar and pestle" activity, where indicated for efficiency, would be absent. *E*, escapement spaces. (See also Figs. 16–45 and 16–46.)

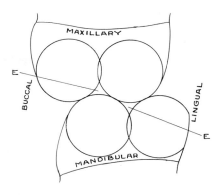

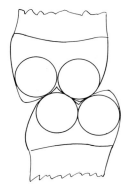

Figure 16–43. Schematic drawing of the mesial aspect of maxillary and mandibular first molar crowns in centric relation. Circles have been placed within the outlines of cusp forms to emphasize the curvatures.

Figure 16–44. Schematic drawing of the buccal aspect of maxillary and mandibular first molar crowns, separated as in jaw opening. Circles have been placed within the outlines of cusp forms to emphasize curvatures. Note the adaptability of the circles to the actual occlusal outline of the mandibular first molar.

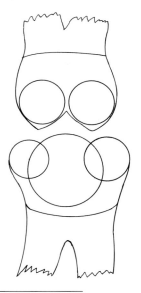

Figure 16–41. *Continued.*

The most desirable supplement, of course, would be a good skull specimen or accurate casts reproducing the natural teeth faithfully. Reference to them could be repeated, returning to the three-dimensional material for study whenever desired.

2. The lingual aspect of the teeth as illustrated buccally in 1. Drawings such as these two do not show any free interdental spacing or any overjet relationships. Escapement spaces are necessary requisites for efficient occlusion. Therefore, when maxillary and mandibular teeth fit together so that all contacting cusp slopes ("planes") are parallel and closed, a pathological situation exists with occlusal trauma to be expected.

3. Schematic drawings of first molars drawn with geometric effect. The occlusal surfaces fit tightly together without relief. If occlusal planes were like this on natural teeth, the teeth would have to be placed in one position only in the jaws, allowing for no flexibility in tooth movement. Needless to say, the "potato masher" effect would increase occlusal pressures and interfere with good tooth maintenance.

the investing tissues of the teeth are completed, the conclusion should be that the jaws and their articulation will coincide with the requirements of the occlusal design of the teeth.

Paradoxically, the occlusal curvatures of the tooth crowns are the *foundation* of *occlusion,* and the *investing tissues* of the teeth, which include the alveolar process of the jaw bones and the temporomandibular articulation, are the *superstructure* of *occlusion.*

Because jaw relations are dependent upon the form and alignment of the teeth, loss of one or more of the teeth will change jaw relations ultimately, along with the compensatory action and reaction of the temporomandibular articulation. The changes and adaptations will be affected by the number of dental units lost or missing, and by physical changes in functioning teeth brought on by accident, excessive wear or disease. Each unit plays its part as a stabilizer of occlusion; the instability of the occlusion is affected in direct ratio to the number of stabilizers missing. The temporomandibular articulation will adjust (within limitations) in order to accommodate any damaged arches; by virtue of this adaptability *relative* efficiency is maintained by the damaged masticatory mechanism.

The movements of the condyles over the meniscus in the glenoid fossa are regulated by the alignment and the occlusion of the teeth.

The ligamentous attachments to the condyles allow a greater range of movement than the occlusion of the teeth usually requires.

When all of the teeth are lost, the mandible loses the terminals of movement which are established by the teeth. The limitation of mandibular movement after the loss of teeth is governed by the extent of flexibility and elasticity of the ligamentous attachments and by the tonicity of muscles.

The curved surfaces of the occlusal surfaces of tooth crowns allow adjustment with a minimum of placement and displacement of the individual teeth during the alignment of the dental arches during jaw development.

If occlusal thirds possessed plane surfaces, these plane surfaces would require the teeth to be placed in one position only. If that position were not attained, *i.e.,* if the plane surfaces of one tooth did not adapt themselves perfectly to the plane surfaces of its antagonists in the opposite jaw, the position of the tooth would not be stabilized until the counterplanes became parallel to each other. No flexibility of adjustment would be permitted. Plane surfaces would adapt themselves to each other so closely that there would be little or no spacing between cusps and marginal ridges. This arrangement would produce a mashing rather than a cutting effect, decreasing the efficiency for our purposes, not to mention the tremendous increase in occlusal pressure which would have to be accommodated by a more secure periodontal anchorage and attachment (Fig. 16–41).

Escapement spaces are needed for efficient occlusion because of the nature of the duties the teeth must perform during mastication.

The human being is omnivorous. His teeth are designed to reduce the varied food material to a consistency which fits the requirements of his digestive system. His dental mechanism does not reduce food material to a pulpy mass. The teeth cut, shred or crush food into particles which are small enough to enable the digestive system to continue the reduction without strain and within a normal time limit for proper nourishment of the individual.

The cusps and incisal ridges of the teeth act as cutting blades when they are brought into contact with opposing cusps and incisal ridges or into contact with the concave surfaces of opposing teeth. These concavities may be natural or they may be created by wear. When curved surfaces of different planes come together at any

Figure 16–45.   Sectional drawing of a typical mortar and pestle. The convex end of the pestle is in contact with the concave floor of the mortar chamber. The surfaces are in contact in a small circumscribed area, with escapement space appearing around the area of contact. Some of the occlusal contacts of the human teeth resemble this working arrangement. *C,* contact; *E,* escapement.

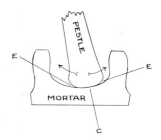

point, they touch in circumscribed points or areas, and spaces appear all around the points of contact where the curved surfaces do not fit together (Figs. 16–44 and 16–45). These spaces, when relating the process to the occlusal surfaces of the teeth, act as escapement spaces or spillways.

Escapement space is provided in the teeth by the form of the cusps and ridges, the sulci and developmental grooves, and the interdental spaces or embrasures when teeth come together in occlusion.

Although the teeth when in centric occlusion seem to intercuspate rather closely, on examination it is found that escapements have been provided. When occluding surfaces come together, some escapement spaces are so slight that light is scarcely admitted through them; they vary in degree of opening from such small ones to generous ones of a millimeter or more at the widest points of embrasure (Fig. 16–38).

The *location* and *form* of the escapement spaces are immediately changed when the occlusal relation is changed. When the occlusion is *normal,* the teeth fit together or intercuspate with *less escapement space* available in *centric* occlusion than in any other occlusal relation. As soon as the mandibular teeth are moved out of centric relation with the maxillary teeth, the *escapements are enlarged,* since the intercusping relation is not so complete.

When the teeth are occluding in the lateral relation or in protrusive relation, the escapement space is *increased* but the number of spotted areas or points of occlusal contact between the teeth of the two arches is *decreased.* This variation in the number of contacting areas of the teeth during the various occlusal relations may be demonstrated by markings made by the teeth of one jaw on the teeth of the opposing jaw, registered by carbon "articulating" paper held between the teeth during the movements (Fig. 16–47). As the teeth are brought back from lateral or protrusive toward centric occlusion, the spotted areas of contact increase in number as the teeth approach centric. Simultaneously the escapement space is reduced in direct ratio to the increase in occlusal contact (Fig. 16–91).

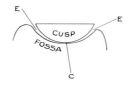

Figure 16–46.   Schematic drawing of "mortar and pestle" design of some of the occlusal contacts of the teeth. Examples: buccal cusps of mandibular molars in contact with central sulci of maxillary molars; incisal ridges of mandibular incisors in contact with lingual fossae of maxillary incisors. *C,* contact; *E,* escapement.

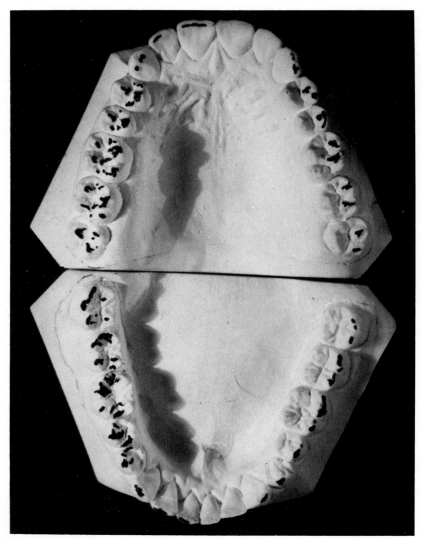

Figure 16–47. Casts of maxillary and mandibular teeth showing the occlusal contacts. The side showing buccal markings only demonstrates the contacting areas in left lateral relation for this individual. The opposite side with many more registered markings shows the contacting areas in centric occlusal relation. Note all of the unmarked areas on occlusal surfaces. These areas represent escapement spaces existing at the same time spotted areas were in contact.

The functional value of the system just described is obvious: *The number of cutting blades is reduced when the position of the teeth places them at a greater disadvantage to the resistance of force, as experienced in a lateral relation; and at the same time the escapement spaces, which serve to decrease pressure, are multiplied or enlarged. The opposite arrangement is countenanced only as the teeth return to centric occlusion, where their form and their alignment with each other offer combined resistance to the maximum forces of mastication.*

6. THE FACIAL AND LINGUAL RELATIONS OF EACH TOOTH IN ONE ARCH TO ITS ANTAGONIST IN THE OPPOSING ARCH IN CENTRIC OCCLUSION

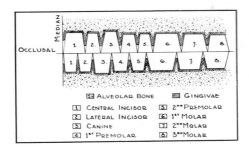

In the centric occlusal relation, facial views of the normal denture show each tooth of one arch in occlusal with portions of two others in the opposing arch with the exception of the mandibular central incisors and the maxillary third molars. Each of the exceptions named has one antagonist only in the opposing jaw (Fig. 16–48 and 16–49). To repeat: each tooth in one jaw will contact two teeth in the opposing jaw when in centric relation (except for the two just mentioned). This does not mean that the teeth are "offset" one-to-two like standard bricks in a wall. An individual tooth, a posterior especially, will have most of its occlusal surface in contact with its namesake and adversary in the opposite jaw, *i.e.*, first molar against first molar. There will always be a portion, however, of the occlusal surface left over to contact the tooth next to its main antagonist (Fig. 16–71 and 16–72).

This scheme serves to equalize the forces of impact in occlusion, thereby distributing the work. The arrangement helps in another way to preserve the integrity of

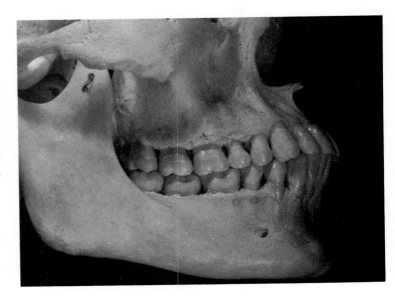

Figure 16–48. View of specimen with normal occlusion from the right side in line with first molars. Note the shadows cast by posterior teeth caused by overjet of maxillary versus mandibular arches. This picture serves as a good example of facial relationships of maxillary and mandibular teeth.

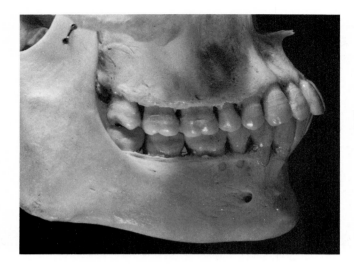

Figure 16–49. Close-up of specimen shown in Fig. 16–48. The lighting was varied for additional study.

the denture: the loss of a tooth in one jaw does not immediately disturb the alignment in the opposing jaw.

Since each tooth has two antagonists, the loss of one still leaves one antagonist remaining which will keep the tooth in occlusal contact with the opposing arch and keep it in its own arch relation at the same time by preventing elongation and displacement through the lack of antagonism. Actually, the loss of one or more teeth ultimately precipitates a gradual disintegration of the occlusal relation of the dental arches unless a prosthetic replacement is made. The permanency of the arch forms depends upon the mutual support of the teeth in contact with each other. The normal tooth arrangement minimizes the loss, however, and serves to resist *immediate* disintegration of the alignment.

When a tooth is lost, the adjoining teeth in the same arch usually migrate in an effort to fill the void. The migration of adjoining teeth disturbs the contact relationships in that vicinity. In the meantime, tooth movement changes occlusal relations with antagonists in opposing dental arches. The common result is elongation of the tooth opposing the space left by the lost tooth. Elongation of one or more teeth in one arch breaks up occlusal contacts in both upper and lower arches over a period of time. This could result in total physical collapse of an entire side of the mouth (Fig. 16–50). The ultimate result, if uninterrupted, would be a gradual breakdown of the whole dental mechanism right and left owing to mechanical and pathologic changes.

The only way to avoid possible premature loss of all of the teeth is to avoid any permanent change in the original normal arrangement of them.

If one of the maxillary central incisors is lost, the mandibular central incisor on the same side is left without an opposing tooth. The same situation exists regarding the maxillary third molar if the mandibular third molar is lost.

The offset arrangement of the teeth, demonstrating one against two (alternating from one dental arch to the other), is attained by an ingenious manipulation of the form and dimensions of each tooth involved (Figs. 16–50, 16–51, and Figs. 16–52 to 16–55).

First the dental arches are composed throughout by teeth in pairs, starting at the median line, one right, one left. Each pair is made up of two teeth alike in form and dimension, but since one is right and the other left, the outline form is reversed from one side to the other to accommodate the situation. Central incisors only are in con-

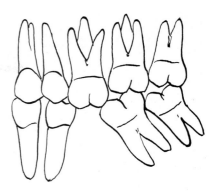

Figure 16–50. This illustration demonstrates a typical clinical picture showing elongation, migration and improper contact and occlusal relation resulting from neglect after the loss of a mandibular first molar.

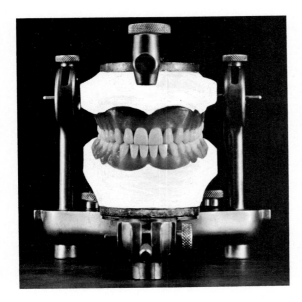

Figure 16–51. Carvings in ivorine of individual teeth set up into complete dental arches on an anatomic articulator (See also Fig. 1–19).

Figure 16–52. Another view of the carving shown in Fig. 16–51.

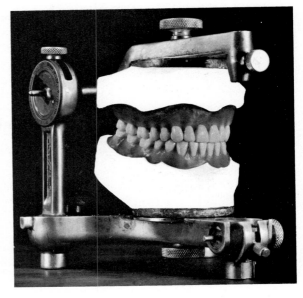

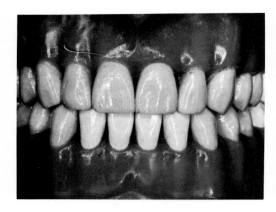

Figure 16–53. *Close-up Views of Carvings Illustrated in Figs. 16–51 and 16–52.*

Labial aspect of the teeth in centric occlusion. This aspect is taken from a position directly in alignment with the median line.

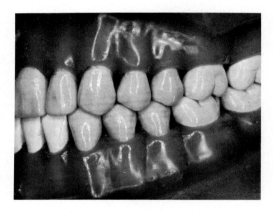

Figure 16–54. Labiobuccal aspect of the teeth in centric occlusion. This aspect is taken from a position directly in line with the labial surface of the maxillary canine.

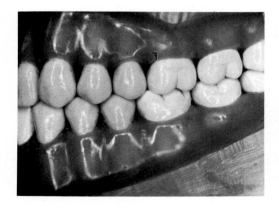

Figure 16–55. Buccal aspect of the teeth in centric occlusion. This aspect is taken from a position directly buccal to the contact of maxillary premolars.

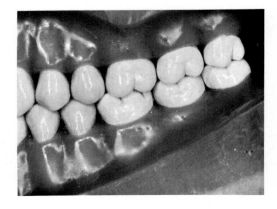

Figure 16–56. Buccal aspect of the teeth in centric occlusion. This aspect is taken from a position directly buccal to the mesiobuccal cusp of the maxillary first molar.

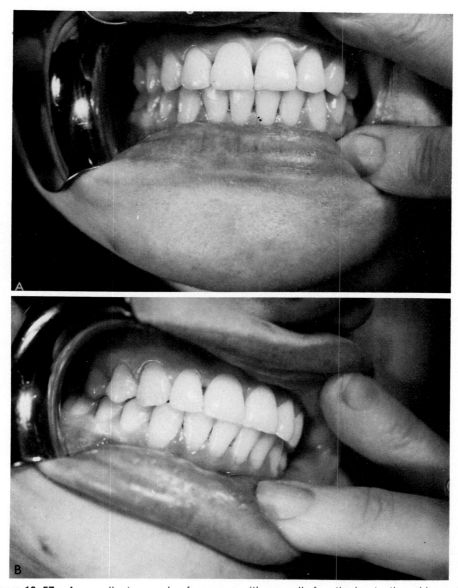

Figure 16–57. An excellent example of a person with normally functioning teeth and jaws. *A.* Centric occlusal relation—frontal view. *B.* Centric relation—lateral view.

tact with each other at the median line; other pairs are divided distal to the centrals and each member of each pair will be to the left or to the right and will be in contact on both of its sides with other members of other pairs. To repeat: the right and left central incisors are together at the median line; right and left lateral incisors are placed distal to them. The lateral incisors will contact central incisors, as well as canines. Right and left canines are distal to lateral incisors, contacting them, as well as first premolars, etc.

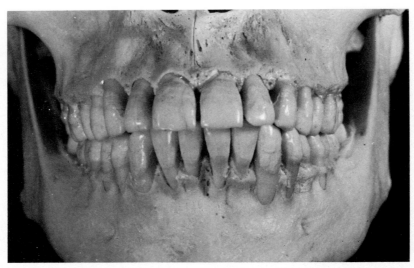

Figure 16-58. A photograph of the model skull taken from a direct view opposite to the median line, and approximately at the occlusal level. This is the same specimen as that shown in Item 6, Figs. 16–59 and 16–60. Other aspects at various levels are to follow this one illustrating normal occlusion. The spacing between the anterior teeth was physiological in character because there was no evidence present in the specimen to suggest the possibility of pathological involvement. It must be remembered that occlusion can be normal and functional without being able to qualify as ideal.

This illustration and photographs to follow will be useful for continuous reference while reading the text on occlusion.

Each arch is symmetrical bilaterally. The division into halves occurs at the median line. Both maxillary and mandibular central incisors are in contact at this point, the only teeth in both arches with contact areas and embrasures directly in line with each other. All the other points of contact with associated embrasures, when located in one arch, are offset mesially or distally from contact and embrasure locations in the opposing arch. The contacts and embrasures of one arch are not equally measured from those in the opposing arch at any one location because of variations in the relative size of teeth.

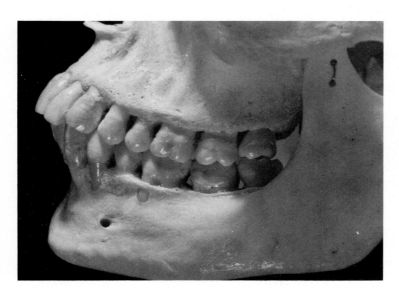

Figure 16-59. This view of the specimen shows the occlusion in centric from the left side opposite the first molars and at the occlusal level of the molars. Note the overjet displayed.

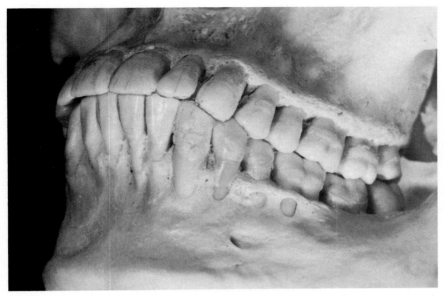

Figure 16–60.   The angle for the photograph is to the left side and considerably below the occlusal level. Some details of occlusal contact that might otherwise escape notice may be observed in this manner. The teeth are in centric relation. Although it is not apparent because of photographic difficulties, there is just as much interdental spacing under the left incisors as that which shows clearly on the right side.

The maxillary arch is larger in outside measurement than the mandibular arch, yet the difference in arch length is slight, the distal margins of maxillary and mandibular third molars appearing almost flush with each other when the teeth are in centric occlusion.

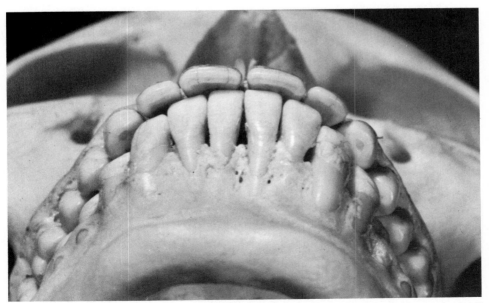

Figure 16–61.   An extreme angle, looking under the incisal edges of maxillary anterior teeth and noting the inter-digitation of all the teeth in view. Take particular note of the overjet of maxillary canines, premolars, and first molars.

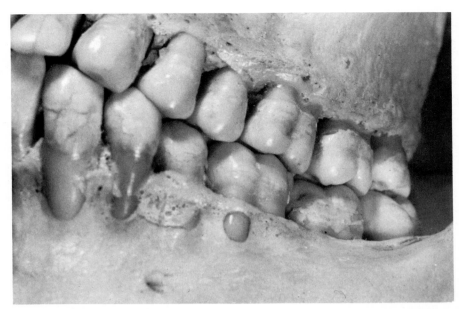

Figure 16–62. Looking at the tooth arrangement and occlusion from a vantage point opposite the mandibular canine and first premolar. Discounting the mandibular central incisor and the maxillary third molar, each tooth in one dental arch will contact two teeth in the opposing arch. This contact, however, is not evenly divided between teeth. The major portion occlusally of each *molar* or *premolar* will be in contact mainly with its namesake in the opposite jaw (See also Figs. 16–71 and 16–72).

The mandibular arch is narrower when calibrated at the buccal surfaces of posterior teeth than is the maxillary arch. This relation is brought about by the differences in mesiodistal width between mandibular and maxillary anterior teeth (particularly the incisors) and by the lingual projection of mandibular posterior tooth crowns, an arrangement which brings about proper intercuspation.

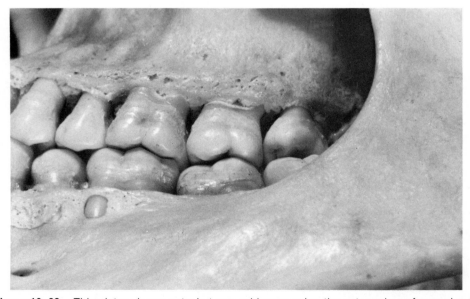

Figure 16–63. This picture bears out what was said concerning the antagonism of opposing teeth. It also shows in a very graphic way the occlusal contact system of posterior teeth creating escapement spaces even after reaching the terminus of centric relation. This specimen continues to demonstrate the system even though the teeth are worn considerably. Earlier in life this individual would have shown more elaborate free space in centric relation.

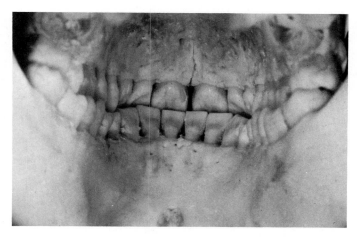

Figure 16–64. Lingual views of the teeth in centric relation. A view in line with the suture of the maxillae showing no evidences of periodontal destruction of bone around the anterior teeth. These teeth show the wear of usage, but in centric with good jaw support posteriorly, the anteriors are at rest with some interdental spacing.

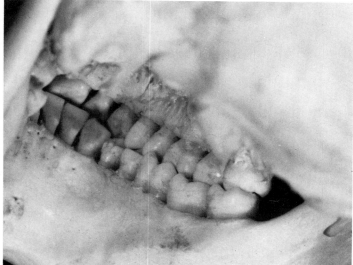

Figure 16–65. Another view of the teeth from the lingual anteriorly and to the right. Again, the abrasion of anterior teeth would indicate that they have not avoided work. Although they seem to be free of contact when jaws are closed in centric relation, a slight protrusion of the mandible upon opening would activate these teeth as incisors. The relationship of anterior vs. posterior teeth as depicted here might serve as an indicator of treatment advisable in clinical cases. Treatment should endeavor to relieve anterior teeth so that they do not have to assume the responsibility for jaw support.

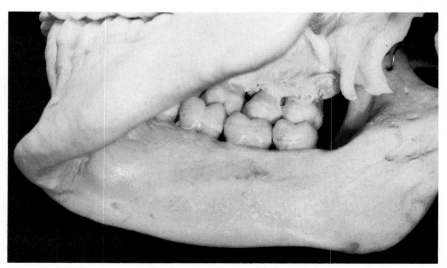

Figure 16–66. An unusual picture taken at a most advantageous angle, which serves to emphasize the value of molars as the intended jaw supporters and the guide to normal occlusion. The molars have the advantage of form, structure, anchorage and placement (See also Fig. 16–29).

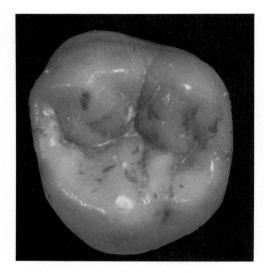

Figure 16–67.   Natural occlusal third surface of maxillary second molar. The occlusal surface contour illustrated here is a good example of the irregular contour of cusps and ridges to be found on all maxillary molars.

Note rounded cusp tips and cusp ridges; also note the rounded and turned "triangular" ridges folding into the generous central fossa and into the smaller mesial and distal fossae as well.

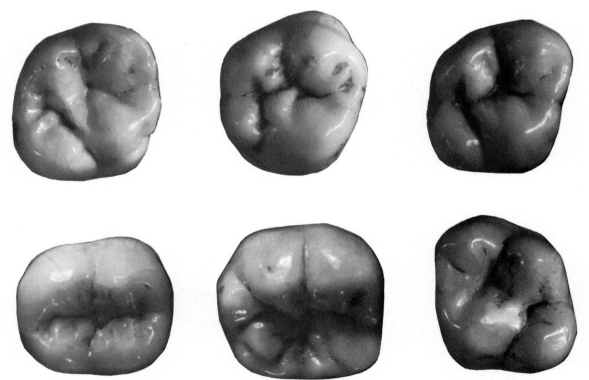

Figure 16–68.   Occlusal aspects of several fine specimens of molars. These teeth suggest the possibility that during development, the smooth contoured enamel was "folded" into the developmental grooves.

It is quite apparent that rounded contours and cusp formations of similar design will strike opposing teeth with like surfaces in points and constricted areas only.

No flat surfaces are to be found on occlusal third portions of posterior teeth unless they are caused by wear or accident.

The normal limits on occluding surfaces are illustrated. The registration of all occlusal contacts, including centric relation, should be held within these limitations in order to establish physiological activity.

7. THE OCCLUSAL CONTACT AND INTERCUSP RELATIONS OF ALL THE TEETH OF ONE ARCH WITH THOSE IN THE OPPOSING ARCH IN CENTRIC OCCLUSION (Figs. 16–71 and 16–72)

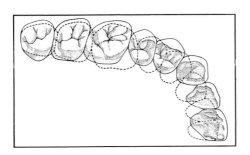

Item 7, on occlusal contact and intercusp relations, is the most difficult section to study, and also the most difficult one to illustrate. However, it must be kept in mind that the knowledge acquired in the study of this item has practical application in any phase of daily practice. It might be said that a working knowledge of occlusal contact and intercusp relations of both dental arches in centric occlusion is the final summation of what one has learned about occlusion (Fig. 16–47).

Centric occlusal relation, when development of the entire dental mechanism has been normal, is the terminus of occlusal movement. When the teeth of both jaws come together in centric relation, forces have been equalized so that the teeth are stabilized by all the forces operating favorably toward them. Details were discussed previously in this chapter under the heading, "Eight Items Which Must Be Included In The Study Of Occlusion" (Fig. 16–6). When jaws are closed and the two dental arches are brought together in definite centric relations, the teeth are said to be in the *physical rest position.* When the muscles of mastication are relaxed, the jaws may seem closed but actually the teeth are not in contact. This jaw relation is called the *physiologic rest position,* but the teeth are not involved.

Item 7 is by far the most intricate section in the study of occlusion. Item 8, though complicated, when explained illustrates the adaptation of the tooth form *to* and *from* centric relation during the various occlusal movements. Every detail of Item 7 must be recognized in order to have an understanding of *all* occlusal problems. The terminus of physiologic jaw movement is always *centric relation.*

In order to obtain a clear understanding of occlusal contacts and the inter-relations of the cusps of teeth in centric occlusion, the surfaces involved must be observed from three points of view; facially, lingually and occlusally.

The apposition of occlusal surfaces from facial and lingual aspects was explained in Item 6. The study of occlusal surfaces of the teeth and their design for service has to be accomplished with the arches separated. A partial perspective of the true state of affairs when jaws are closed may be observed by superimposing outlines of the occlusal surfaces of one dental arch over those of the opposing arch, charting the points of contact and the cusp relationships (Figs. 16–71 and 16–72).

PHASES IN THE DEVELOPMENT OF THE DENTAL ARCHES

The written word even though accompanied by good two-dimensional illustrations, is deficient when dealing with a subject that is clearly three dimensional in character. Therefore one who is conscientious about learning all of the aspects of three-dimensional occlusion will lose no time in applying this study to good skull specimens or at least to good casts of teeth made from impressions of normal mouths. Even more instructional would be to compare mouth examinations with casts of the same individuals.

A well-established truism states that the occlusal relationship of the mandibular and maxillary first permanent molars marks the key to other occlusal patterns in the permanent dentition. In describing that relationship it is taken for granted in the study that the development of the teeth and jaws has been normal; that the teeth are truly anatomical dimensionally; and that normal development has permitted their placement in proper relation to one another.

First molar relations are observed foremost because they are so important developmentally. They lead in the eruption sequence, taking their places immediately posterior to the second deciduous molars and apparently using them as a guide to determine their proper places in the developing jaws. (See Phase 1, page 420.) The mandibular molar erupts first and the maxillary molar moves down against it to establish the *initial occlusal relation of the permanent dentition.*

If the first molars attain proper occlusal contact and intercusping relations, and if the jaw development cooperates and is normal, the teeth erupting anterior to the first molars can come into proper alignment in due time, and molars posterior to them will find their proper places also. The ultimate result should be *normal placement and occlusion of all of the teeth of both jaws.*

Before a description of the details of occlusal apposition is made, certain fundamentals in occlusal relations between maxillary and mandibular teeth must be established in the mind.

The background for study should be the realization that occlusion, dental maintenance, and even jaw relations are established by the molars and premolars. The canines certainly help in providing anchorage anteriorly, but they, along with the incisors, have simpler occlusal relations than posteriors, and as a consequence were never expected to assume the responsibility of jaw support.

An observation often overlooked is that each premolar or molar tooth is in contact mainly with its namesake in the opposite jaw in unworn teeth (first molar to first molar, etc.) (Fig. 16–71). Especially is this true of the lingual portions of maxillary teeth and the buccal portions of mandibular teeth. This is difficult for the uninitiated in dental physiology to understand, because labial and buccal views of the teeth in occlusion impress them as being offset to one another rather evenly (Figs. 16–51 and 16–52).

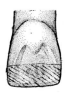   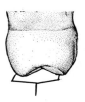 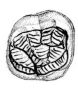

Figure 16–69. Maxillary teeth.

Figure 16-70. Mandibular teeth.

The location and the limitation of occlusal apposition depends upon the type of tooth being considered (incisors, premolars, maxillary or mandibular, etc.) (Figs. 16–69 and 16–70).

A mental picture to be acquired is one depicting the way mandibular and maxil-

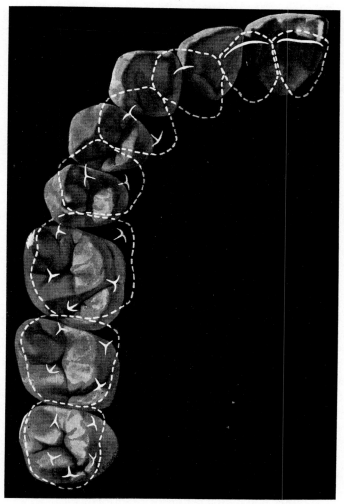

Figure 16-71. Contact relation of human teeth—maxillary teeth with dotted lines of mandibular teeth superimposed in occlusion. Heavy lines and T's within dotted outlines denote incisal ridges and summits of cusps. (Courtesy of Sheldon Friel, Dublin.)

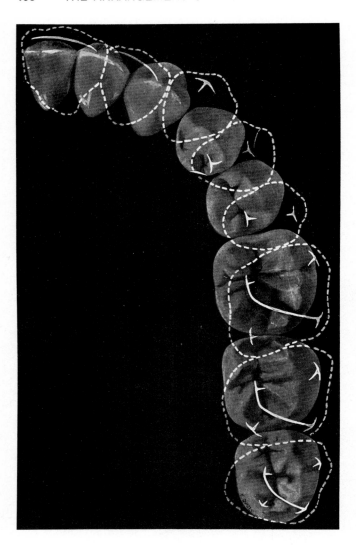

Figure 16–72. Contact relation of human teeth—mandibular teeth; with dotted lines of maxillary teeth superimposed in occlusion. Note the slanted heavy lines of maxillary molars which mark the shape and location of oblique ridges. (Courtesy of Sheldon Friel, Dublin.)

lary posterior teeth differ when a comparison is made between the respective forms of crowns and their alignment with root bases (Fig. 16–73).

Maxillary and mandibular posteriors differ from each other anatomically but each includes a certain fundamental form which through cooperation they share in use. In each case the portion to be in contact with its antagonist is placed squarely on the root base. This conforms to good principles of engineering by directing forces in line with the anchorage. This remarkable crown design arranges for the intercuspation of the *lower buccal working portion* into the *centralized intercusp portion of the upper* without cusp interference, keeping the forces in line with root bases at the same time.

Hard contact registrations when opposing teeth meet are important in the study of occlusion, but they do not complete the picture of *physiologic occlusion*.

The occlusal process makes use of other functional tooth form besides the constricted areas of enamel which complete the final punching and cutting operation. Actually, the *major* portion of areas of the occlusal third of opposing teeth never register

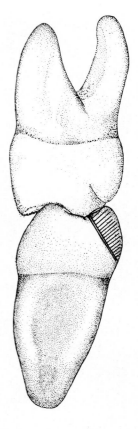

Figure 16–73. First molars in occlusion. The shaded portion representing the lingual cusps are out of occlusal contact on all mandibular posterior teeth, especially during lateral movements. The distolingual cusps of the second premolar and those of all mandibular molars are often in partial contact in centric, but even then the tip portions of the cusps are usually free.

After removing the cusp in this manner, the remaining part of the functioning tooth bears a close resemblance to the mandibular premolar form with buccolingual measurement increased. The lingual cusps out of contact function by broadening the "food table" during mastication.

actual contact. Escapement form includes spacing in sulci, fossae, cusp tips, crown form creating embrasures, etc.

Therefore the old methods of describing occlusal relations by emphasizing planes and points of contact will be discarded. Following suggestions made many years ago by Friel, the technique of description will be borrowed from Gregory and Hellman as told in their reports on comparative anatomy and paleontology.

Their plan in describing occlusion of the teeth was to list the prospective occluding surfaces into the following divisions:

A. Surface contact
B. Cusp and fossa contact
C. Ridge and embrasure contact
D. Ridge and groove contact

It must be remembered that when this listing was made (50 or more years ago), the investigators were primarily interested in descriptions of functional form and development and not in the details required for dental treatment or restoration.

Since the purpose of this book is to focus on the latter activities, the author has taken the liberty of adding to the above list some minor changes in nomenclature that are intended to be of assistance in understanding the detailed description. The listing of the occluding parts will help in describing centric relation and "eccentric" occlusal relations as well when Item 8, which follows, is covered.

The list, as it was changed for the purpose at hand, is as follows:

A. Interocclusal offset relationship of opposing teeth

B. Surface contact
C. Cusp and fossa apposition
D. Cusp and embrasure apposition
E. Ridge and sulcus apposition. (Includes ridge and developmental groove apposition.)

An earlier statement bears repeating, and that is that all occlusal apposition (including its effect on jaw relations) is affected and supported by the posterior teeth. The inter-relationship of premolars and molars is quite involved and will require the major portion of the description under the above headings.

Figures and legends featuring landmarks on posterior teeth are to be repeated for use in ready reference during the reading (Fig. 16–71, Fig. 16–75, Figs. 16–76 and 16–77). Many illustrations have been added for reference also, including close-up photographs of specimen teeth in occlusion (Figs. 16–80 through 16–89). It would be well to emphasize again the unyielding, hard, rounded surfaces to be seen everywhere on the occlusal "working surfaces" of the teeth (Figs. 16–67 and 16–68).

Interocclusal Offset Relationship of Opposing Teeth

This subject was discussed at length under Item 6. To summarize: each premolar or molar tooth is in contact mainly with its namesake in the opposite jaw in unworn teeth. (First molar to first molar, etc. See Fig. 16–71.)

Surface Contact

This category assumes the contact of flattened or essentially level surfaces. These occlusal surfaces are found at *incisal portions* of *mandibular anteriors* which become functional when they come into contact with the *lingual surfaces* of *maxillary anterior teeth*. However, even these contacting areas exhibit some curvature (Figs. 16–69 and 16–70).

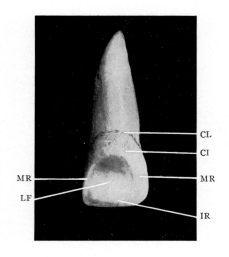

Figure 16–74. Maxillary right central incisor (lingual aspect). *CL,* Cervical line; *CI,* cingulum; *MR,* marginal ridge; *IR,* incisal ridge; *LF,* lingual fossa.

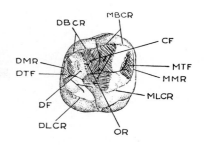

Figure 16–75. Maxillary right first molar—occlusal landmarks. *MBCR,* Mesiobuccal cusp ridge; *CF,* central fossa (shaded area); *MTF,* mesial triangular fossa (shaded area); *MMR,* mesial marginal ridge; *MLCR,* mesiolingual cusp ridge; *OR,* oblique ridge; *DLCR,* distolingual cusp ridge; *DF,* distal fossa; *DTF,* distal triangular fossa (shaded area); *DMR,* distal marginal ridge; *DBCR,* distobuccal cusp ridge.

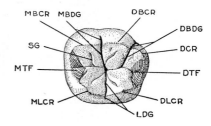

Figure 16–76. Mandibular right first molar—occlusal aspect. *DBCR,* Distobuccal cusp ridge; *DBDG,* distobuccal developmental groove; *DCR,* distal cusp ridge; *DTF,* distal triangular fossa (shaded area); *DLCR,* distolingual cusp ridge; *LDG,* lingual developmental groove; *MLCR,* mesiolingual cusp ridge; *MTF,* mesial triangular fossa (shaded area); *SG,* a supplemental groove; *MBCR,* mesiobuccal cusp ridge; *MBDG,* mesiobuccal developmental groove.

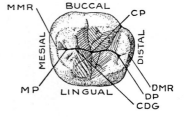

Figure 16–77. Mandibular right first molar—occlusal aspect. Shaded area—central fossa; *CP,* central pit; *DMR,* distal marginal ridge; *DP,* distal pit; *CDG,* central developmental groove; *MP,* mesial pit; *MMR,* mesial marginal ridge.

Cusp and Fossa Apposition

The outstanding examples under this heading are the massive and pointed mesiolingual cusp portions of the maxillary molars that fit into the major fossae of lower molars in centric relation. This occlusal design is not only useful in the act of chewing; it is most effective as a stabilizer of alignment because of the way the cusps "key into" the fossae. The manner in which these parts fit together in centric relation is more important than the relationship of buccal cusps of maxillary molars to buccal grooves of mandibular molars. The latter has always been the key to the initial observations on normal alignment (Figs. 16–81, 16–81, A and 16–82, A).

The position of first molars in apposition to each other is regarded as the key to occlusion. This statement might be qualified even further; the key to occlusion might very well be dependent upon the placement of the mesiolingual cusp of the maxillary first molar into the central fossa of the mandibular first molar (Figs. 16–81 *C,* and 16–82 *A*).

The distolingual cusps of maxillary molars are in apposition to the distal triangular fossae and marginal ridge of mandibular molars and often to the mesial marginal ridge of the molar distal to their namesakes. (Maxillary first molar distolingual cusp to mesial of mandibular second molar, etc.) (Fig. 16–79).

Another *cusp-fossa* relationship to be noted is the contact of relatively sharp lingual cusps of *maxillary premolars* with triangular fossae of *mandibular premolars.*

(*Text continued on page 474.*)

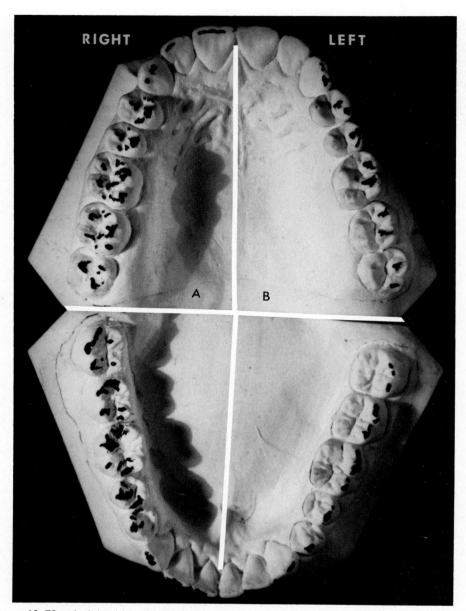

Figure 16–78.   *A,* right side, and *B,* left side. This is a photograph of the casts of the individual shown in Fig. 16–108 and 16–115. *LLOR,* Left lateral occlusal relation in contrast with *RCOR,* right centric occlusal relation. In any lateral relation the occlusal contacts are reduced markedly. Black spots represent the markings of occlusal contacts. (See also, pages 502, 503.)

Figure 16–79.   An interesting approach which is designed to illustrate proportional contact in centric occlusal relation.

The occlusal aspect of one half of the mandibular arch of the carved reproduction shown in Fig. 16–52 is displayed. These carvings were designed to show "ideal" normal relationships, including centric relation.

It was thought that the study of centric relation could be simplified if the mind of the viewer was not burdened by an overall picture which would be difficult to grasp before certain details were explained. Therefore, two figures are presented that show mesial and distal outlines only of opposing teeth with cusp tip markings included within the outlines of each tooth.

The study is made even more graphic by separating the tooth outlines to illustrate the contact relations of every other maxillary tooth with free space between that shows no contact. This portrayal requires two figures.

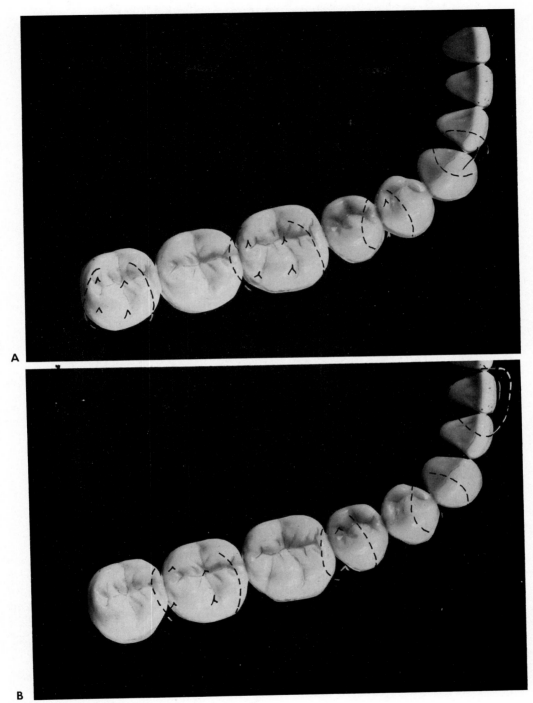

Fig. 16–79. *Continued.*

A. The study should begin with the mesial and distal borders of the *maxillary first molar* with its cusp tip markings. The first molar relationship affects dental arch alignment during development and should continue to have an important role in occlusion in later years.

The *other* maxillary tooth outlines shown here are the *laterial incisor*, the *first premolar*, and the *third molar.*

B. This picture shows the mesial and distal outlines with cusp tip markings of the following maxillary teeth: *Central incisor, canine, second premolar, second molar.*

A   B

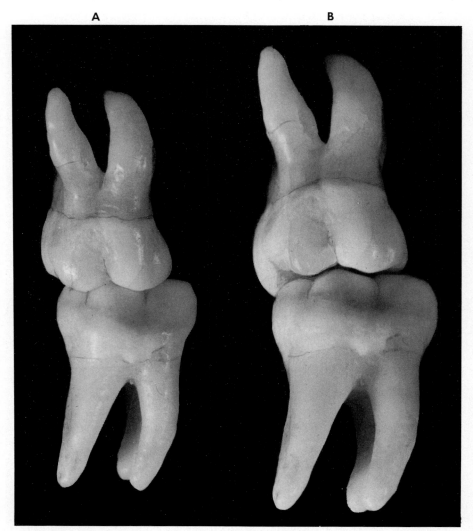

Figure 16–80. *First Molars in Centric Occlusal Relation.*

Because the first molars are instrumental in establishing occlusal relations anterior to them—and posterior to them as well—their study should receive special attention in order to facilitate understanding of the fundamentals of occlusion generally.

Here are four unusual photographs of natural first molars placed in occlusal relations.

A. This view is at right angles to facial portions about level with occlusal surfaces. This is the classic view, giving the impression (held by most observers) of the mesiobuccal cusp of the maxillary molar fitting snugly into the sulcus of the mesiobuccal groove of the mandibular first molar.

B. The combination has been tipped so that one is able to peer under the buccal cusps of the maxillary molar. It is apparent that the triangular ridge of the mesiobuccal cusp is slightly distal to the groove mentioned previously.

(*Illustration continued on opposite page.*)

This association is not as stable as the association of molar contacts just described, because the fossa areas are shallow. Just the same, this relationship of cusp to tooth is an important feature of good alignment (Fig. 16–86, *A*).

The *cusp-fossa* apposition, including the *buccal cusps* of *mandibular posterior teeth,* follows:

The *mesiobuccal* cusps of *mandibular molars* are in apposition to the distal fossa,

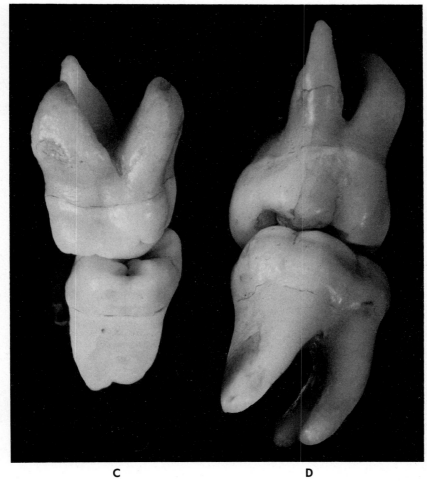

C   D

Figure 16–80. *Continued.*

C. This view is directly mesial to the combination and considerably above the level of the occlusal surface of the mandibular molar. Note the escapement provided by the tooth form of the crowns when in centric relation.

D. A perspective view from an odd angle that portrays the efficiency of the occlusal form of the molars.

The rounded folds of ridges and cusp forms contact opposing teeth without rigid interlocking. This formation permits some adjustment in alignment without trauma. Yet the cusp-fossa and ridge-sulcus arrangement still fits well enough to promote stability.

or the marginal ridge bordering it, of the tooth above, mesial to its namesake (first molar mandibular to distal of second maxillary premolar, etc.).

The *distobuccal cusps* of *mandibular molars* are accommodated by the central fossae of their namesakes in the opposite jaw.

The *buccal cusp point* of the *second mandibular premolar* approaches the *mesial occlusal fossa* of the *opposing second premolar*, while the *first mandibular premolar* occludes partly with the *first premolar* above and partly with the *maxillary canine* (Fig. 16–85, *A, B* and *C*).

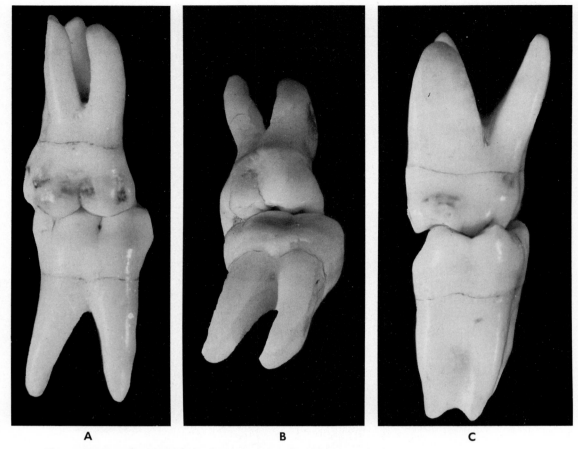

Figure 16–81. *Occlusion of First Molars in Centric Relation.*

A. The arrangement of first molars in centric relation usually accepted as normal. Actually the arrangement of this traditional relationship is not what it should be; the close contact of the mesiobuccal cusp of the maxillary molar, with its triangular ridge centered in the mesiobuccal groove of the mandibular molar, would hamper escapement and would not allow for proper angulation during lateral jaw movements.

B. The first molars arranged in a more ideal relation than that of *A.* The view is looking up under the buccal cusps of the maxillary molar with the two teeth posed in the proper relation for efficiency. Note the distal relationship of the mesiobuccal cusp and its triangular ridge of the maxillary molar with the mesiobuccal developmental groove of the mandibular molar. The distobuccal cusp and triangular ridge of the maxillary molar have a distal relationship with the distobuccal developmental groove of the mandibular molar. Note that there is some open space created for escapement purposes.

Since these are right first molars, a right lateral occlusal movement of the jaw would aim the triangular ridges of the buccal cusps of the maxillary first molar toward the sulci of the mesial and distal developmental grooves between the buccal cusps of the mandibular first molar. Lateral occlusal movements are oblique in relation to buccal surfaces of molars (Fig. 16–93).

C. A view from the mesial showing the first molars in centric relation. Note the freedom of the tip of the mesiobuccal cusp of the maxillary molar; the close apposition of the mesiobuccal cusp of the mandibular molar to the marginal ridge of the maxillary molar; the entire mesiolingual cusp of the mandibular molar is out of contact; and even the tip of the distolingual cusp of the mandibular first molar lacks contact.

Cusp and Embrasure Apposition

Under this heading some description is made that is often omitted when defining normal occlusion in centric relation. Some *cusp points* are actually *opposed* to *embrasure spaces.* Other cusps are in partial contact with marginal and cusp ridges, in

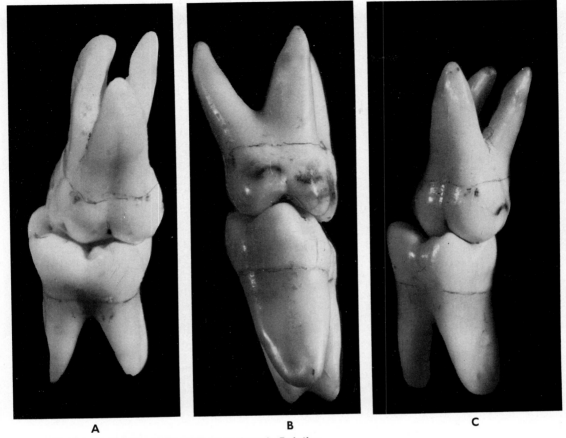

A   B   C

Figure 16–82. *Occlusion of First Molars in Centric Relation.*

    A. Above and lingual to occlusal surface of mandibular first molar. Relation of the two teeth showing considerable escapement mesially—close adaptation distally near the distal marginal ridge of the maxillary molar.
    B. Articulation of the first molars distally. Note the close adaptation of the distolingual cusp of the maxillary molar to the distolingual and distal cusps of the mandibular molar. Also note the lack of contact of the distobuccal cusp of the upper molar, creating escapement space. Lateral relation of the jaw would put the upper molar triangular ridge of the distobuccal cusp in contact.
    C. Distolingual view of first molars in centric relation. Compare this aspect with *A.* Note the spacing which has opened up mesially and the close adaptation of the distolingual cusp of the upper molar with the distal marginal ridge and the distal cusp of the lower molar. The distolingual cusp of the mandibular molar opposes the lingual sulcus of the lingual developmental groove.

    addition to straddling the embrasure spaces created by the ridges. (Study Figures 16–71 and 16–72 and Figures 16–80 through 16–89, which show specimen teeth articulated in centric relation.)
    Outstanding examples of cusps out of hard contact and in apposition with embrasure space, while in centric occlusal relation, may be listed as follows:
    Mesiolingual cusp—all mandibular molars (Figs. 16–71, 16–89)
    Distobuccal cusp—maxillary first molar; second molar sometimes (Fig. 16–82)
    Lingual cusp—mandibular first premolar (Figs. 16–71, 16–86)
    Mesiolingual cusp—mandibular second premolar (Figs. 16–72, 16–86)
    Buccal cusp tips—both maxillary premolars (Figs. 16–72, 16–85)

A   B   C

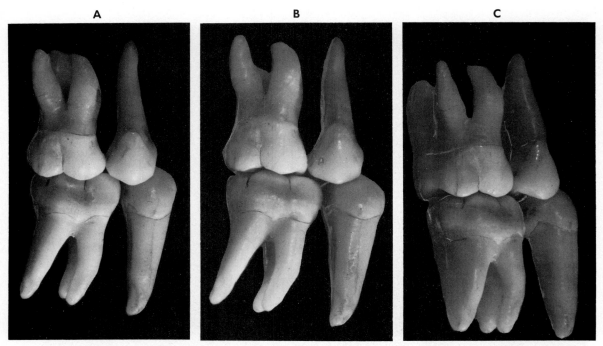

Figure 16–83. The specimens shown in occlusal contact in centric relation are second premolars and first molars, maxillary and mandibular. They were photographed from the buccal aspect.

A. The sighting of the aspect is about 90°, with the buccal surfaces of the molars approximately level with the tips of the buccal cusps of the mandibular teeth.

B. Without changing occlusal relations the specimens were tipped so the view was directed somewhat under the maxillary teeth occlusally. Note the actual distal relationship of cusp tips and triangular ridges of the maxillary molar to the buccal developmental grooves of the mandibular molar. This relationship was not apparent in *A.*

C. From the viewpoint farther distally, the cusp tips and grooves seem to be more in line with each other. Note the lack of occlusal contact in some areas that promotes escapement by creating free space even in centric relation.

The maxillary canine cusp must be included because this canine has to be aligned with the maxillary posterior teeth in order to complete the picture of all posterior teeth in occlusion (Fig. 16–85).

The embrasure spaces these free cusps approach are given the names of tooth combinations which form the space (*buccal embrasure, first* and *second mandibular molar,* etc.).

Ridge and Sulcus Apposition

A short reminder of the parts under discussion: *"triangular" ridges,* a continuation of prominently formed enamel which extends from cusp tips toward the center of occlusal surfaces, usually ending in fossae or developmental grooves (Figs. 16–75 through 16–77).

Sulci are linear depressions between these enamel ridges with developmental grooves at the bottom of the enamel valleys; the grooves extend at times on to buccal and lingual surfaces.

The main ridge and sulcus occlusion which dominates discussion is that of the triangular ridges of the buccal cusps of maxillary molars as they are accommodated into buccal grooves with their sulci in mandibular molars (Figs. 16–75, 16–80).

Another important combination is that of the triangular ridge of the distolingual

A   B   C

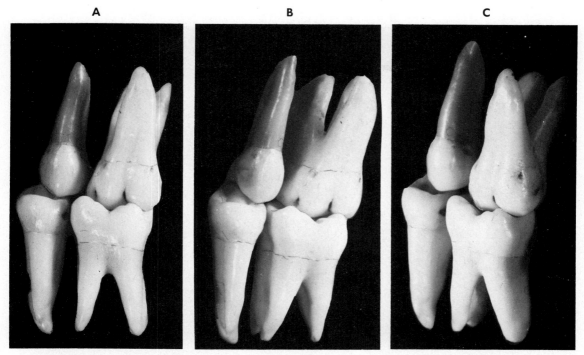

Figure 16–84.   The specimens shown in occlusal contact include the maxillary second premolar and first molar and the mandibular second premolar and first molar.

A. The teeth were posed so that the view was almost directly opposite the lingual surface of the maxillary molar. The occlusal relationship of first molars here is interesting, as it is assisted by the inclusion of second premolars.

B. Compare *B* with *A* and notice how a slight change in angle clarifies the study. The view is now almost from directly opposite the mandibular premolar and from slightly above its occlusal surface. Note particularly the cusp-fossa relationship.

C. This is a distolingual view with the occlusal relationship comparable to *B*. Note how escapement spacing varies and cusp relations are clarified when the teeth are studied from more than one aspect.

cusp of the mandibular first molar as it fits into the lingual groove sulcus of the maxillary first molar (Fig. 16–82, *C*).

The ridge and sulcus contact of note that is significant in lateral occlusal movements, as well as in centric relation, is the *oblique transverse ridge* of the *maxillary first molar*, a triangular ridge extending obliquely from the distobuccal cusp to the mesiolingual cusp. This ridge fits into the sulcus formed on the occlusal surface of the mandibular first molar, marked by the junction of *distobuccal, central,* and *lingual developmental grooves. Normally, the direction the oblique ridge of the maxillary tooth takes in sliding through the angled sulcus of the mandibular molar governs the angle at which mandibular posterior teeth cross and contact the maxillary teeth during lateral movements in mastication* (Fig. 16–93).

Taking these most important ridge-sulcus listings as starting points, it is possible to formulate many other combinations if a complete and ideal picture of occlusion is desired.

Hellman listed 138 points of possible occlusal contacts to be observed and tabulated in a complete description of occlusion. The tabulation included thirty-two teeth. The list of points is as follows:

a. Lingual surfaces of upper incisors and canines.. 6
b. Labial surfaces of lower incisors and canines 6
c. Triangular ridges of upper buccal cusps of premolars and molars................ 16
d. Triangular ridges of lingual cusps of lower premolars and molars............... 16

A

B

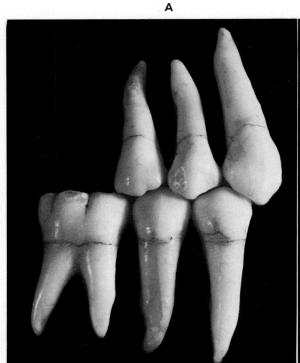

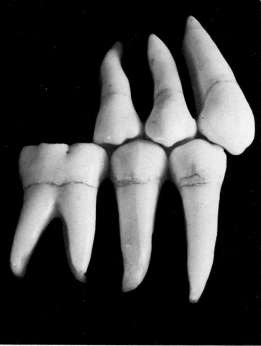

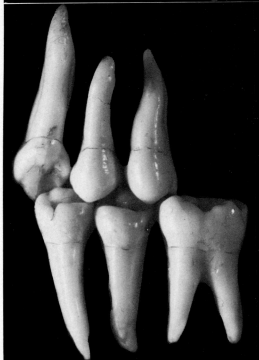

C

Figure 16–85. Natural tooth specimens set up to show occlusal relations. The teeth displayed include the maxillary canine, the maxillary first and second premolars; the mandibular first and second premolars and the first molar.

A. View at right angles to facial surfaces. This is the typical aspect made in occlusal studies that gives the impression of surfaces fitting rather tightly together with little apparent open relief.

B. The arrangement was tipped so the camera was allowed to see under the facial cusps of maxillary teeth. Note the point contact effect in occlusion of lowers with marginal ridge areas of uppers and the creation of escapement spaces.

C. A distolingual view of the same arrangement of teeth as seen in *A* and *B*. This view is often neglected in studies of occlusion. It illustrates occlusal contact and emphasizes the additional escapement space created by the tooth form lingually.

A   B

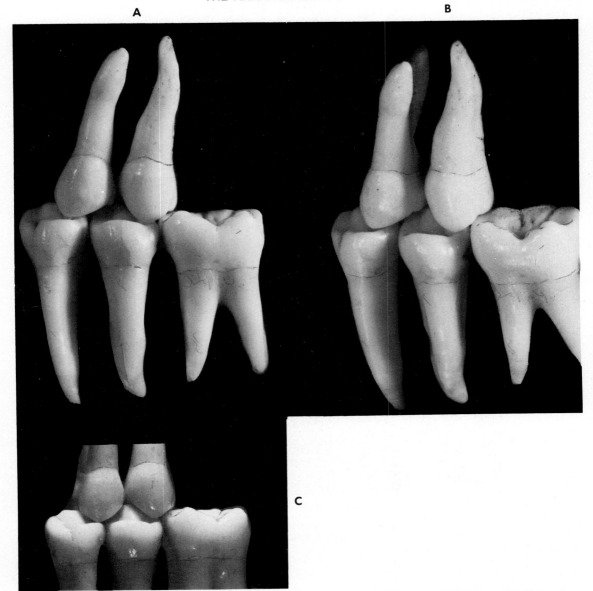

C

Figure 16–86.   The photos of specimen teeth are made from four separate angulations lingually. The specimen teeth show the occlusal relations of maxillary premolars in contact with mandibular premolars and first molar.
    A. Viewed from directly opposite the lingual surface of the mandibular second premolar; the viewer is to make his own analysis.
    B. A view of the occlusal relations taken distolingually above the occlusal surfaces of the mandibular teeth. Note particularly the occlusal contact of the lingual cusps of the maxillary premolars.
    C. The picture of the crowns exclusively may be compared with *A;* there is a slight variation in angle and lighting.

e. Buccal embrasure of lower premolars and molars 8
f. Lingual embrasures of upper premolars and molars (including the canine and first premolar embrasure accommodating the lower premolar).................... 10
g. Lingual cusp points of upper premolars and molars................................. 16
h. Buccal cusp points of lower premolars and molars.................................... 16
i. Distal fossae of premolars... 8
j. Central fossae of the molars 12
k. Mesial fossae of the lower molars 6

A   B

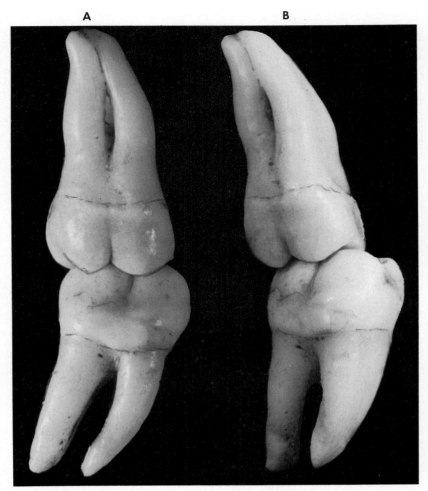

Figure 16–87. *The Apposition of Second Molars in Occlusion.*

A. Occluded in centric relation. Note the variation in cusp design between the two molars. The maxillary molar has a relatively small distobuccal cusp, whereas the mandibular molar distobuccal cusp development is featured.

B. The angle usually displayed when looking at second molar articulation. The molars appear to be fitted together very closely, which is actually not the case.

(Illustration continued on opposite page.)

l.	Distal fossae of the upper molars	6
m.	Lingual grooves of the upper molars	6
n.	Buccal grooves of the lower molars *	6
	Total	138

Therefore if a complete description without the omission of any detail of ideal occlusion is desired, close scrutiny of a good skull or cast showing thirty-two teeth would make possible a list of all ridge-sulcus combinations, all cusp embrasure combinations, and so on. Usually, if the combinations of points that have been mentioned in the last few pages can be established, some details, such as the approximate location of hard contact in occlusion, are automatic.

---

* Hellman did not list the distobuccal groove of the lower first molar, possibly because it is normally out of occlusal contact.

C   D

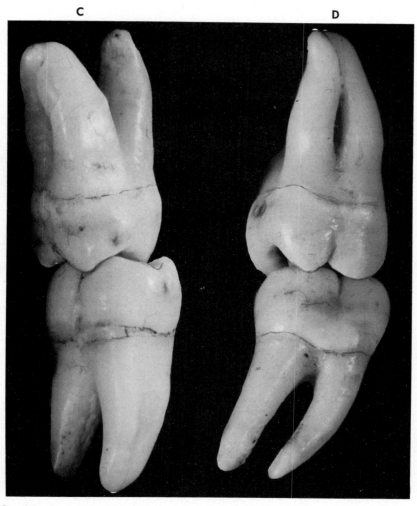

Figure 16–87. *Continued.*
  C. A change in angulation with the specimens in the same relationship as in *B.* From this slight change of view some spacing is apparent.
  D. An odd angle was obtained by lifting the maxillary molar buccal cusps ever so slightly, and aiming the camera up under its occlusal anatomy. In this way the "potential" of occlusal contact and escapement may be observed.

  The remarkable funtional form of the occlusal portions of the posterior teeth permits adjustment in angulation and alignment without loss of function when it is found necessary in individual cases. Consequently, it is very unlikely that two individuals will be found who have identical markings on the occlusal surfaces when occlusal registrations are made clinically. Nevertheless, these markings need to be located within certain limits occlusally, determined by the functional form of the teeth (architecture) and by their alignment and periodontal attachment (foundation).
  Because there can be variations in the actual placement and quality of markings, it is only necessary to realize the apposition of parts of opposing teeth in occlusion when describing the activity taking place. At the same time, one must be able to notice any straying of contacts beyond the normal limitations. These details were discussed in this chapter under Item 5. There will be no further attempt to locate circumscribed occlusal contacts as having to conform to any one design.

(*Text continued on page 486.*)

A   B

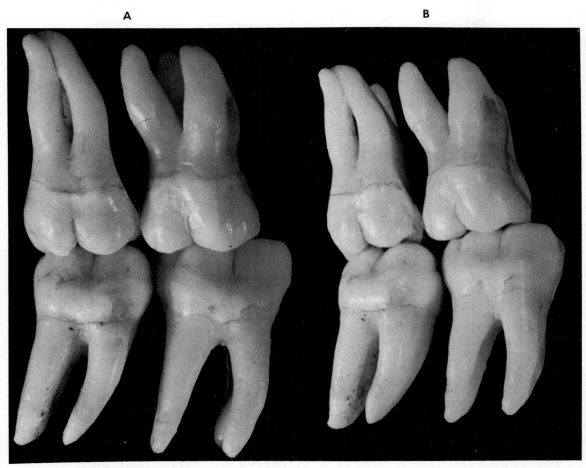

Figure 16–88. These photos of specimen teeth include maxillary first and second molars and mandibular first and second molars as they might appear in centric relation.

A. This view shows the teeth from directly opposite the mandibular first molar. The mesiobuccal cusp of the maxillary first molar appears to be directly above the mesiobuccal developmental groove of the mandibular first molar. The same arrangement seems to be comparable in second molar relations. Note the liberal escapement space showing over proximal contact areas.

B. Compare this view with *A*. The combination was tipped so that it was possible to make comparisons by looking underneath the buccal cusps of the maxillary molars. Spacing is opening up, hard contact may be seen, and it will be noticed that although triangular ridges of cusps are located within sulci, they do not fit down in tight formation against developmental grooves.

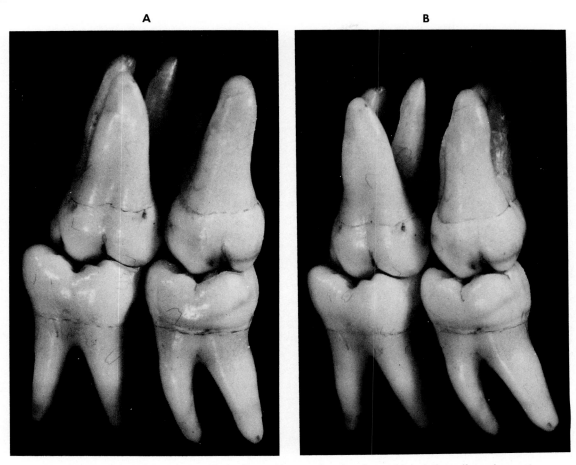

Figure 16–89.   Maxillary and mandibular first and second molars in centric relation—lingual aspect.
    A. This view of the lingual aspect was taken from slightly distal and above the occlusal surfaces of the mandibular teeth.
    Note the relationship of cusps to fossae. Mesiolingual cusps of mandibular molars are entirely free. Although distolingual cusps of all the molars are in contact, the very tip ends of the mandibular cusps are free.
    The lingual views of molars in centric relation display a greater degree of escapement design than any other aspect.
    B. A more extreme camera angle for comparison with *A.*

8. THE OCCLUSAL CONTACT AND INTERCUSP RELATIONS OF ALL THE TEETH DURING THE VARIOUS FUNCTIONAL MANDIBULAR MOVEMENTS

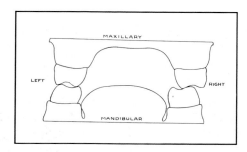

Centric occlusal relation, just described, is the terminus of all functional jaw movements. Rarely, however, is the jaw opened from centric relation and closed in centric with a perfectly straight hinge movement. The normal activity of the mandible is a rotating movement to the right or left before a return to centric relation, or a forward movement and return. These masticatory movements of the mandible are named as follows:

1. Right lateral movement
2. Left lateral movement
3. Protrusive movement

Each of these movements is but part of a cycle which has *centric relation as starting point and terminus.*

Therefore the functional occlusal contact relation of the teeth of one arch with those of the other have been named according to the relative position of the mandible which governs the relations. They are:

1. Centric occlusal relation
2. Right lateral occlusal relation
3. Left lateral occlusal relation
4. Protrusive occlusal relation

Although the mandible is capable of extreme extensions out of range of dental relations when it relaxes toward functional dental occlusal relations the extent of the movement of mandibular teeth over their opponents in the maxillary arch is rather limited. Therefore *the physiologic form of the teeth, their alignment and their anchorage are concerned with final short arcs of movement only, near the terminus of centric relation.*

During the *right lateral movement,* the mandible is depressed and the dental arches are separated, the jaw moves to the right and brings the teeth together at points to the right of centric relation, called *right lateral occlusal relation.* The return movement bears left, sliding the teeth over each other until centric relation is re-established (Figs. 16–90 and 16–91).

The *left lateral movement* is similar, except that the initial action is to the left, causing the teeth to come into contact in a *left lateral occlusal relation,* and the return movement to centric bears right.

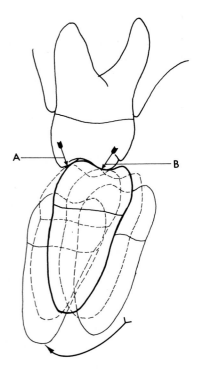

Figure 16–90. The cycle of occlusal movements, represented by a schematic drawing of first molar relations—mesial aspect. The heavy outline of the mandibular molar represents it to be in centric occlusal relation with the maxillary molar. The shadow outlines represent the mandibular molar in various relations during the cycle of mandibular movement during mastication. The two short arrows, *A* and *B*, at right angles to the occlusal surface of the maxillary molar, measure the extent of movement between them over the occlusal surface from the first contact of the mandibular molar to the last contact before continuing another cycle.

During the *protrusive movement,* the mandible is depressed, then moves directly forward, bringing the anterior teeth together at points most favorable for the incision of food. After contact has been established, the jaw is retruded, returning to centric occlusion. Protrusive movement is followed by a retrusive movement to centric (Fig. 16–114).

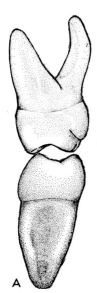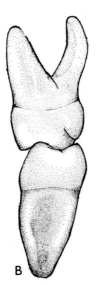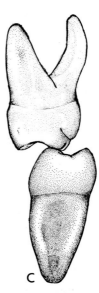

Figure 16–91. Occlusal relations of first molars during the cycle of occlusal movements (See also Fig. 16–90). *A,* Initial occlusal contact in right lateral occlusal relation. *B,* Centric occlusal relation. *C,* Final contact after leaving centric relation before the mandible drops away to begin another cycle. This is also the balancing contact for the left lateral occlusal relation.

It is possible to retrude the mandible to a point slightly posterior to centric relation, dependent entirely upon the compressibility of the soft tissues posterior to the condyle heads. Since this places the teeth in a nonfunctional occlusal relation, *retrusive relation* is not considered to be a physiologic occlusal relation.

To repeat: The range of movement of the mandible may appear quite extensive while one is watching the complete displacement during lateral excursions, but, from the time the opposing teeth come into contact, the extent of movement of the mandibular teeth over the maxillary teeth is very limited.

The teeth do not mill together from side to side in the manner of small millstones.

The rolling and rounded occlusal surfaces come into contact during a rotary movement of the mandible with a cutting thrust as the teeth approach centric relation; then there is a momentary *mortar and pestle* action in a narrow range before the mandibular teeth drop away to begin another excursion.

The compensating curvature of the dental arches is intended to achieve *occlusal balance* throughout the range of mandibular movements. Occlusal balance is apparently a definite part of the plan in occlusion of the teeth, but ideal occlusal balance as anatomists conceive it is rare. Nevertheless, many people may be found who have teeth in good alignment and occlusion, passing all of the requirements necessary for efficient performance including some balancing of occlusal contacts.

Occlusal balance is achieved when one section of the arch is supported by one or more other sections, each section having *some contact* simultaneously. The more nearly these sections are opposite one another in the arches, the more nearly perfect the balance. As an example, if the molars on one side of the jaws are at some point of occlusal contact during lateral mandibular movement, the occlusion is balanced by simultaneous contact at some points in the molar areas on the opposite side of the jaws. If, at the same moment on the balancing side, additional contact is made in the canine and premolar area, the balance is improved. During the return to centric occlusion, a rapid assumption of efficient cooperation by respective dental units favors balanced support for that person (Figs. 16–78 and 16–110).

When the mandible is making a protrusive movement during the incisive action of the anterior teeth, good balance requires simultaneous contact of some posterior teeth on each side at the moment the anterior teeth make actual contact; some balancing contacts on each side should be maintained until centric relation is re-established.

LATERAL OCCLUSAL RELATIONS OF THE TEETH

When the mandibular teeth make their initial contact with the maxillary teeth in right or left lateral occlusal relation, they bear a right or left lateral relation to centric position. The canines, premolars and molars of one side of the *mandible* make their occlusal contact facial (labial or buccal) to their facial cusp ridges at some portion of their occlusal thirds (Fig. 16–78, LLOR). Those points on the mandibular teeth make contact with *maxillary* teeth at points just lingual to their facial cusp ridges. The central and lateral incisors of the working side are not usually in contact at the same time; if they are, the labioincisal portions of the mandibular teeth of that side are in contact with the linguoincisal portions of the maxillary teeth.

During the sliding contact action, from the most facial contact points to centric relation, the teeth intercuspate and slide over each other in a *directional line approximately parallel with the oblique ridge of the upper first molar* (Fig. 16–93). The combined sulci of the distobuccal and lingual developmental grooves of the occlusal surface of the *mandibular* first molar are counter in form generally to the oblique ridge of

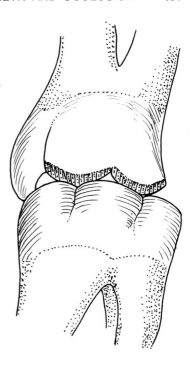

Figure 16–92. First molars in centric relation, demonstrating escapement. The camera approach was at an odd angle while photographing specimens which served as models for this drawing. (See Fig. 16–80D.) The drawing represents a maxillary first molar with the buccal surface ground away to the level of occlusal contact with the mandibular first molar. It shows escapement space occlusally where the two teeth do not touch. Even where triangular ridges of buccal cusps are in contact, they do not fit tightly into the bucco-occlusal developmental grooves of the mandibular molar, nor are they shaped and pointed for that purpose.

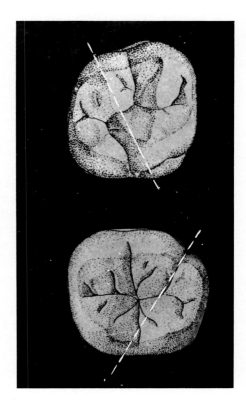

Figure 16–93. Drawings of the occlusal surfaces of the first molars, showing the directional path traveled by the teeth during lateral occlusal movements. The path follows the general direction of the alignment of the oblique ridge of the maxillary first molar and the occlusal sulci of the distobuccal and lingual developmental grooves of the mandibular first molar. Straight lines were drawn to emphasize the angulation. Actually, the sulcus formation in the lower molar is shaded to show the accommodation of the curved transverse ridge of the upper molar.

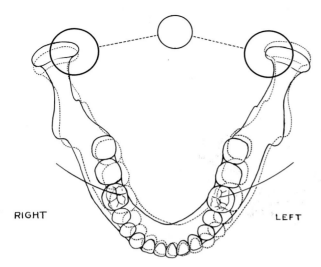

RIGHT   LEFT

Figure 16–94. Tracing of actual photograph of a mandible (from Fig. 16–2) taken from a point directly above the first molar. The heavy outline denotes centric occlusal relation; the dotted outline denotes the approximate position of the mandible during left lateral occlusal relation. The dotted outline represents a tracing which was superimposed over the other drawing in centric relation, then rotated in such a manner that the *heavy arc lines to central fossae of first molars,* of both the drawings, *were kept in the same arc of rotation.* The pivotal center of the first molars is somewhere within the area of the small circle between, and posterior to, the condyles. The pivotal center of either condyle in right or left lateral relation is somewhere within the circles drawn over the medial portion of the condyles. Evidently all points on the mandible or on the teeth move in concentric circular motions which make it difficult if not impossible to locate pivotal points in single planes.

the *maxillary* first molar. The sulci and ridge fit together loosely, the sulci encompassing the ridge during the lateral occlusal movement somewhat in line with the oblique ridge longitudinally (Figs. 16–72, 16–93 and 16–94).

From the foregoing it is evident that the *mandibular teeth do not ride over the maxillary teeth at right angles to the buccal surfaces but at an acute angle to them.*

At this point the reader should have his three-dimensional model of occlusion at hand in order properly to study the subsequent details of tooth relations during the mandibular movements.

As the teeth of one side move from lateral relation to centric relation, the cusps and ridges bear a certain relationship to each other; the cusps and ridges (including marginal ridges) of the canines and posterior teeth of the *mandibular* arch have an ·intercusping relationship to the cusps and ridges of the teeth of the *maxillary* arch. The crowns of the teeth are formed in such a way that cusps and ridges may slide over each other without mutual interference. In addition, the crowns of the teeth are "turned" on the root bases to accommodate the angled movement across their opponents (Fig. 16–95).

The cusp tip of the mandibular canine moves through the linguoincisal embrasure of the maxillary lateral incisor and canine. The cusp tip is often in contact with one of the marginal ridges making up the lingual embrasure above it. Its mesial cusp ridge is usually out of contact during the lateral movement. Its distal cusp ridge contacts the mesial cusp ridge of the maxillary canine.

The cusp tip of the mandibular first premolar moves through the occlusal embrasure of the maxillary canine and first premolar (Figs. 16–96 and 16–97). Its mesiobuccal ridge contacts the distal cusp ridge of the maxillary canine, its distobuccal cusp ridge the mesio-occlusal slope of the buccal cusp of the maxillary first premolar.

The mandibular second premolar buccal cusp tip moves through the occlusal embrasure and then over the linguo-occlusal embrasure of the maxillary first and second premolars. Its mesiobuccal cusp ridge contacts the disto-occlusal slope of the buccal cusp of the maxillary first premolar, its distobuccal cusp ridge the mesio-occlusal slope of the buccal cusp of the upper second premolar.

The lingual cusps of all premolars are out of contact until centric relation is attained. Then the only lingual cusps in contact are those of the maxillary premolars,

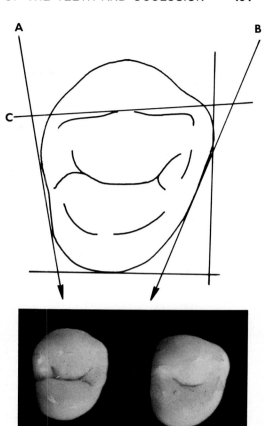

Figure 16–95. An outline of the occlusal aspect of the right maxillary first premolar with its distal and lingual surfaces surveyed by a right angle disto-lingually (see Figure 9–14).

A. A line following the angulation of the mesial surface is not too far removed from parallelism with the vertical line of the right angle distally. This formation allows a proper contact relationship with the distal proximal surface of the maxillary canine; simultaneously it cooperates with the canine in keeping the lingual embrasure design within normal limitations.

B. Line B demonstrates a more extreme angulation of the distal portion of the first premolar. This form allows cusp and ridge by-pass by mandibular teeth over the distal marginal ridge surface of the maxillary tooth with normal jaw movements during lateral occlusal relations.

C. Line C, aligned with mesiobuccal and distobuccal line angles, demonstrates the adaptation of the form of the buccal surface of the crown to dental arch form without changing the functional position of crown and root.

D. Two natural specimens of the maxillary right first premolar that display similar characteristics when compared to the accented drawing above them.

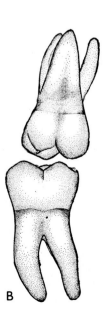

D

Figure 16–96. Cusps and cusp ridges, embrasures, and so forth, bear an interrelationship to each other. *A,* Mandibular first premolar relation to maxillary canine and first premolar on the verge of occlusal contact. Lingual aspect. *B,* Mandibular first molar relation to the maxillary first molar on the verge of occlusal contact. Lingual aspect.

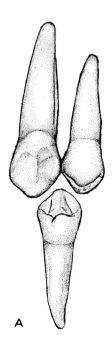

A

B

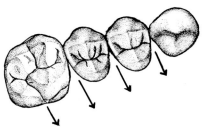

Figure 16–97. Assembly of the maxillary canine, first and second premolars and the first molar as they appear in the maxillary arch. The arrows indicate the direction of movement of the mandibular teeth over the maxillary teeth during the masticatory cycle. The major embrasures of canines and premolars are above marginal ridges occlusally. The arrows are on a line approximately parallel to the oblique ridge of the maxillary first molar.

with the possible addition of the distolingual cusp of a mandibular second premolar of the three-cusp type (Fig. 16–84, *B*).

The molars have a more involved *lateral occlusal relation* because of their more complex design. Their *occlusal form* and their *other occlusal relations* have been described in detail under Items 5, 6 and 7.

It has been determined previously, while describing the lateral occlusal relations of canines and premolars, that cusps, cusp ridges, sulci, and embrasures bear an interrelationship to each other. Cusps and elevations on the teeth of one arch pass between or over cusps and through embrasures or sulci. The tooth form and the alignment of the opposing teeth of both jaws make this possible. The cusps of the teeth of one jaw simply do not ride up and down the cusp slopes of the teeth in the opposing jaw. This explanation of the occlusal process has created wide misunderstanding.

The misconception at fault was the creation of the term "planes of occlusion," locating them on occlusal surfaces as real entities. Flat planes on the occlusal surfaces of posterior teeth would limit their adaptability and their function during developmental years and on to the time of maturation of all dental tissues. The cusp, ridge, fossa and embrasure form of occlusion allow interdigitation without a "locked-in" effect. There is no clashing of cusp against cusp or any interference between parts of the occlusal surfaces if the development is proper (Figs. 16–92 and 16–96).

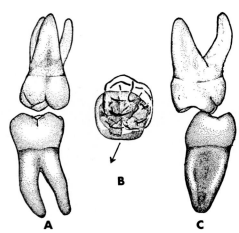

Figure 16–98. *A*, Maxillary and mandibular first molars as they are related just before contact during the occlusal cycle. *B*, Shadowed maxillary molar superimposed over the mandibular molar in the relation they bear to each other in centric relation contact. *C*, The final contact relation upon completion of the occlusal cycle.

A DESCRIPTION OF THE OCCLUSAL CYCLE IN THE MOLAR AREAS DURING RIGHT OR LEFT LATERAL OCCLUSAL RELATIONS

In lateral movements during mastication (*Bennett movements*), the mandible drops downward and to the right or left of centric relation. As it continues the cycle of movement and returns toward centric relation, the bucco-occlusal portions of mandibular molars come into contact with the occlusal portions of the maxillary molars lingual to the summits of buccal cusps and in contact with their triangular ridges of the slopes on each side of them, continuing the sliding contact until centric relation is accomplished (Figs. 16–90 and 16–91).

From these first contacts the mandibular molars slide into centric relation with maxillary molars, coming to a momentary rest following a mortar and pestle action.

The movement continues with occlusal surfaces in sliding contact until the linguo-occlusal slopes of the buccal portions of the mandibular molars pass the final points of contact with the linguo-occlusal slopes of the lingual portions of the maxillary molars (Fig. 16–90). When the molars lose contact, the mandible drops away in a circular movement to begin another cycle of lateral jaw movement (Fig. 16–91).

The actual distance traveled by mandibular molars in contact across the occlusal surfaces of maxillary molars, from first contacts to final contacts at separation, is very short, probably not more than 3 to 5 mm. in most instances. The measurement on the maxillary molars from first to final contact may at times be a little more than this, but it must be noted that the first contacts on lower molars, buccal to the summits of buccal cusps, have final contact lingual to the same summits. The lower molars, which are the moving antagonists, are taken out of contact before the first contact location on their buccal cusps reaches the final points of contact on the maxillary molars. (Compare A and C in Fig. 16–91.)

Maxillary molars will measure buccolingually from cusp tip to cusp tip a little more than half (on the average) their buccolingual overall measurement. The crown of a large molar will calibrate no more than 14 mm. buccolingually. Its occlusal surfaces from cusp tip to cusp tip would measure about 8 mm. Therefore, with large molars to be taken as examples, the distance from contact to contact against the occlusal surfaces of maxillary molars during lateral jaw movements would approximate 5 mm. only (Fig. 16–90).

When the complications in the plan of occlusion are discussed in detail, it should convince any serious-minded investigator that the physiologic form of the individual tooth in each dental arch must be recognized as an important link in the chain of occlusion. There are no unimportant units.

MECHANISM OF MASTICATION

During the masticatory process, the individual chews on one side only at any one chewing stroke. Most of the work is done by shifting material from one side to the other when convenient; the shifting is confined generally to the molar and premolar regions. Occasionally, for specific reasons the shift of mastication may be directed anteriorly. Nevertheless, the posterior teeth, of right or left side, are depended upon by the host to do the major portion of the work of mastication. The posteriors are aided, of course, in various ways by the canines; but the latter do not possess the broad occlusal surfaces required for chewing efficiency overall.

The food is manipulated by the tongue, lips and cheeks so that it is thrown between the teeth continuously during the mandibular movements which bring the

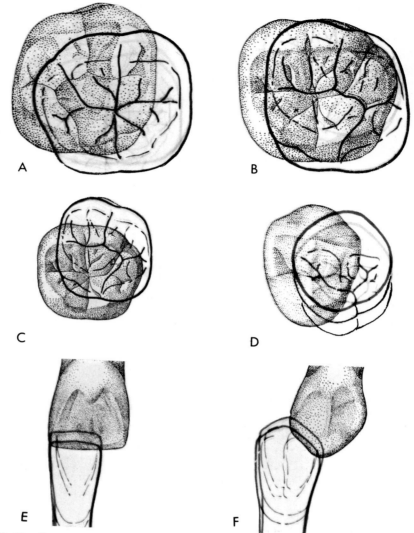

Figure 16–99. Illustrations made by superimposition of outlines over rendered drawings, attempting to show occlusal relations between some maxillary and mandibular teeth.

A. The relation between first molars when the mandibular first molar (outline) contacts the maxillary first molar in a lateral relation.

Note the alignment of the oblique ridge of the maxillary first molar with the distobuccal groove of the mandibular molar.

B. This illustration reverses the example in *A.* The outline is maxillary over the mandibular rendered drawing. The effect is that of looking through a transparent occlusal surface of the maxillary first molar as the mandibular molar strikes it underneath in lateral relation. This is equivalent to example *A.*

C. Maxillary first molar over mandibular first molar in centric relation.

D. This example attempts to show occlusal movement. The completed outline of the mandibular first premolar has its buccal cusp tip inside the mesiobuccal cusp ridge of the maxillary first premolar and on or slightly distal to the mesial marginal ridge. That contact represents the extreme lateral relation.

The "double lines" lingually represent movement in that direction. The first one (center) represents the lingual surface position in centric relation and the second and last outline shows the position of the lingual surface of the mandibular tooth in relation to the maxillary premolar in the balancing occlusal relation.

E. The shadow outline of the mandibular central incisor is superimposed over the rendered drawing of the maxillary central incisor. When incisal edges are in contact, the representation is that of central incisors in protrusive relation. In centric relation the mandibular central will approach the maxillary tooth higher up on its lingual surface.

F. Canine occlusal relations. Lateral relation is represented by cusp ridges in contact. The lingual slope of the mesial cusp ridge of the maxillary canine is in contact with the labial slope of the distal cusp ridge of the mandibular canine. In centric relation the same cusp ridges are involved, but the contact is higher on the maxillary canine.

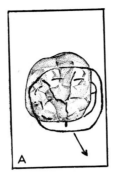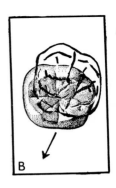

Figure 16–100. Shadow drawings of opposing first molars superimposed so that centric relation may be studied in detail. The arrows show the angle at which the *mandibular* molar crosses over the *maxillary* molar in a lingual direction during *lateral occlusal movements. A,* Centric relation of mandibular first molar to maxillary first molar. *B,* Centric relation of maxillary first molar to mandibular first molar.

teeth together in their various relations. To repeat: the major portion of the work is accomplished in the *premolar* and *molar* regions, while the mandible is making right lateral and left lateral movements, bringing the teeth into right lateral and left lateral occlusal relation, terminating the strokes in centric relation.

Most people enjoy a tactile sense in their teeth and this enables them to place the mandibular teeth into a contact relationship which promotes efficiency during mastication. It is admitted, however, that ordinarily the masticatory act is carried on subconsciously.

When a bolus of material is placed between the teeth, it separates mandibular and maxillary teeth on both sides of the jaws. When the material is penetrated there is occlusal contact on the *working side;* when the contact is operative on that side,

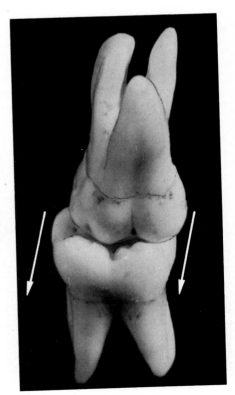

Figure 16–101. Natural specimens of first permanent molars related as they would be in centric occlusion. The view is directly opposite the lingual aspect of the mandibular molar, sighted above the level of its occlusal surface. Actually the viewer is looking down on the whole combination from the lingual aspect.

The arrows indicate the angle at which the lower molar slides over the upper during the lateral occlusal relation. Apparently the line of direction is parallel to or in line with the oblique ridge of the occlusal surface of the maxillary molar. (See also Fig. 16–93.)

occlusal balance requires some occlusal contact on the opposite side. In technical parlance, this activity indicates cooperation of the *balancing side* with the *working side*.

Without this bilateral contact, produced simultaneously on both sides of the jaws, traumatic stresses are created. The single bow-like bone of the mandible with its two joints of attachment would suffer through torsion produced by the lack of balance. It is true that imbalance during jaw activity can produce discomfort, as well as pathologic change.

OCCLUSAL CONTACT AND OCCLUSAL BALANCE

Dental arches in good alignment and occlusion will show a balanced situation during right and left lateral occlusal relations (Fig. 16–111). The occlusion may be considered normal and effective and still fail to be "ideal." Investigation will show that an effective "setup" possesses certain fundamental physiologic requisites. (More of this subject will follow in a discussion of occlusal requisites in a summary concluding Chapter 16.) Because of the possibility of misunderstandings in a discussion of this complicated subject, some repetition may be acceptable in explaining occlusal values.

Good occlusal balance should register as follows: when the buccal cusps of the posterior teeth of both jaws on one side (the right side, for instance), achieve their initial contact in their extreme lateral relation, there is a balancing relationship on the opposite side (the left side in this instance). The balancing contacts on the left side are the *linguo-occlusal* slopes of the *buccal cusps* of *mandibular teeth* in balancing contact with the *linguo-occlusal* slopes of *lingual cusps* of *maxillary teeth*. The return to centric relation during this masticatory cycle proceeds immediately (Figs. 16–107 and 16–108).

In cases which may be classified as normal, occlusal balance is present, but all of the teeth supposedly involved may not take part according to plan, especially on the balancing side. Apparently, perfection is not a requirement, as long as the balancing side furnishes enough occlusal contact, especially molar contact, to avoid torsion of the mandible. The pathologic result could be traumatic symptoms in the temporomandibular joints and occlusal trauma in the teeth themselves.

The molars make the best balancers because of their size, anchorage and location. They are placed closer than others to the rotation points of the mandible, and this location posteriorly indicates their choice as being better able to withstand the forces of the powerful muscles of mastication (Figs. 16–65 and 16–66).

(Text continued on page 500.)

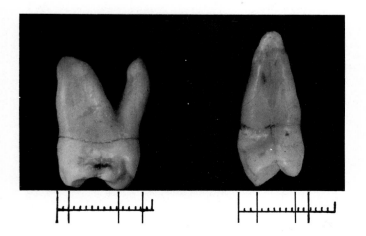

Figure 16–102. Photographs of specimen teeth with calibrations below, showing the relationship between the buccolingual calibration of the posterior tooth crowns and the measurements from cusp tip to cusp tip occlusally. The calibrations in millimeters of maxillary posteriors will always exhibit the following approximation: the measurement from cusp tip to cusp tip buccolingually will be a trifle more than half the calibration of the crown buccolingually. (See Figs. 9–9 and 11–13).

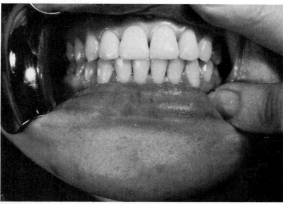

Figure 16–103. Centric occlusal relation—anterior view.

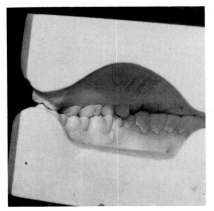

Figure 16–104. Centric occlusal relation—lateral view.

Figure 16–105. Casts of the person's teeth shown in Figs. 16–103 and 16–104. Centric occlusal relation—right side.

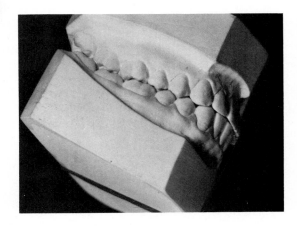

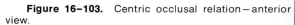

Figure 16–106. Looking at the casts from the lingual on the left, one may see normal intercusping in centric fashion.

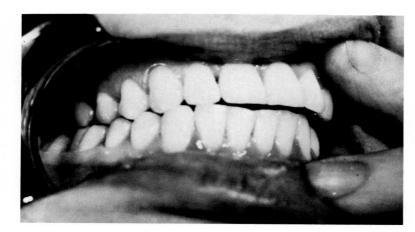

Figure 16–107. Right lateral occlusal relation. Balancing contacts on the left side shown in a cast of the individual in Fig. 16–108.

Figure 16–108. Balancing contacts on the left side shown from the lingual aspect. The casts were made from accurate impressions of the teeth shown in Fig. 16–107.

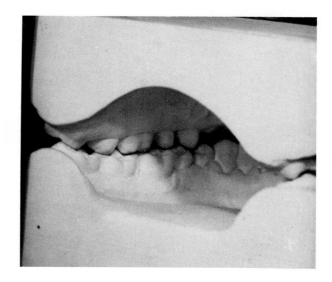

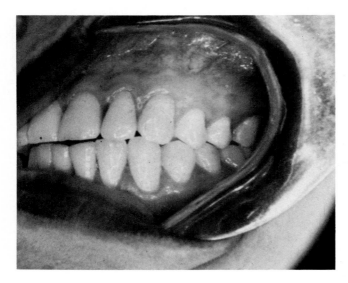

Figure 16–109. Left lateral occlusal relation. The left lateral incisor was not in contact as it seems in the photograph. Note the contact posteriorly including the canine. Incisors should be out of contact in a normal lateral occlusal relation.

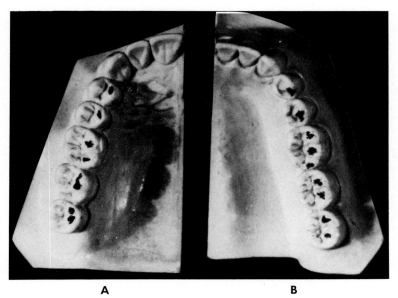

A   B

Figure 16–110.   The spotted contacts on lingual cusps of right maxillary teeth and the buccal cusps of right mandibular teeth represent the approximate balancing contacts for the left lateral occlusal relation. *A.* Right maxillary teeth. *B.* Right mandibular teeth. Associate these balancing occlusal contacts with the illustration of the left lateral occlusal relation in Fig. 16–111.

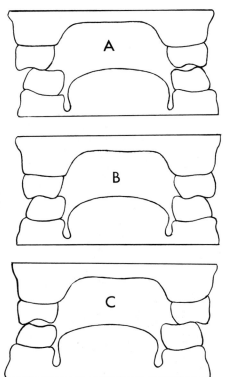

Figure 16–111.   Schematic drawing of posterior view of molars. *A,* Right lateral occlusal relation. *B,* Centric occlusal relation. *C,* Left lateral occlusal relation.

THE OCCLUSAL CYCLE OF THE POSTERIOR TEETH WITH THEIR CANINES: A SUMMARY

The occlusal cycle of the posterior teeth, accompanied by the canines during the right and left lateral occlusal relations, with balancing contacts to be looked for, may be summarized as follows:

1. There are right lateral and left lateral relations to be observed, depending on which is to be called the working side.
2. If the right side is the working side, the first occlusal contact is said to put the teeth in right lateral occlusal relation. Buccal cusps of the posterior teeth of both jaws will be in contact, including some contact of canine to canine on the working side (Figs. 16–107 and 16–116). The balancing contacts on the left side are buccal cusps of mandibular teeth against lingual cusps of maxillary teeth (Fig. 16–108).
3. From right lateral relation the teeth slide into centric occlusal relation, and this relationship includes both the right and the left sides (Fig. 16–111, *B*).
4. Left lateral occlusal relation will be a duplication of the description above for right lateral relation, except for substitution of the word *left* where the term *right* was used and vice versa (Figs. 16–109, 16–110 and 16–111, *C*).
5. From left lateral relation the teeth return to centric relation, the occlusal terminus (Fig. 16–111, *B*. See also Figs. 16–103 to 16–106).

PROTRUSIVE OCCLUSAL RELATIONS OF THE TEETH

The process of *biting* or *shearing* food material is negotiated by the *protrusive occlusal relation.*

Although the mandible may be lowered considerably in producing a wide opening of the mouth, the occlusion of the anterior teeth is not concerned with any arrangement very far removed from centric relation.

When the jaw is opened and moved straight forward to the normal protrusive

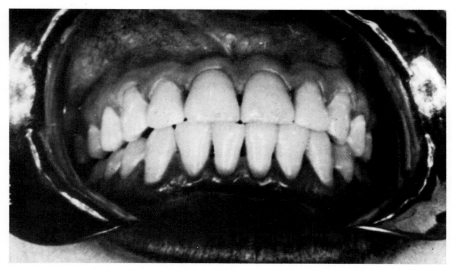

Figure 16–112.   Protrusive occlusal relation. Anterior view of natural teeth.

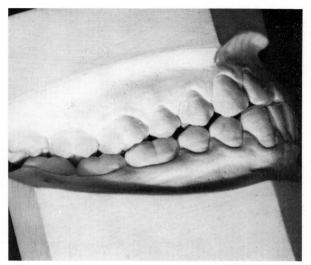

Figure 16–113. Protrusive occlusal relation. Lateral view of all of the teeth of one side as shown by a cast of the individual in Fig. 16–112.

relation, the mandibular arch bears a forward, or anterior, relation of only 1 or 2 mm. in most cases to its centric relation with the maxillary arch (Fig. 16–114).

The protrusive occlusal relation places the labioincisal areas of the incisal ridges of the mandibular incisors in contact with the linguoincisal areas of the incisal portions of the maxillary incisors. The mesiolabial portion of the mesial cusp ridge of the mandibular canine should be in contact with the maxillary lateral incisors distolinguoincisally.

As soon as food has been penetrated during the incisive movement, the anterior teeth come into contact in the protrusive occlusal relation which has just been noted. At the same moment occlusal balance requires occlusal contact of the posterior teeth. The buccal cusps of posterior teeth furnish the balancing contacts posteriorly, although rarely does one find all of the posterior teeth co-operating in protrusive balance. Naturally, in the occlusal balance requirement during protrusion, the mandibular posterior teeth are placed anteriorly to their centric relation with the maxillary posterior teeth.

(*Text continued on page 505.*)

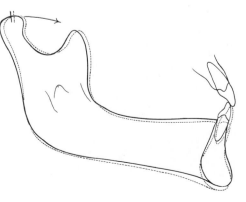

Figure 16–114. Outline tracing of the left portion of a human mandible sectioned at the median line. The maxillary central incisor is also outlined. The unbroken outlines illustrate the central incisors in centric occlusal relation. The broken outline illustrates the approximate relation of the central incisors and the mandible in protrusive relation. Note the relative positions of the condyle, the coronoid process and the body of the mandible on the two outline drawings.

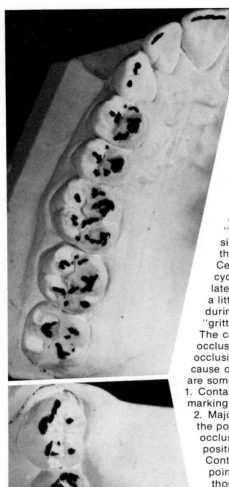

Figure 16–115.   Enlarged photo of the right side of casts shown in Fig. 16–78. The accurate casts show occlusal markings as they were registered on the right side of the mouth of the person shown in Figs. 16–103 and 16–104.

The occlusal markings to be seen at left are registrations of "hard contact" during centric occlusal relation. It must be remembered that markings for a completed centric relation are registered during a full cycle of movement. Therefore, the markings for extreme lateral relation buccally will be included and so will markings showing their relationship to occlusal balance at the end of the chewing cycle (Fig. 16–117C).

The breadth of the markings shown here is greater than a registration of hard contacts of teeth brought together with a straight up and down "tap-tap" movement. That kind of registration may be valuable on occasion, but it would not be a portrayal of occlusal contact relations during the masticatory cycle.

Centric occlusal relation does represent the terminus of the occlusal cycle. But it does not represent a "locked in" position which allows no lateral or protrusive adjustment. In order to avoid trauma, there must be a little play in the contact relationship. This allows compensatory reaction during the application of jaw forces. In common parlance, the teeth may be "gritted" in centric, without "rocking" the teeth in their respective alveoli.

The casts of the individual pictured here display the normal alignment and occlusion of teeth as perfectly as any that might be found. Although the occlusion does not qualify as "ideal," still, it deserves a high qualification because of the placement of occlusal markings within functional borders. Here are some of the observations to be made in an analysis of occlusal markings:

1. Contact markings on incisors and canines. They are made up of linguoincisal markings on the maxillary, and labioincisal markings on mandibular teeth.

2. Major occlusal markings registering the occlusal cycle will show only on the posterior teeth. They will include initial contacts made during the lateral occlusal relation for that side; additional markings register the terminal positions in centric relation.

Continuing the observations, one sees markings which represent contacts pointing to the end of the occlusal cycle; these markings are identical with those made as balancing contacts during lateral occlusal relations involving the opposite side of the mouth (Figs. 16–107 and 16–108).

3. *Note the surfaces that are unmarked. These areas represent escapement spaces.*

4. The actual tip formation of the lingual cusps of mandibular molars are unmarked. An ideal arrangement would show lingual cusp contacts distolingually only, including second premolars and each of the mandibular molars. However, even then the tips of those cusps should be free of contact.

5. The tips of buccal cusps of the maxillary molars and premolars are free of contact. Note the location of the occlusal contacts on triangular ridges, lingual to buccal cusp tips.

6. Occlusal embrasures located over contact areas *should show* no marks on the marginal ridges; thus, some escapement is automatic.

7. Crests of buccal cusps of all mandibular posterior teeth show very definite broad markings, identical with lateral occlusal contact markings for that side before the teeth glided into centric relation.

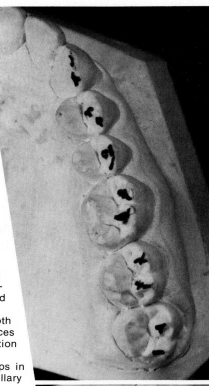

Figure 16–116. This represents the contact markings as registered for the initial occlusal contact in *left lateral relation*. Notice that no markings appear at all on incisors. The progression of the occlusal cycle will multiply the markings as shown in Fig. 16–115.

8. Variation occurs from the usual standard of the ideal in centric relation; there are no contact markings within the central occlusal fossae of the mandibular molars. Although some mouths might show marks closer to the center of the fossae than this example, none will show marks centered. The fossae are deep with pointed pit formations in their centers. This formation allows escapement spaces and a rough ''mortar'' effect when contacted from above by the blunted but effective ''pestles,'' namely, the well-developed mesiolingual cusps of the maxillary molars. Only *unnatural,* sharply pointed cusps of upper molars could mark the centers of fossae of lower molars.

9. Note the limited buccolingual occlusal contact areas in teeth of both jaws; also note the way markings are centered, mostly in occlusal surfaces between cusps of upper molars, but mainly over the buccal cusp formation of lower molars. (Figs. 16–70, 16–73).

10. Generally speaking, the hardest working and most efficient cusps in mandibular teeth are buccal, whereas the lingual cusp forms of maxillary teeth will qualify in that category.

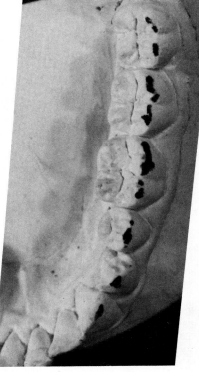

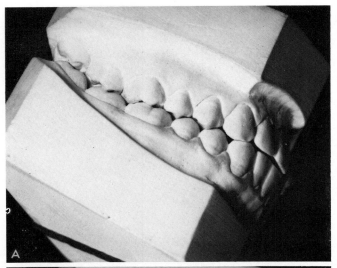

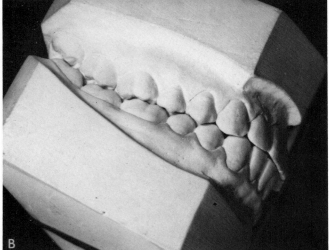

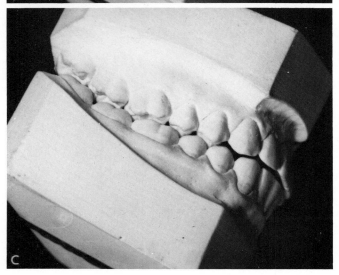

Figure 16–117. The occlusal cycle as demonstrated on one side. These casts, here put into occlusal relations, are shown with their occlusal markings in Fig. 16–78.

A. Right lateral occlusal relation.

B. Centric occlusal relation.

C. End of occlusal cycle with buccal cusps of mandibular teeth in contact with lingual cusps of maxillary teeth before separating for another cycle. This contact relation also serves as the balancing contact for the lateral occlusal relation when registered on the opposite side, the *left* lateral occlusal relation in this instance.

From the protrusive occlusal relation the teeth glide over each other in a *retrusive* movement of the mandible, a movement which terminates in centric occlusal relation. During this final shearing action, the incisal ridges of the lower incisors are in continuous contact with the linguoincisal third portions of the maxillary incisors, from the position of protrusive occlusal relation to the return to centric occlusal relation.

The maxillary canines may assist in the balancing relation by having their distal cusp ridges in contact with the mesial cusp of the mandibular first premolar. They may not assist in a specialized, straightforward incisive action; nevertheless, their form and anchorage prove their design as prehensile members of the dental arches. Consequently, they cooperate with the incisors most of the time in one way or another. A slight movement to right or left during protrusion will bring canines together in a "biting" manner. In addition, at the end of the incisive cycle, the contact of the canines with each other in centric relation lends final effectiveness to the process.

Occlusal balance posteriorly during the protrusive relation is required in order to insure the stability of the incisors. It must be remembered that their angulation in the jaws makes them unable to withstand the forces of occlusion without the assistance of the posterior teeth as stabilizers. Therefore, lack of posterior support, such as premature loss of posterior teeth, affects the security of the anterior teeth, the incisors in particular (Figs. 16–29 and 16–63).

OCCLUSAL CYCLE OF ANTERIOR TEETH

The occlusal cycle of the anterior teeth (protrusive relation to centric relation) with the accompanying occlusal balance may be summarized as follows:

1. The anterior teeth come together with the mandibular dental arch a bit depressed and a bit forward of its centric relation with the maxillary dental arch.

2. When the anterior teeth come into contact, the mandibular arch is in protrusive occlusal relation; the posterior teeth furnish a balancing contact on both sides, mainly with their buccal cusps.

3. The mandible is retruded and slides the teeth over each other in a movement which is upward and backward ending at centric relation.

4. The opening movement of the mandible downward and forward to the protrusive occlusal relation, combined with the closing movement backward and upward to centric relation, completes a cycle of rotation known as the protrusive and retrusive occlusal cycle.

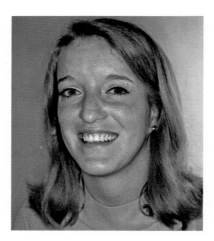

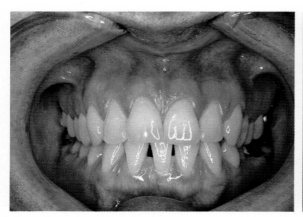 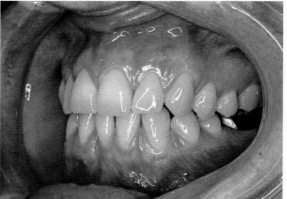

The photographic record above is a fine representation of what good dental treatment can accomplish. Two examples of treatment are in view. Signs of orthodontic treatment appear anteriorly and a complete restoration of the mandibular first molar is on the left. The interest in meticulous home care is obvious. Without it the gingiva would not show such perfection.

Above all, the patient is clearly happy.

Epilogue — Occlusion

Normal occlusion in the permanent dentition comes about as a result of many factors which control growth and development of body tissues. These are nutrition, internal secretions, environment and so on. Therefore considerable thought should be appropriated to diagnostic questions in the effort to decide what is best in a given situation.

Changes are to be expected during the various stages in life from youth to advancing age. There are no changes macroscopically in tooth form (except from wear or accident), but all of the tissues lending support are subject to change in form and function, especially when those tissues contend with metabolic and circulatory problems.

Although we may postulate an hypothetically ideal occlusion (one that is said to be normal), observation of tooth relationships in numbers of people emphasizes a common problem: over a period of years, occlusion changes slowly and imperceptibly, even when dental arches are intact and the teeth are anchored in healthy tissue. Naturally, tooth movement and deterioration are much more rapid when conditions governing stability are unfavorable. The thought is ever present that occlusion in the adult mouth is bound to the general biologic principle of potential change and adjustment. One of the functional responses mentioned earlier in this book was "physiological mesial drift," the tendency of posterior teeth to drift mesially. The form of the mature tooth is static, but its periodontal investment is not.

Fortunately, the tooth crowns are wondrously designed for adaptation to alignment problems. To illustrate: the teeth in one jaw do not fit into or against the teeth in the opposing jaw in a manner which prevents mobility. There is no interlocking of cusps. Instead, hard, rounded surfaces resistant to wear in one jaw interdigitate loosely with accommodating hard, curved surfaces of opponents in the opposite jaw. Thus, the crown forms with their occlusal portions allow for considerable variation in alignment and occlusal contact during jaw development and even after the maturation of parts.

Adjustments are limited, of course, by the static, unyielding form of the tooth units making up the two dental arches. In clinical diagnosis and in the prognosis of treatment, no hard and fast rules of procedure seem acceptable. It is common knowledge that there are many people in every age group whose dental apparatus fails to qualify as ideal, but who are nevertheless happy with their teeth and jaws. Their mouths seem to function well and they enjoy healthy periodontal tissues also. Usually such fortunate though variable situations may be explained by pointing out that certain fundamentals governing good occlusion and jaw relations are present. In all of these cases, bone and soft tissue metabolism are cooperating. The following observations should be made in any examination for problems in occlusion:

Proximal contacts (continuous alignment) must be maintained; restoration in some form may be advisable.

Occlusal contacts should be held within normally narrow limits faciolingually; and lines of forces (translated by the occlusal markings) should be confined within the periphery of root bases.

When occlusal surfaces of opposing teeth fit together too closely, as in those cases where the units are flattened by undue wear, some means must be employed in order to relieve traumatic pressures. It is possible, usually, to create spillways and escapement by reshaping the occlusal contact in some manner. The teeth seem to prosper when occlusal contacts qualify as *minimal* rather than *maximal*.

Hygiene

A simple definition is *the science of health and its maintenance*. All dental treatment, preventive or restorative, is expected to conform to the rules of hygiene. Normal tooth form and tooth alignment, placed in a proper setting, will foster cleanliness. This fortunate situation helps in making the state of dental health autogenous.

References

Alldritt, W. S.: The Epithelia in the Dentogingival Junction. Dent. Pract. *11*:213, 1961.

Arnim, S. S., and Hagerman, D. A.: The Connective Tissue Fibers of the Marginal Gingiva. J. Am. Dent. Assoc. *47*:271, 1953.

Bauer, W.: Z. Stomat. *30*:1136, 1932.

Black, G. V.: Dental Anatomy. S. S. White Mfg. Co., Philadelphia, 1902.

Bonwill, W. G. A.: Scientific Articulation of Human Teeth as Founded on Geometrical Mathematical Laws. Dental Items of Interest. *21*:817, 1889.

Brauer, J. C., Higley, L. B., Massler, M., and Schour, I.: Dentistry for Children. The Blakiston Co., Philadelphia, 1947.

Brodie, A. G.: Temporomandibular Joint. Illinois Dent. J. 8:2, 1939.

Carabelli, G.: Anatomie des Mundes. Braumuller & Seidel, Vienna, 1842.

Chissin, C.: Ueber die Offhungbewegung des Unterkiefers und die Beteiligung der ausseren ptergoidmuskein bei derselben. Arch. f. Anat. u. Entwickelungsgesch, 1906.

Coolidge, E. D.: Anatomy of Root Apex in Relation to Treatment Problems. J. Am. Dent. Assoc. *16*:1456, 1929.

Cunningham, D. S.: Textbook of Anatomy, 8th Ed. Oxford University Press, London, 1943.

Deaver, J. B.: Surgical Anatomy of the Human Body, 2nd Ed. P. Blakiston's Son Co., Philadelphia, 1926.

Dewey, M.: Dental Anatomy. C. V. Mosby Co., St. Louis, 1916.

Dewey, M., and Thompson, A. H.: Comparative Dental Anatomy, 2nd Ed. C. V. Mosby Co., St. Louis, 1920.

Diamond, M.: Dental Anatomy. The Macmillan Co., New York, 1929.

Dingman, R. O., and Natvig, P.: Surgery of Facial Fractures, W. B. Saunders Co., Philadelphia, 1964.

Easlick, K., and Moyers, R. E.: Chapter XII in Watson, E. H., and Lowery, G. H.: Growth and Development of Children, 2nd Ed. Year Book Publishers, Inc., Chicago, 1954.

Freil, S.: Occlusion—Observations on Its Development from Infancy to Old Age. Internat. J. Orthodontia and Oral Surgery, *13*:322, 1927.

Gottleib, B.: Tissue Changes in Pyorrhea. J. Am. Dent. Assoc. *14*:2178, 1927.

————————: The Gingival Margin (Pathological, Normal). Odonto. Sec. Royal Soc. Med. Trans. *20*:51, 1926–27.

Gregory, W. K.: The Origin and Evolution of the Human Dentition. Williams and Wilkins Co., Baltimore, 1922.

Gregory, W. K., and Hellman, M.: Paleontology of the Human Dentition. The First International Dental Congress. C. V. Mosby Co., St. Louis, 1927.

Grossman, L. I.: Root Canal Therapy. Lea & Febiger, Philadelphia, 1946.

Hemley, S.: Fundamentals of Occlusion. W. B. Saunders Co., Philadelphia, 1944.

Hess, W., and Zürcher, E.: The Anatomy of Root Canals. William Wood & Co., Baltimore, 1928.

Higley, L. B.: Some Controversies Over the Temporomandibular Joint. J. Am. Dent. Assoc. *27*:594, 1940.

Hogeboom, F. E.: Practical Pedodontia, 5th Ed. C. V. Mosby Co., St. Louis, 1946.

Johnston, H. B., and Orban, B.: Interradicular Pathology as Related to Accessory Root Canals. J. Endodont. 3:21, 1948.

Klatsky, M.: A Cinefluorographic Study of the Human Masticatory Apparatus in Function. Am. J. Orthodontics *26*:664, 1940.

Kornfeld, M.: Mouth Rehabilitation. Vol. 1, Vol. 2. C. V. Mosby Co., St. Louis, 1967.

Kraus, J. A.: Dental Anatomy and Occlusion. Williams and Wilkins Co., Baltimore, 1969.

Kronfeld, R.: Dental Histology and Comparative Dental Anatomy. Lea & Febiger, Philadelphia, 1937.

Kurth, L. E.: Mandibular Movements in Mastication. J. Am. Dent. Assoc. *29*:1769, 1942.

Logan, W. H. G., and Kronfeld, R.: Development of the Human Jaws and Surrounding Structures from Birth to Age of Fifteen Years. J. Am. Dent. Assoc. 20:379, 1933.

Lord, F. P.: Movements of the Jaw and How They Are Effected. Internat. J. Ortho. 23:557, 1937.

MacMillan, H. W.: Foundations of Mandibular Movement. J. Am. Dent. Assoc. 21:429, 1934.

McBride, W. C.: Juvenile Dentistry, 4th Ed. Lea & Febiger, Philadelphia, 1945.

McCall, J. O., and Wald, S. S.: Clinical Dental Roentgenology, 2nd Ed. W. B. Saunders Co., Philadelphia, 1947, Chaps. XI, XII, and XIII.

Massler, M., and Schour, I.: Atlas of the Mouth. Bureau of Public Relations and Council on Dental Health, American Dental Assoc., Chicago.

Maximow, A. A., and Bloom, W.: Textbook of Histology, 7th Ed. W. B. Saunders Co., Philadelphia, 1957.

Monson, G. S.: Architectural Bone Changes of Face and Cranium. J. Am. Dent. Assoc. 14:828, 1927.

——————: Occlusion as Applied to Crown and Bridgework. J. Nat. Dent. Assoc. 7–399, May, 1920.

Morris, H.: Human Anatomy, 10th Ed. The Blakiston Co., Philadelphia, 1942.

Mueller, E., and Orban, B.: The Gingival Crevice. J. Am. Dent. Assoc. 16:1206, 1929.

Nolla, C.: Studies, Child Development Laboratories, University Elementary School, Development of the Permanent Teeth. J. Dentistry Children 27:254, 1960.

Noyes' Oral Histology and Embryology. Edited and revised by I. Schour, 8th Ed. Lea & Febiger, Philadelphia.

Noyes, F. B., Schour, I., and Noyes, H. J.: Dental Histology and Embryology, 5th Ed. Lea & Febiger, Philadelphia, 1938.

Okumura, T.: Anatomy of the root canals. J. Am. Dent. Assoc. 14:632, 1927.

Orban's Oral Histology and Embryology. Edited by H. Sicher, and S. N. Bhaskar. 7th Ed. C. V. Mosby Co., St. Louis, 1972.

Orban, B.: Biologic Considerations in Restorative Dentistry. J. Am. Dent. Assoc. 28:1069, 1941.

——————: A Contribution to the Knowledge of the Physiologic Changes in the Periodontal Membrane. J. Am. Dent. Assoc. 16:405, 1929.

——————: Dental Histology and Embryology. P. Blakiston's Son Co., Philadelphia, 1930.

Orban, B., et al.: Periodontics. C. V. Mosby Co., St. Louis, 1958.

Orthodontic Congress: The First International. Records published in book form by C. V. Mosby Co., St. Louis, 1927.

Pappas, G.: Dental Radiography and Photography. Eastman Kodak Co., Vol. 43, No. 2, page 29.

Permar, D.: Oral Embryology and Microscopic Anatomy, 4th Ed. Lea & Febiger, Philadelphia, 1967.

Prentiss, H. L.: Regional Anatomy Emphasizing Mandibular Movements with Specific Reference to Full Denture Construction. J. Am. Dent. Assoc. 15:1085, 1923.

Prinz, H.: The Etiology of Pyorrhea Alveolaris. Dental Cosmos. 68:1, 1926.

Ramfjord, S. P., and Ash, M. M.: Occlusion, 2nd Ed. W. B. Saunders Co., Philadelphia, 1971.

Riethmüller, R. H.: The Filling of Root Canals with Prinz' Paraffin Compound. Dental Cosmos. 56:490, 1914.

Robinson, H. B. G.: Some Clinical Aspects of Intra-oral Age Changes. Geriatrics. 2:9, 1947.

Robinson, M.: The Temporomandibular Joint: Theory of Reflex Controlled Nonlever Action of the Mandible. J. Am. Dent. Assoc. 33:1260, 1946.

Sherrington, C. S.: Proc. Royal Soc. Lond. 92:245, 1921.

Sicher, H., and DuBrul, E. L.: Oral Anatomy, 5th Ed. C. V. Mosby Co., St. Louis, 1970.

Sicher, H., and Tandler, J.: Anatomie fur Zahnarzte. Julius Springer, Vienna and Berlin, 1928.

Simpson, C. O.: Advanced Radiodontic Interpretation, 3rd Ed. C. V. Mosby Co., St. Louis, 1947.

Skillen, W. G.: Normal Characteristics of the Gingiva and Their Relation to Pathology. J. Am. Dent. Assoc. 17:1088, 1930.

Skillen, W. G., and Lindquist, G. R.: An Experimental Study of Periodontal Membrane Reattachment in Healthy and Pathologic Tissue. J. Am. Dent. Assoc. 24:175, 1937.

Spee, F. Graf von: Die Verschiebungsbahn des Unterkiefers am Shadel. Arch. f. Anat. u. Physiol., 1890.

Stimson, L. A.: Treatise on Dislocations. Lea Brothers & Co., 1907.

Thompson, J. R.: Cephalometric Study on Movements of the Mandible. J. Am. Dent. Assoc. 28:750, 1941.

Thompson, J. R., and Brodie, A. G.: Factors in the Position of the Mandible. J. Am. Dent. Assoc. 29:915, 1942.

Tims, H. W., and Henry, C. B.: Tomes' Dental Anatomy. The Macmillan Co., New York, 1923.

Turner, C. R.: American Textbook of Prosthetic Dentistry. Lea & Febiger, Philadelphia, 1931.

Updegrave, W. J.: Dental Radiography and Photography. Eastman Kodak Co., Vol. 31, No. 4, Figs. 1, 2, 3, 4.

——————: Dental Radiography and Photography. Eastman Kodak Co., Vol. 43, No. 2, Figs. 1, 2, 3, 4.

Wheeler, R. C.: A Comparison of Periodontal Attachment Levels. Dental Digest 41:261, 1935.

——————: An Atlas of Tooth Form, 4th Ed. W. B. Saunders Co., Philadelphia, 1969.

_____: Evidences of Compensating Occlusal Curvature in the Anatomy of Individual Units of the Human Dental Arch. Research report, International Association of Dental Research, Columbus, Ohio. March, 1932.

_____: Normal Tooth Form and Dental Maintenance. Journal, Southern California State Dental Assoc. Vol. XXXI, No. 12, December, 1963.

_____: Restoration of Gingival or Cervical Margins in Full Crowns. Dental Cosmos. 73: 238, 1931.

_____: Some Fundamentals in Tooth Form. Dental Cosmos. 70:889, 1928.

_____: Dental Restoration And Dental Maintenance: Conservation Of Tissue. J. Am. Soc. Preventive Dentistry. Vol. 3, No. 4, 1973.

Index